Lecture Notes of the Institute for Computer Sciences, Social Informatics and Telecommunications Engineering 297

More information about this series at http://www.springer.com/series/8197

Lorenzo Mucchi · Matti Hämäläinen ·
Sara Jayousi · Simone Morosi (Eds.)

Body Area Networks

Smart IoT and Big Data for Intelligent Health Management

14th EAI International Conference, BODYNETS 2019
Florence, Italy, October 2–3, 2019
Proceedings

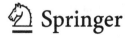 Springer

Editors
Lorenzo Mucchi (iD)
Department of Information Engineering
University of Florence
Florence, Italy

Matti Hämäläinen (iD)
Centre for Wireless Communications
University of Oulu
Oulu, Finland

Sara Jayousi (iD)
University of Florence
Florence, Italy

Simone Morosi (iD)
University of Florence
Florence, Italy

ISSN 1867-8211   ISSN 1867-822X (electronic)
Lecture Notes of the Institute for Computer Sciences, Social Informatics
and Telecommunications Engineering
ISBN 978-3-030-34832-8   ISBN 978-3-030-34833-5 (eBook)
https://doi.org/10.1007/978-3-030-34833-5

This Springer imprint is published by the registered company Springer Nature Switzerland AG
The registered company address is: Gewerbestrasse 11, 6330 Cham, Switzerland

Preface

We are delighted to introduce the proceedings of the 14th edition of the 2019 European Alliance for Innovation (EAI) International Conference on Body Area Networks (BodyNets). This conference has brought together researchers, developers, and practitioners from around the world who are leveraging and developing in- and on-body sensors and applications for human health. The theme of BodyNets 2019 was "Smart IoT and Big Data for Intelligent Health Management."

The technical program of BodyNets 2019 consisted of 32 full papers in 3 different tracks. The conference technical sessions were

- Sensors
- Systems and Medical Applications
- Physical Activity Monitoring
- In-body Communications
- On-body Communications
- Security, Privacy, and Performance Evaluation
- ICT Solutions for Diagnosis and Social Inclusion
- Propagation

Aside from the high-quality technical paper presentations, the technical program also featured two keynote speeches, four invited talks, and two special tracks. The two keynote speeches were given by Prof. Ari Pouttu from Oulu University, Finland, and Dr. Sandro Carrara from EPLF, France. The invited talks were presented by Prof. Paolo Lucattini from Agazzi Rehabilitation Centre "Madre Divina Provvidenza" of Passionisti, Italy, by Prof. Malin Olsson from Lulea University, Sweden, by Dr. Marco Manso from EDGE Technology, Portugal, and by Prof. Massimiliano Pierobon from Nebraska University, USA.

The two special tracks were the International Workshop on Smart Body Area Networks for e-health and the International Workshop on ICT for Social/Sport Re-inclusion of People with Impairments. The first special track aimed to address the European vision for the standardization of body area networks, while the second addressed the importance of ICTs for disable people.

Coordination with the Steering Committee, I. Chlamtac, A. V. Vasilakos, J. Suzuki, and G. Fortino was essential for the success of the conference. We sincerely appreciate their constant support and guidance. It was also a great pleasure to work with such an excellent Organizing Committee team and we thank them for their hard work in organizing and supporting the conference. In particular, the Technical Program Committee, led by our TPC Co-chairs: Prof. Matti Hamalainen, Prof. M. Pierobon, Dr. D. Nguyen, and Prof. J. Iinatti, completed the peer-review process of technical papers and made a high-quality technical program. We are also grateful to conference manager, Radka Pincakova, for her support and all the authors who submitted their papers to the BodyNets 2019 conference and workshops.

We strongly believe that the BodyNets conference series provides a good forum for all researcher, developers, and practitioners to discuss all science and technology aspects that are relevant to body area networks. We also expect that future BodyNets conferences will be as successful and stimulating, as indicated by the contributions presented in this volume.

September 2019   Lorenzo Mucchi
                                                Matti Hämäläinen
                                                   Sara Jayousi
                                                 Simone Morosi

Organization

Steering Committee

Chair

Imrich Chlamtac   University of Trento, Italy
(Bruno Kessler Professor)

Members

Athanasios V. Vasilakos   National Technical University of Athens, Greece
Jun Suzuki   University of Massachusetts, USA
Giancarlo Fortino   University of Calabria, Italy

Organizing Committee

General Chair

Lorenzo Mucchi   University of Florence, Italy

General Co-chair

Giancarlo Fortino   University of Calabria, Italy

Program Chairs

Matti Hamalainen   University of Oulu, Finland
Massimiliano Pierobon   University of Nebraska-Lincoln, USA
Diep Nguyen   University of Technology Sydney, Australia
Jari Iinatti   University of Oulu, Finland

Publicity and Social Media Chair

Raffaele Gravina   University of Calabria, Italy

Local Chair

Sara Jayousi   University of Florence, Italy

Publications Chair

Simone Morosi   University of Florence, Italy

Web Chair

Stefano Caputo   University of Florence, Italy

Conference Manager

Radka Pincakova   EAI

Technical Program Committee

Ahmed Khorshid	University of California, Irvine, USA
Heikki Karvonen	University of Oulu, Finland
Huan-Bang Li	NICT, Japan
John Farserotu	CSEM, Switzerland
Lin Wang	Xiamen University, China
Marcos Katz	University of Oulu, Finland
Mariella Särestöniemi	University of Oulu, Finland
Mohammad Ghavami	London South Bank University, UK
Qiong Wang	Dresden University of Technology, Germany
Sen Qiu Dalian	University of Technology, China
Takahiro Aoyagi	Tokyo Institute of Technology, Japan
Timo Kumpuniemi	University of Oulu, Finland
Xinrong Li	University of North Texas, USA
Valeria Loscri	Inria, France
Rossi Kamal	Kyung Hee University, South Korea

Contents

In-body Communications

On-body Communications

Sensors

A Portable Continuous Wave Radar System to Detect Elderly Fall

Muhammad Arslan Ali, Malikeh Pour Ebrahim,
and Mehmet Rasit Yuce[✉]

Department of Electrical and Computer Systems Engineering,
Monash University, Melbourne, Australia
mehmet.yuce@monash.edu

Abstract. Fall is the leading cause of death among elderly people worldwide. In this work a low power portable continuous wave radar (CWR) system is proposed to detect elderly fall. This paper presents experimental evaluation of the system to detect human fall motion among various sitting, standing and walking activities. Signals from three subjects with different heights and weights engaged with the different movement activities including walking, sitting, standing and fall in front of the proposed radar system are analyzed. Overall, 60 fall and 180 non-fall activities were recorded. The Short-time Fourier Transform (STFT) is employed to obtain time-frequency Doppler signatures of different human activities. Radar data is analysed by using MATLAB and an algorithm is employed to classify the fall on the basis of analysed data. The results show that the proposed portable CWR can be used to detect fall from non-fall activities with almost 100% accuracy.

Keywords: Fall detection · CWR · STFT

1 Introduction

In recent years average life expectance of human beings has increased unprecedently. By 2050 more than 50% of the total population of the world will be over 60+ age [1]. Each year approximately 37.3 million falls occur which require intense medical attention. Approximately 646,000 deaths occur every year due to fall and majority of these are above age of 60 years [1]. In United States, unintentional fall of elderly people above 65 age is the leading cause of death. This situation is same among the less developed countries [2]. Besides fatal injuries, fall also causes serious implications which affect the quality of life of elderly people. Fractures resulted from a fall can reduce the mobility of elderly people to bed only and most of them die within 1 year of fall [3]. Early and accurate fall detection can significantly contribute towards immediate response and proper care of the elderly people which will alleviate the risk of mortality [4].

Wearable and non-contact devices are the two most competing technologies for fall detection. Wearable devices like accelerometer sensors can detect a fall by calculating the vertical acceleration of the body [5]. Although wearable technologies; accelerometer sensors or emergency push buttons are widely used, the major drawbacks of such devices are that they have to be worn by a person all the time which may

L. Mucchi et al. (Eds.): BODYNETS 2019, LNICST 297, pp. 3–11, 2019.
https://doi.org/10.1007/978-3-030-34833-5_1

impede one's daily routine. Moreover, elderly people are required to remember wearing them all the time and they must be mentally conscious after the fall to press the push button. Furthermore, these devices suffer from intrusiveness, fragility and degradability. Cameras can be used to monitor movements of the elderly but in this way, their privacy is compromised. The striking attributes of a radar system include nonintrusive sensing, immune to lighting and weather conditions and preservation of privacy [6].

Radar back scatter by a moving object changes the frequencies of the radar signal and this phenomenon is called Doppler Effect. A fall motion can be detected by a radar by analyzing the back scattering caused by a fall. In literature target back scatterings have been recorded for different types of motion [7–9]. To analyze these back-scatter signals different processing techniques such as STFT [10], Wavelet Transforms [11] and Fractional Domain Fourier Transform (FrFT) [12] have been employed. Depending on the operating frequency and power of the equipment, unique Doppler signatures have been achieved for different type of motions. Once the radar signals are analyzed, their unique features are extracted and a fall is determined by using different classifiers. Most common classifiers used are Support Vector Machine used in [13], k-nearest neighbours used in [7] and machine learning based on Hidden Markov model has been used in [14].

In this work a low power, low frequency, portable yet efficient Doppler radar system to detect a human fall is proposed. In [6–14] the radar systems used were quite large and expensive. A comparatively portable Doppler radar system was proposed in [15] but for physiological parameter measurements. This paper presents experimental evaluation of the system to detect fall motion in various sitting, standing and walking activities. The proposed portable Doppler radar system can detect a fall very efficiently from other human motions even with the events which involve immediate falls during walk activity. Radar data is analysed by using MATLAB and an algorithm is employed to classify the fall on the basis of analysed data.

The rest of the paper is divided in the following sections. Section 2 describes signal model. Section 3 explains hardware model. Section 4 deals with signal processing. Section 5 includes results and discussions. Section 6 concludes the paper followed by references.

2 Signal Model

The signal transmitted by the radar is given by

$$T_x(t) = A \cos(\omega_c t) \tag{1}$$

where $\omega c = 2\pi fc$ is the central operating frequency of the CWR. The signal received by the radar at any time interval t is given by

$$R_x(t) = T_x(t - \phi(t)) \tag{2}$$

where

$$\phi(t) = \frac{2}{c}(d_o - vt) \tag{3}$$

Where d_0 be the distance of the body from the radar at time t_0 and v is the target velocity component. Substituting (1) and (3) in (2)

$$R_x(t) = M\cos\left[2\pi\left(f_c t - f_c \frac{2d_o}{c} + \frac{2f_c vt}{c}\right)\right] \tag{4}$$

where M is a constant and the phase given by

$$\Theta = 2\pi f_c \frac{2d_o}{c} \cdots \tag{5}$$

The doppler frequency is given by

$$f_D = \frac{2f_c v}{c} \tag{6}$$

The in-phase and quadrature components are given by

$$I(t) \approx \cos(\omega_o + \Theta + f_D t) \tag{7}$$

and

$$Q(t) \approx \sin(\omega_o + \Theta + f_D t) \tag{8}$$

STFT is computed by

$$R(a,b) = \sum_{n=1}^{m} x[n]\omega^*(nT - aT)e^{-i\omega t}bFn\ldots \tag{9}$$

where a is the time index, b is the frequency index, T is sampling period, F is frequency step size, ω (.) is Hamming window function, and * denotes complex conjugate [14].

3 Hardware Model

Radar hardware is shown in Fig. 1.

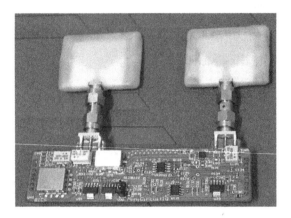

Fig. 1. Radar hardware

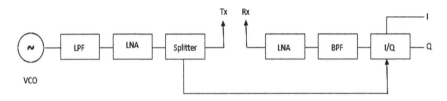

Fig. 2. Radar hardware block diagram

As described in Fig. 2, an 887 MHz signal was generated using a voltage control oscillator (VCO) with 10dBm power. The signal is then passed through a low pass filter (LPF) to remove high frequency noise components of the VCO, which may cause non-linearity at the receiver side. The signal is then amplified by a low noise amplifier (LNA) and split by using a two-way power splitter. One part of the signal goes to transmitter antenna while the other goes to a local oscillator (LO) input of an in-phase-quadrature (I/Q) demodulator. Radar back scatter received by the receiver antenna are very low in power, so an amplifier of 16 dB gain is applied. Finally, to eliminate unwanted frequency components the signal is passed through a bandpass filter (BPF) before down-converted to baseband signal.

Ultrawideband (UWB) patch antennas are used for transmitter and receiver purposes with return loss lower than −10 dB at operating frequency.

3.1 Data Experimental Setup

Figure 3 shows the experiment setup. Radar uses 887 MHz center frequency, as the system is portable it can be placed anywhere in a room. For this setup, the antennas were setup at a height of 2 m above the ground. Three subjects with different heights and weights volunteered for different movement activities including walking, sitting, standing and fall in front of the radar. All of these activities are monitored within a distance of four meters in front of the Radar. Four different experiments were conducted involving the above-mentioned activities. In the first experiment the subjects were asked to stand in front of the radar system and fall on a mattress, then stand up and again perform fall. Ten number of falls for each subject were recorded. In the second experiment the subjects were asked to walk in front of the radar and then fall on the mattress, again ten number of falls for each subject were recorded. To distinguish between walk and sit with a fall, in the third experiment the volunteers were asked to sit on a chair in a fast manner while walking. Each subject was asked to sit ten times while walking. Finally, in the fourth experiment the subjects were asked to sit and stand quickly on the chair, again each subject was asked to sit and stand ten times. Overall, 60 fall and 180 non-fall activities were recorded.

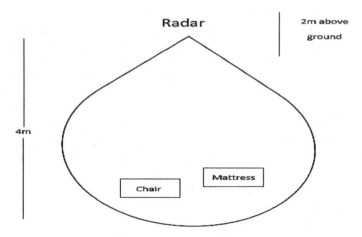

Fig. 3. Experimental setup

In all these experiments the data was recorded for a duration of three minutes for each experiment and activities were performed at different locations in front of the radar system.

4 Signal Processing

Figure 4 surmises the signal processing unit. A MATLAB program was developed to fetch data from the radar system. The in-phase (I) and quadrature (Q) data were sampled at 1000 samples per second and stored in a m.file for signal processing.

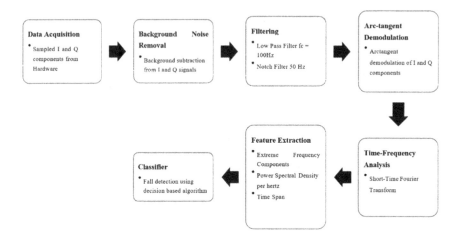

Fig. 4. Signal processing flow chart for fall detection

First of all, in order to remove background noise or dc level, the I and Q signals were subtracted with the data recorded without any activity and sampled at same rate i.e. 1000 samples per second. As STFT proved to be very effective in obtaining time-frequency signatures of Doppler radars [16], the main goal was to get the time- frequency signature of the radar by applying STFT. To do so, different filtering techniques were applied to remove additional frequency components from the signals. At the end an algorithm was developed to detect fall on the basis of features generated by STFT. Power spectral density in dB/Hz was extracted from STFT and an algorithm was applied making decision based on the value of dB/Hz on extreme frequency components. For instance, a low pass infinite-impulse response IIR filter was first applied with cut-off frequency of 100 Hz. After that a constant noise was noticed at 50 Hz, so a notch filter with 50 Hz center frequency was applied on I and Q channels.

Once the noise components were filtered then the arctangent demodulation was performed to get the best of I and Q signals. Finally, for linear time-frequency analysis STFT was employed. The results from the spectrogram obtained clearly distinguished a fall from other non-fall activities.

For STFT following settings were employed: window size of 1024, 1000 non-overlap, sampling frequency of 1000 samples per second and minimum threshold of 0db were set. The values of window size and non-overlap sample were set to get best temporal resolution. The threshold level was set to eliminate weak reflections as we were concerned with only gross motor activities to detect fall.

For fall classification features such as, extreme frequency components, power spectral density per frequency and time span of event were extracted and sent to a decision-making algorithm.

5   Results and Discussions

Figure 5 shows different time-frequency Doppler signatures of human activities in the form of the spectrogram. The spectrogram is computed using Hamming window of 1024 point, logarithm scale and 0 dB power/frequency threshold. This threshold is set to record only those reflections which contain sufficient amount of energy. The highest frequency component with at least 0 dB power is below 25 Hz because at low center frequency, 887 Hz in our case, most of the energy is reflected back by the target on lower frequency components [14]. The results of all the spectrograms in Fig. 5 are consistent with previous works [10–14] yet with low power, low frequency and portable equipment.

Figure 5(a) represents the spectrogram of the first experiment. The peaks in the spectrogram at different time intervals are the falls in the experiments. The reflected energies are concentrated to lower frequencies but at the time of fall maximum displacement can be observed in the frequency axis with at least 0 dB power. As described in [17], after a fall no higher energy was received due to negligible movement. Figure 5(b) represents the spectrogram of the second experiment in which falls during walk were detected. The peaks in the spectrogram at different time intervals are the falls in the experiments. The reflected energies are concentrated to lower frequencies but again at the time of every fall maximum displacement can be observed on the frequency axis.

As explained in [16], detecting a fall from walk is very challenging due to movement of the whole body. It can be seen in the Fig. 5(b) that due to acceleration of a fall high Doppler frequency components can still be easily distinguished from high energy walk t-f signatures.

Figure 5(c) shows the spectrogram of third experiment. It can be easily observed that sitting after walk generates high Doppler frequency but these are low as compared to fall during walk motion, hence can easily be distinguished from each other. Figure 5(d) is the spectrogram based on the fourth experiment. First spike represents sitting followed by standing and the subsequent spikes follow the same pattern. The Doppler frequencies of these motions are less than the ones of fall.

Based on the frequency components having high power spectral density and time information obtained from spectrogram an algorithm is developed to classify a fall from non-fall activities. Table 1 shows the fall detection based on the extracted features. Accuracy is determined by dividing the correctly detected activities with total activities.

Table 1. Fall detection based on extracted features

Experiment	Total activities	Actual falls	Detected fall	% Accuracy
1. Stand and Fall	60	30	30	100
2. Walk and Fall	60	30	33	95
3. Walk and Sit	60	0	2	96.6
4. Stand and Sit	60	0	0	100

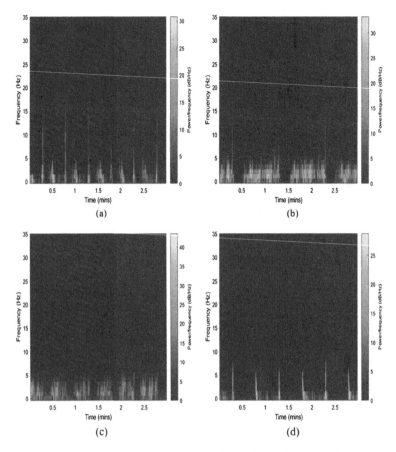

Fig. 5. Spectrogram of experiments: (a) Stand and Fall (b) Walk and Fall (c) Walk and Sit (d) Stand and Sit

6   Conclusion

This work demonstrates that a low power and portable CWR can be effectively used to detect fall among other human activities. Unique time-frequency signal for a fall are obtained by applying STFT on radar's sampled data. Based on the power spectral density and time information of the spectrogram, an algorithm analyzing radar signals has been developed to classify a fall. The results verified that a fall can be classified with high accuracy from the proposed system and processing techniques.

All of the experiments are conducted within a distance of four meters from the radar system and the classification algorithm makes decision on the basis of power spectral density and time information only. High gain amplifiers and appropriate filters can be used to maximize the fall detection range. A more powerful and efficient classification algorithm utilizing more features can be trained to minimize false detection of the system.

References

1. UN Population Prospects. https://www.un.org/development/desa/publications/world-popula tion-prospects-the-2017-revision.html. Accessed 12 May 2019
2. CDCP. https://www.cdc.gov/injury/wisqars/index.html. Accessed 12 May 2019
3. Carneiro, M.B., Alves, D.P., Mercadante, M.T.: Physical therapy in the postoperative of proximal femur fracture in elderly. Literature review. Acta Ortop Bras. **21**(3), 175–178 (2013)
4. Moran, C.G., Wenn, R.T., Sikand, M., Taylor, A.M.: Early mortality after hip fracture: is delay before surgery important. J. Bone Joint Surg. **87**(1), 483–489 (2005)
5. Giansanti, D., Maccioni, G., Macellari, V.: The development and test of a device for the reconstruction of 3-D position and orientation by means of a kinematic sensor assembly with rate gyroscopes and accelerometers. IEEE Trans. Biomed. Eng. **52**(1), 1271–1277 (2005)
6. Tivive, F.H.C., Amin, M.G., Bouzerdoum, A.: Wall clutter mitigation based on eigen-analysis in through-the-wall radar imaging. In: 17th International Conference on Digital Signal Processing (DSP), pp. 1–8. IEEE (2011)
7. Liu, L., Popescu, M., Skubic, M., Rantz, M., Yardibi, T., Cuddihy, P.: Automatic fall detection based on Doppler radar motion. In: Proceedings of 5th International Conference on Pervasive Computing Technologies for Healthcare, pp. 222–225, Dublin, Ireland (2011)
8. Tomii, S., Ohtsuki, T.: Falling detection using multiple Doppler sensors. In Proceedings of IEEE International Conference e-Health Networking, Applications and Services, Beijing, China, pp. 196–201 (2012)
9. Wang, F., Skubic, M., Rantz, M., Cuddihy, P.E.: Quantitative gait measurement with pulse-Doppler radar for passive in-home gait assessment. IEEE Trans. Biomed. Eng. **61**(9), 2434–2443 (2014)
10. Gadde, A., Amin, M.G., Zhang, Y.D., Ahmad, F.: Fall detection and classification based on time-scale radar signal characteristics. In: Proceedings of SPIE, Baltimore, MD, vol. 9077, pp. 1–9 (2014)
11. Mallat S.: A Wavelet Tour of Signal Processing: The Sparce Way, 3rd edn. AP Professional, London (2009)
12. Almeida, B.L.: The fractional Fourier transform and time-frequency representations. IEEE Trans. Signal Process. **42**(11), 308–3091 (1994)
13. Kim, Y., Ling, H.: Human activity classification based on micro-Doppler signatures using a support vector machine. IEEE Trans. Geosci. Remote Sens. **47**(5), 1328–1337 (2009)
14. Wu, M., Dai, X., Zhang, D.Y, Davidson, B., Zhang, J., Amin, M.G.: Fall detection based on sequential modelling of radar signal time-frequency features. In: Proceedings of IEEE International Conference on Healthcare Informatics, Philadelphia, PA, pp. 169–174 (2013)
15. Pour Ebrahim, M., Sarvi, M., Yuce, M.: A Doppler Radar system for sensing physiological parameters in walking and standing positions. Sensors **17**(3), 485 (2017)
16. Amin, M.G., Zhang, Y.D., Ahmad, F., Ho, K.D.: Radar signal processing for elderly fall detection: the future for in-home monitoring. IEEE Signal Process. Mag. **33**(2), 71–80 (2016)
17. Wu, Q., Zhang, Y.D., Tao, W., Amin, M.G.: Radar-based fall detection based on Doppler time–frequency signatures for assisted living. IET Radar Sonar Navig. **9**(2), 164–172 (2015)

A Piezoelectric Heart Sound Sensor for Wearable Healthcare Monitoring Devices

Zhenghao Chen, Dongyi Chen[(✉)], Liuhui Xue, and Liang Chen

School of Automation Engineering,
University of Electronic Science and Technology of China, Chengdu 611731,
People's Republic of China
dychen@uestc.edu.cn

Abstract. Heart disease is the leading cause of death all around the world. And heart sound monitoring is a commonly used diagnostic method. This method can obtain vital physiological and pathological evidence about health. Many existing techniques are not suitable for long-term dynamic heart sound monitoring since their large size, high-cost and uncomfortable to wear. This paper proposes a small, low-cost and wearable piezoelectric heart sound sensor, which is suitable for long-term dynamic monitoring and provides technical support for preliminary diagnosis of heart disease. First, the theoretical analysis and finite element method (FEM) simulation have been carried out to determine the optimum structure size of piezoelectric sensor. Subsequently, the sensor is embedded into the fabric-based chest strap to verify the detection performance in wearable scenarios. An existing piezoelectric sensor (TSD108) is used as reference. The designed sensor can acquire complete heart sound signals, and its signal-to-noise ratio is 2 dB higher than that of TSD108.

Keywords: Wearable · Heart sound sensor · Finite element method · Signal-to-noise ratio

1 Introduction

1.1 A Subsection Sample

Nowadays, heart disease is the leading cause of death all around the world [1]. In 2016, heart diseases killed 17.9 million people, i.e. three in every ten deaths [2]. The heart sound signal contains a lot of heart information, giving a preliminary suggestion for further diagnosis. Long-term and dynamic monitoring of early and sudden heart attacks to capture transient, non-sustainable abnormal heart sounds play a crucial role in diagnosis [3]. The stethoscope are widely used in auscultation, however it has many limitations for continuous monitoring. For instance, the stethoscope is difficult to be wearable and the hand-held measurement introduces friction noise. Echocardiography (echo), cardiac magnetic resonance images (other diagnostic equipment such as MRI) and computed tomography (CT) have high cost and high requirements for medical personnel. Therefore, providing economical and accurate long-term dynamic monitoring methods is an urgent task for researchers.

© ICST Institute for Computer Sciences, Social Informatics and Telecommunications Engineering 2019
Published by Springer Nature Switzerland AG 2019. All Rights Reserved
L. Mucchi et al. (Eds.): BODYNETS 2019, LNICST 297, pp. 12–23, 2019.
https://doi.org/10.1007/978-3-030-34833-5_2

Heart sound sensors play a vital role in heart sound detection systems, and many researchers are currently engaged in the research and exploration of heart sound sensor. Chen et al. designed a heart sound detection system based on the new XH-6 sensor, it collected the slight heart sound signals, displayed in real-time and saved the Phono-cardiography (PCG) [4]. Hu et al. designed a chest-worn accelerometer for cardio-respiratory sound monitoring based on the asymmetrical gapped cantilever, the cantilever was composed of bottom mechanical layer and a top piezoelectric layer separated by a gap [3]. Ou et al. presented a novel electronic stethoscope based on micro-electro-mechanical-system (MEMS) microphone. The heart sounds were recorded and displayed with mobile APP [5]. Zhang et al. proposed the double-beam-block microstructure heart sound sensor based on the piezoresistive principle and MEMS technology [6]. Malik et al. utilized a high quality Littmann chest piece to pick up body sounds and then fed into a microphone sensor for conversion to electrical signals. The converted signals were processed by the signal conditioning circuit, and the external speaker was used to amplify the processed signals [7]. Above all, the sensor can be divided into two categories: piezoelectric-based and microphone-based according to the principle of sensor [8–12]. However, the microphone-based method is usually easy to pick up excessive ambient noise, and requires a higher frequency response range of microphone. The piezoelectric-based overcomes this problem, and the energy loss during the sound propagation is small.

2 Sensor Design

2.1 System Design

Considering the practical application scenarios, the system should be portable and wearable for long-term monitoring. A completed heart sensing system is composed of chest strap embedded with sensor, acquisition module, display module and analysis system. The overall system is shown in Fig. 1. First, the piezoelectric sensor is embedded into the chest strap with a fixed structure. During the auscultation process, the users wear the strap where the sensor position keep contact with the chest wall. The acquisition module consists of a microcontroller, signal conditioning circuit and a Bluetooth 4.0 unit, which samples the heart sound signals and transmits the data to the software for real-time display. Besides the heart sound can be listened using the earphone.

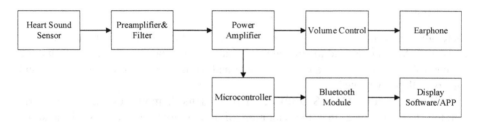

Fig. 1. Schematic block diagram of the heart sound sensing system

In this paper, the piezoelectric vibrator is selected as the sensitive component of the heart sound sensor. Based on the positive piezoelectric effect, while receiving external force of the chest wall vibration, the internal charges on both sides move relatively, resulting in potential difference. The change of potential difference reflects as the strength of heart sound signal.

Based on the principle of heart sound detection, this paper improves some existed sensors on the market, in order to design a smaller, thinner heart sound sensor which is suitable for long-time wearing. According to the prior knowledge, the structure diagram of the designed sensor is shown in Fig. 2, which consists of piezoelectric vibrator, cavity, protective shell and flexible film. The influence of piezoelectric vibrator and cavity size on the sensitivity of heart sound detection is the focus of this chapter. The real working environment of piezoelectric sensor will be simulated to determine the optimum size of piezoelectric vibrator and cavity. And then a sensor that meets the needs of comfort and long-term monitoring of heart sounds will be designed and implemented.

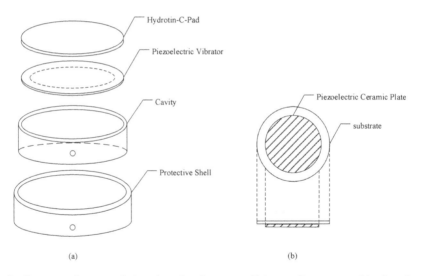

Fig. 2. Structure diagram of the piezoelectric sensor ((a) overall structure (b) piezoelectric vibrator structure)

2.2   Modelization

There are some limitations in the scientific theory and experiment. The infinite element method (FEM) can be used to simulate and analyze the structure of sensors so that the mechanical performance parameters are obtained. And then the designed heart sound sensors will be evaluated [13].

We first use the ANSYS software to build a mesh model of the piezoelectric vibrator. It is assumed that the vibration of the piezoelectric vibrator is a small deflection bending problem. When establishing the mesh model, the piezoelectric vibrator is divided into two parts: piezoelectric ceramic plate and metal substrate. The piezoelectric material (ceramic plate) is solid 5, which is a hexahedral element with 8 nodes. The substrate unit is solid 45, which is a commonly used structural element. They are bonded together by Glue command. The mesh model of the piezoelectric vibrator is shown in the Fig. 3.

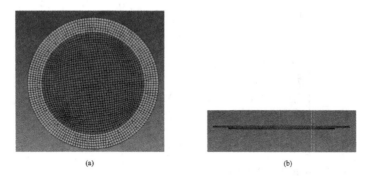

(a)   (b)

Fig. 3. Mesh model of the piezoelectric model (a) vertical veiw (b) front view

2.3 Simulation

The piezoelectric vibration is composed of a substrate made of H65 brass and a piezoelectric ceramic plate of PZT-4. And the material of cavity is also H65 brass. They are bonded together with polyurethane glue. The material properties used in the simulation are shown in Table 1. In order to determine the size of piezoelectric vibrator and cavity, the influence of the parameters of the substrate and the piezoelectric ceramic plate on the sensitivity of the piezoelectric sensor are respectively compared and analyzed; then the influence of the sensitivity on the piezoelectric sensor was verified by changing the cavity height. According to the simulation results, the parameters of heart sound sensors are determined. Finally, to verify the feasibility of the piezoelectric vibrator, the static and dynamic simulation of the selected piezo-electric vibrator are tested.

Table 1. Material properties

Material	H65 Brass	PZT-4	H62 brass	Polyurethane
$Density(g/m^3)$	8.5	7.5	8.5	1.07
Young's modulus $(10^{11}N/m^2)$	1.3	–	–	0.13
Poisson's ratio	0.3	–	0.30	0.42
Tensile strength (MPa)	≥ 390	–	410-630	–
Extensibility (A%)	≥ 25/20	–	15.0	–

The material parameters of piezoelectric ceramic plate are as follows: dielectric constant is ε, piezoelectric constant matrix is $d \times 10^{10} \mathrm{C/m^2}$, stiffness matrices is $K \times 10^{10} \mathrm{N/m}$ [14].

$$\text{where } \varepsilon = \begin{bmatrix} 804.6 & 0 & 0 \\ 0 & 804.6 & 0 \\ 0 & 0 & 804.6 \end{bmatrix}, d = \begin{bmatrix} 0 & 0 & -4.1 \\ 0 & 0 & -4.1 \\ 0 & 0 & 14.1 \\ 0 & 0 & 0 \\ 0 & 10.5 & 0 \\ 10.5 & 0 & 0 \end{bmatrix},$$

$$K = \begin{bmatrix} 13.2 & 7.1 & 7.3 & 0 & 0 & 0 \\ 7.1 & 13.2 & 7.3 & 0 & 0 & 0 \\ 7.3 & 7.3 & 11.5 & 0 & 0 & 0 \\ 0 & 0 & 0 & 3 & 0 & 0 \\ 0 & 0 & 0 & 0 & 2.6 & 0 \\ 0 & 0 & 0 & 0 & 0 & 2.6 \end{bmatrix}$$

Parameters of Piezoelectric Sensors
First, the size of the circular piezoelectric vibrator is determined, the vibrator is composed of a piezoelectric ceramic plate and substrate. Therefore, the influence of the diameter of piezoelectric ceramic plate and substrate on its sensitivity are studied. In the simulation, the diameter of substrate ranges from 10–50 mm, and the diameter of piezoelectric ceramic plate ranges from 10–30 mm (the diameter of the substrate does not exceed that of the ceramic plate). The thickness of the substrate and the ceramic plate is 2 mm. A uniform load of 2 kPa is applied to the surface of piezoelectric vibrator [15]. The sensitivity is reflected by the displacement of the center point of the piezoelectric vibrator as shown in Fig. 4. It is not difficult to see from the figure that the displacement of the center point of the piezoelectric vibrator decreases with the increase of the diameter of the piezoelectric ceramic plate and increases with the increase of the diameter of the substrate.

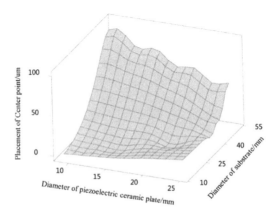

Fig. 4. Influence of different diameters of substrate and piezoelectric ceramic on the sensitivity of heart sound detection

When designing a circular piezoelectric vibrator, if a relatively larger diameter substrate and a smaller diameter ceramic plate are used, the output displacement is larger, but the rigidity is lowered as well as the output load is reduced. Meantime the larger diameter of the substrate is not conducive to the wear-ability. Considering the practicability and wear-ability, the center point of the figure is selected, that is, the diameter of piezoelectric ceramic plate is 15 mm, and the diameter of substrate is 27 mm.

Subsequently, whether the cavity height affects the deformation of the piezoelectric vibrator is verified. According to the single variable principle, the piezoelectric vibrator selected previously is used in this experiment. The single variable is the height of the cavity (the cavity diameter is consistent with the piezoelectric vibrator). The cavity height varies from 2–10 mm, and a uniform load of 2 kPa is applied to the piezoelectric vibrator. And then we observe the change of sensitivity of the piezoelectric vibrator with the height of cavity. As displayed in Fig. 5, the height of the cavity has little effect on the displacement output of the circular piezoelectric vibrator, which is almost negligible.

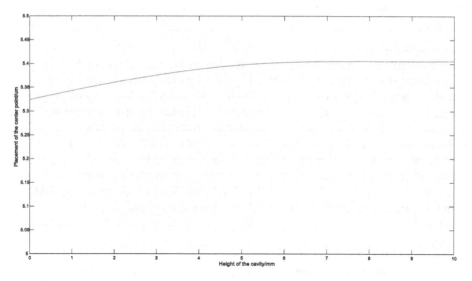

Fig. 5. Cavity height and center point displacement curve of piezoelectric vibrator

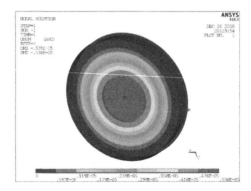

Fig. 6. Deformation diagram of piezoelectric sensor (Color figure online)

In summary, the size of the sensor designed in this paper is as follows: the diameter of the substrate is 27 mm, the diameter of piezoelectric ceramic piece is 15 mm, the height of the cavity is 3 mm, and the outer diameter is the same as the substrate. The deformation diagram is shown in Fig. 6 and the colors represent the displacement of the sensor.

Dynamic Simulation

To avoid resonance caused by the close working frequency and natural frequency of piezoelectric sensors, the dynamic characteristics of piezoelectric sensors are analyzed, including natural frequency and modal analysis, which is only related to the structure of piezoelectric sensors regardless of external loads. Considering that the behaviors such as speaking, breathing and exercise are unavoidable during their daily life, the frequency range of this dynamic characteristic experiment is set from 10–20000 Hz.

The first to 6th order modal shape diagram obtained by simulation (the corresponding natural frequencies are shown in Table 2.) show that the first mode of the piezoelectric sensor is similar to its static displacement under uniform load, and the corresponding natural frequency is 2236.1 Hz. The clinically valuable frequency range of heart sound is usually 10–600 Hz, so the sensor meets the application requirements.

Table 2. 1st–6th order natural frequencies of piezoelectric vibrator

Order	1	2	3	4	5	6
Frequency (Hz)	2236.1	4524.5	4534.2	8422	8457.3	10447

Static Simulation

To verify the performances of stress concentration, the static simulation has been carried out. The 2 kPa load has been applied to the piezoelectric vibrator. The stress distribution diagram is shown in Fig. 7(a). By defining the path, the stress distribution curve in the X direction has been extracted, as shown in Fig. 7(b). The unit of the vertical axis in Fig. 7(b) is Pa, and the horizontal axis corresponds to the external diameter length of the sensor.

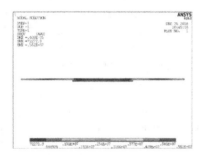
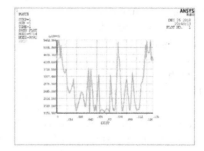

Fig. 7. (a) Stress distribution diagram (b) Stress distribution curve

From the results of the static simulation, it can be seen that the maximum stresses occur in the stress concentration areas, this is, the position of the piezoelectric ceramic plate. The detection sensitivity can be guaranteed.

2.4 Fabrication

After determining the size of sensor components, it needs to be packaged according the designed structure. The piezoelectric vibrator is bonded to the cavity with reference to the traditional stethoscope structure; the flexible film made of Hydrotin-C-Pad [16] material is covered on the surface of the vibrator considering the performance of piezoelectric vibrator and the transmission quality of heart sound, so as to improve the wear-ability of the sensor; The PVC plastic shell is used as the protective layer to prevent sweat corrosion. Finally, the above components are adhered by the polyurethane glue to ensure the sensor sealing property (Fig. 8).

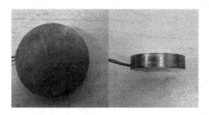

Fig. 8. The designed sensor prototype

3 Experiment and Results

3.1 Preparation

To verify the availability and performance of the designed sensor, TSD108 sensor is selected as the reference group in this chapter, as shown in Fig. 9(b). Piezoelectric sensor and TSD108 sensor are connected to the BIOPAC System (model: MP150, BIOPAC Systems INC., USA) to collect heart sound signals. TSD108 is a physiological sounds microphone developed by the BIOPAC Company. The TSD108 acoustical transducer element is a piezo-electric ceramic disk, which is bonded to the interior of a metallic circular housing. Its similar structure and detection principle with the designed sensor makes it suitable as the reference device in the experiment, besides it has high sensitivity.

The experiment required 6 student volunteers to wear a chest strap at room temperature of 26 °C. The chest strap was fixed at about 2 cm below the chest nipple with a certain initial pressure, requiring the wearer to stand still, the diagram of the acquisition system is shown in Fig. 9(c). The written consent was acquired from each participant before the experiment. And this was a non-clinical study performed on healthy subjects without any harming procedure. Therefore, ethical approval was not sought for execution of this study. According to the Nyquist's sampling law, the sampling frequency was set at 2 kHz and a record of 120 s collection. The collected two groups of heart sound datasets were further compared and analyzed in MATLAB. In this paper, the heart sound signals of one of the volunteers are randomly selected for analysis and comparison.

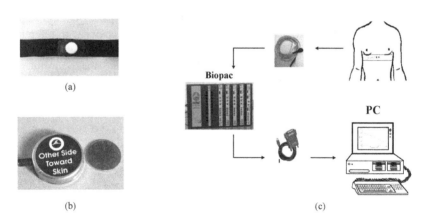

Fig. 9. Diagram of the acquisition system ((a) chest strap with piezoelectric sensor (b) TSD108 sensor (c) acquisition system)

3.2   Results

It can be seen from Fig. 10 that the first and second heart sound (S1 and S2) are obvious and its cardiac cycle is about 700 ms, and the corresponding heart rate is about 85 beats/min. The ratio of the S1S2 interval and S2S1 interval is approximately 1:2, which is consistent with the normal heart sounds standard. In addition, the maximum value collected by the designed sensor and TSD108 is respectively 0.06 V and 0.02 V. Thus the sensitivity of piezoelectric sensor is higher than that of TSD108 sensor under the same conditions.

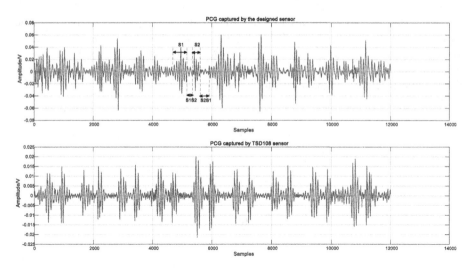

Fig. 10. PCG tested by the designed heart sound sensor and TSD108 sensor

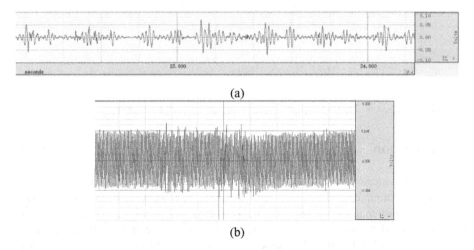

Fig. 11. SNR test of piezoelectric sensor: (a) heart sound signals (b) output without heart sound signals

To further verify the performance of the designed piezoelectric sensor, the signal-to-noise ratio (SNR) testing experiment of the piezoelectric sensor and TSD108 sensor have been conducted. The formula of SNR can be converted into the ratio relation of voltage amplitude, that is, SNR = [20lg(Vs/Vn)] dB.

First the piezoelectric sensor has been tested, and the test results of the heart sound are shown in Fig. 11(a), and it is determined that the maximum value of the heart sound signals is 0.05 V. The output of the sensor without the heart sound signals are shown in

Fig. 11(b), and the noise signals is 4 mV. Therefore, the SNR of the piezoelectric sensor is 21.94 dB. Subsequently, TSD108 sensor has been tested. As shown in Fig. 12 (a), the maximum of heart sound signals is 0.02 V; and the noise signal is 2 mV as shown in Fig. 12(b). So the SNR of TSD108 sensor is 20 dB. The above test results indicate that the SNR of the piezoelectric sensor is 2 dB higher than the TSD108 sensor.

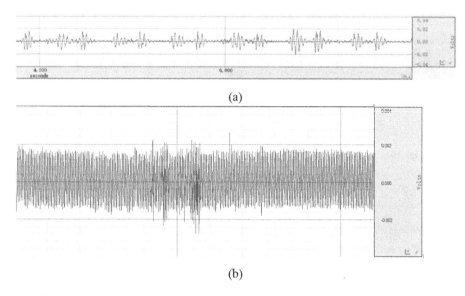

(a)

(b)

Fig. 12. SNR test of TSD108: (a) heart sound signals (b) output without heart sound signals

4   Conclusion

In this paper, a small, low-cost and wearable piezoelectric heart sound sensor has been designed and implemented for long-term dynamic monitoring and preliminary diagnosis. The major contribution includes: the optimum structure design of the sensor has been determined through ANSYS simulation analysis and experimental verification. The sensor is embedded into the fabric-based chest strap to verify the detection performance in wearable scenarios. The test of sensor performance is conducted by using the BIOPAC Systems. The heart sound waveform measured by the designed sensor is significantly correlated with that of the TSD108 sensor. Besides, it exhibits better detection performance, its sensitivity and signal-to-noise ratio are improved.

Acknowledgements. This work is supported by National Key Research & Development Plan of China (NO. 2016YFB1001401) and National Natural Science Foundation of China (NO. 61572110).

References

1. Leng, S., San Tan, R., Chai, K.T.C., et al.: The electronic stethoscope. Biomed. Eng. online **14**(1), 66 (2015)
2. Haoran, R., Hailong, J., Chen, C., et al.: A novel cardiac auscultation monitoring system based on wireless sensing for healthcare. IEEE J. Trans. Eng. Health Med. **6**, 1 (2018)
3. Hu, Y., Xu, Y.: An ultra-sensitive wearable accelerometer for continuous heart and lung sound monitoring. In: 2012 Annual International Conference of the IEEE Engineering in Medicine and Biology Society (EMBC). IEEE (2012)
4. Chen, T., Xing, S., Guo, P., et al.: The design of a new digital collecting system of heart sound signals based on XH-6 sensor. In: International Conference on Measuring Technology & Mechatronics Automation. IEEE Computer Society (2010)
5. Ou, D., Ouyang, L., Tan, Z., et al.: An electronic stethoscope for heart diseases based on micro-electro-mechanical-system microphone. In: IEEE International Conference on Industrial Informatics. IEEE (2017)
6. Zhang, G., Liu, M., Guo, N., Zhang, W.: Design of the MEMS piezoresistive electronic heart sound sensor. Sensors **16**, 1728 (2016)
7. Malik, B., Eya, N., Migdadi, H., et al.: Design and development of an electronic stethoscope. In: Internet Technologies & Applications. IEEE (2017)
8. Grundlehner, B., Buxi, D.: Methods to characterize sensors for capturing body sounds. In: International Conference on Body Sensor Networks. IEEE Computer Society (2011)
9. Popov, B., Sierra, G., Telfort, V., et al.: Estimation of respiratory rate and heart rate during treadmill tests using acoustic sensor. In: International Conference of the Engineering in Medicine & Biology Society. IEEE (2005)
10. Surtel, W., Maciejewski, M., Maciejewska, B.: Processing of simultaneous biomedical signal data in circulatory system conditions diagnosis using mobile sensors during patient activity (2014)
11. Rajala, S., Lekkala, J.: Film-type sensor materials PVDF and EMFi in measurement of cardiorespiratory signals— a review. IEEE Sens. J. **12**(3), 439–446 (2012)
12. Miles, R.N., Cui, W., Su, Q.T., et al.: A MEMS low-noise sound pressure gradient microphone with capacitive sensing. J. Microelectromech. Syst. **24**(1), 241–248 (2015)
13. Jiang, D.-Y., Zheng, Z.-Y., Li, L.: The analyses of the vibration model of piezoelectric ceramic piece based on ANSYS. J. Trans. Technol. **12**(4), 9–16 (2003)
14. Fan, X., Ma, S., Zhang, X., et al.: Simulation analysis of piezoelectric ceramic chip PZT based on ANSYS. Piezoelectrics Acoustooptics **36**(3), 416–420 (2014)
15. Xu, P., Tao, X., Wang, S.: Measurement of wearable electrode and skin mechanical interaction using displacement and pressure sensors (2011)
16. Bail, D.H.L., et al.: Cellulose pads (Hydrotin-C): a new solid coupling agent. Echocardiography **26**(5) 508–512 (2009)
17. BIOPAC. https://www.biopac.com/product/contact-microphone/. Accessed 5 May 2019

Vertical Hand Position Estimation with Wearable Differential Barometery Supported by RFID Synchronization

Hymalai Bello[1]([✉]), Jhonny Rodriguez[1], and Paul Lukowicz[1,2]

[1] German Research Center for Artificial Intelligence DFKI, Kaiserslautern, Germany
bello@dfki.uni-kl.de
[2] Technical University of Kaiserslautern, Kaiserslautern, Germany

Abstract. We demonstrate how a combination of a wrist-worn and stationary barometer can be used to track the vertical position of the user's Hand with an accuracy in the range of 30 cm. To this end, the two barometers synchronized each time an RFID reader detects them being in proximity of each other. The accuracy is sufficient to detect a specific shelve of a cupboard on which something has been placed or determine if the user's hand is touching his/her head or the torso. The advantage of the method over IMU based approaches is that it requires only a wrist-worn sensor (as could be implemented in a smartwatch) and a reference either in an often access location in the environment or a pocket (e.g.in the smartphone) and it does not depend on a stable magnetic environment. The proposed system was tested in two different activities: Shelve recognition in a warehouse picking scenario and movement of the arm to specific body locations. Despite the simplicity of our method, it shows initial results between 55–62% and 73–91% accuracy, respectively.

Keywords: Relative pressure · Barometer · RFID · Order picking · Wearable sensing

1 Introduction and Related Work

Our hands are the primary means of interacting with our physical environment. Thus, the position of user's hands is a crucial piece of information for a broad range of context recognition task. It is made difficult by two considerations. First, in many cases, to be meaningful, the tracking has to be accurate to within 10–50cm. This is, for example, the case when we need to know which object the user has picked from a shelve, which/how she/he has interacted with a household device, or when he/she has taken a piece of food into the mouth. Second, for

---

The research reported in this paper has been partially supported by the BMBF (German Federal Ministry of Education and Research) in the project HeadSense(project number 01IW18001). The support is gratefully acknowledged.

L. Mucchi et al. (Eds.): BODYNETS 2019, LNICST 297, pp. 24–33, 2019.
https://doi.org/10.1007/978-3-030-34833-5_3

many applications, the amount of instrumentation that can be introduced into the environment to facilitate the tracking is limited. In an ideal case, the tracking would be achieved by a sensor that can be easily integrated within a smartwatch or a fitness tracker with no need for further environment instrumentation.

Currently, there are three main approaches to hand tracking. First, are classical object tracking systems. These are either expensive and requiring elaborate infrastructure (such as visual tracking [2], UWB, ultrasound [8]), or have problems achieving the needed accuracy (e.g., Bluetooth [6] or WiFi). Second is the use of RFID tags in the environment combined with a wrist-worn RFID reader (see e.g., [5] as an example of the use of RFID based object interaction detection for activity recognition). The disadvantage is the need to mark every relevant object with an RFID. Also, given the size of the antenna that can be fixed at the wrist there can be problems with the detection of some interactions where the wrist does not approach the tag close enough in the usual interaction mode of the specific object (e.g. tag fixed to the bottom of a cup and the used grabbing the cup by the handle). Finally, IMUs can be used together with appropriate bio-mechanical body models to track the exact position and orientation of the wrist. However, given the degrees of freedom of human joints, this can not be achieved by a wrist-worn sensor alone but requires at least three sensors: one at the wrist, one at the upper arm and one at the torso (at least for an exact solution), under a stable magnetic environment.

This paper focuses on a subset of the hand tracking problem: the detection of the vertical position of the wrist. Specific applications that we consider is detecting which shelve from a cupboard the user has reached to (relevant for household activity monitoring and order picking industrial environments) and the detection of gestures such as reaching to the head/mouth (relevant for example for nutrition tracking). To this end, we propose to use a wrist-worn digital barometer. Such devices are already widely used in smartphones and finding their way into smartwatches. The use of digital barometers has been widely studied in the context of indoor navigation [4]. The idea is that while the absolute air pressure varies too much due to weather conditions to be useful for indoor level estimation, short term changes in the air pressure are a reliable indication of going up or down. Within the accuracy needed to detect going up or down one level in a building drift and other sources of errors [9] have been shown to be manageable. Short term change in air pressure has even been used to distinguish sitting and standing [11] and for fall detection [3].

For the applications envisioned by our work, such as the detection of a specific shelve accessed by the user, such approaches are not directly applicable for two reasons. First, we need to detect not just change in elevation but must somehow translate the measurement to absolute elevation. Second, the envisioned precision of around 30 cm is influenced not just by natural air pressure variations but also by the drift of typical, low-cost sensors. Our solution is based on the observation that in most environments, there is a fixed location with known elevation, which the user's hand frequently approaches. Thus, for example, the hand will often "hang" around the hip. In warehouse picking applications, the user has a pushcart on which items are placed after being taken from the shelves. Such locations can be used to place a reference barometer and an RFID reader while adding an RFID-Tag to the barometer at the user's wrist. Each time the user's hand approaches the location, it is detected by the RFID reader, and the readings of the stationary and the wrist-worn barometer are synchronized. The elevation of the wrist is then tracked by comparing the signal of the wrist-worn barometer to the reference.

In this paper, we describe the implementation of a system based on those ideas and the quantitative evaluation of its performance demonstrating, that given the drift and accuracy of typical low-cost sensors it is indeed a feasible approach.

2   System Description

The prototyping platform used is a combination between the development board STM32L475 DISCOVERY with Arm Cortex-M4, BMP388 Bosch pressure sensor, the RFID PN532 chip, and a firmware development based in MBED OS 5.12. Furthermore, the system is complemented with a fast and straightforward vertical position model using the barometer pressure measurements and RFID detection to signal the reference position. The communication to the sensors is based on I2C port at 400KHz. The data from the platform was obtain using ST-LINK-UART at a baud-rate 1 Mbps. As the firmware is based on a real-time operating system (MBED-OS 5.12), the timing is not sequential, and it depends on the schedule and the total preemptive RTOS. The data of the pressure has a sampling-rate below 62,5 Hz (16 ms) 90% of the time, as shown in Fig. 2, suitable for detecting a picking action(around 1 s). The hardware depicted in Fig. 1 and two systems were built, one of those, used as a reference with the RFID-Reader and the other one assembled on the wrist with RFID-TAG.

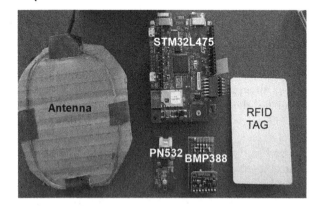

Fig. 1. Hardware: Antenna, STM32L475, PN532(RFID Reader), BMP388, RFID TAG

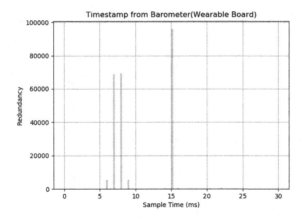

Fig. 2. Sample rate distribution for the pressure

2.1 Vertical Position Model

The vertical position model is based on the well known, and highly used relationship between the barometric pressure and the height as in [4, 7, 12] which is expressed in the following formula 1.

$$H = \frac{Temperature}{Beta} \cdot [\frac{Pressure}{PressureRef}^{\frac{-Beta*R}{g}} - 1] \tag{1}$$

In [12], they used a base barometer and a rover barometer and made the height estimation relative to the sea level pressure. Since the air pressure varies typically between 950 and 1050 hPa during a year, the expected variation in sea level due to air pressure is between +63 cm and −37 cm around mean sea level, which is a situation that we cannot quantify or control. In [9] they studied the sources of errors in the barometer pressure measurements, and they concluded that barometers in differential mode would provide highly accurate altitude solution, but local disturbances in pressure need to be taken into account in the application design. We proposed to apply the formula 1 but, relative to a reference point pressure and a wearable pressure device, removing the sea level pressure dependency entirely, and having access to monitor the changes in the reference height. In the case of temperature on the reference level, the authors in [7] used the temperature as an average of standard atmospheric pressure and current atmospheric pressure, in our case the temperature is considered as the average value between the reference-point and the wearable-device-temperature.

To implement this approach, in the first step two devices equally equipped as described before were placed on the same table (same height) close to each other, and the pressure values were recorded in 3 different days for 20–45 min as depicted in Fig. 3, these recordings were done indoor without interruptions (windows and door closed), this test was done to obtain the static information of the system. The two pressures (in static condition on the same height) and their coherence is depicted in Fig. 4, the coherence result shows that there is a relation between the two pressures in the low-frequency band, which led us to apply exponentially weighted low pass filter with a half-life = 20 samples to both signal with the aims to locate the signals in the area of higher similarity. Increasing the similarity also increase the possibilities of a linear fitting between the two pressures.

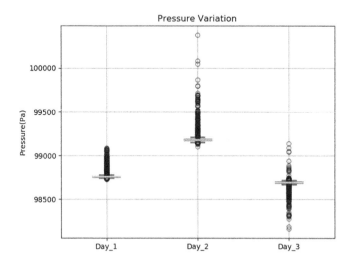

Fig. 3. Pressure variation in 3 days

When the goal is to have a precision of less than one meter it is important to also make the stationary Test (Dickey-Fuller test), because a variation of only 1 Pa in the pressure means an 8 cm difference relative to sea level, and even more with a variable standard deviation, then a linear fitting is only valid in the situation it was calculated. The results of the stationary Test for both signals in Fig. 4 is shown in Table. 1, the Test was applied for the 3 different days in static condition, the Reference-device (RDevice) pressure was 95–99% stationary, ($Test < CriticalValue(1\%)$), and for the Wearable-device (WDevice) pressure was 90–95% stationary ($Test < CriticalValue(5\%)$), despite that the results are almost stationary, we observed that the pressure values were different for each day and that the offset difference between the RDevice and the WDevice is not constant, go to Fig. 3. From the similarity and stationary results, the most simple version for the model will be a linear model, as in Eq. 2.

$$WDevicePressure = a * RDevicePressure + offset \qquad (2)$$

The data in Fig. 4, was divided into 70% training and 30% test, RANSAC, and Polynomial Fit methods were used, and the results are presented in the Table.2. The minimum mean-squared error = 4.27 Pa(an approximated value of

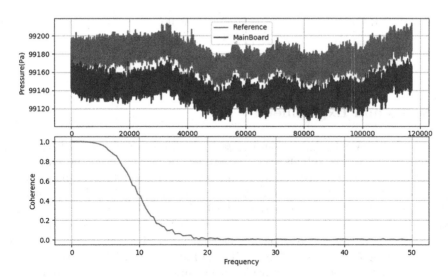

Fig. 4. Reference device pressure(red) and Wearable Device pressure(blue) and the coherence of the signals (Color figure online)

Table 1. Stationary test results

Reference board	Wearable board
Test = −3.44	Test = −3.17
p-value = 0.0096	p-value = 0.022
Lags = 71	Lags = 71
Observations = 118265.0	Observations = 118265.0
Critical-value(1%) = −3.430405	Critical-value(1%) = −3.43
Critical-value(5%) = −2.86	Critical-value(5%) = −2.86
Critical-value(10%) = −2.57	Critical-value(10%) = −2.57

33 cm, relative to the sea level pressure) was from the RANSAC test as shown in Table 2.

$$a = 0.97 \tag{3}$$

Also, the proposed solution for the offset calculation is to use an error-monitor option(RFID-Barometer at reference point), so the difference is measured at the beginning, and then every time the WDevice is in RDevice position. The monitor-error option selected is a simple but widely used RFID Tag-Reader combination for picking order activities like in [1, 10, 13].

Table 2. Linear fitting results

RANSAC	Polynomial
Mean-squared-error = 4.27	Mean-squared-error = 4.47
Variance-score = 0.95	Variance-score: 0.94

3 Setup and Experiments

To evaluate the system, two scenarios were tested, the first one as order-picking inside a warehouse (Warehouse-Box Experiment)which involved the movement of a box between a compartment and a reference position (a table, simulating an order-picking car), and the second scenario as the movement of the arm around the upper, middle and lower part of the body in daily life activities (Body-Experiment). For the Warehouse-Box Experiment, a shelf of six compartments and a table simulating an order picking car was used. Five volunteers were asked at the beginning to go to the reference (RFID-Barometer on the table), and later on to take a box and put the box inside each compartment randomly (10 picking-actions per compartment) and wait there between 3–5 s, each time returning to reference, waiting again on the reference 3–5 s. The maximum compartment height is 28 cm, and the distance of the reference point to the ground is 85.4 cm, the heights of the volunteers in decreasing order were: 197,190,177,170,157 cm. For the Body-Experiment, the reference point was set around the pocket (RFID-Barometer on the pocket), and the person needed to start again at the reference and then go to the upper body part (Head), body middle part (Heart) and body lower part (Foot) randomly (also, 10 repetitions per position), and every time going back to reference. In addition, the use of the RFID as monitor of the reference location, was tested with 3 participants, where two of them pick-up an object 30 times and went back to the table and the third participant did this 50 times, in all of the cases the RFID captured 100% of the picking actions, which means the RFID is a good enough to be a monitor device.

3.1 Identification by Naive Bayes Classifier

To quantify the accuracy of the system a naive Bayes classifier was used, due to the Gaussian behavior shown in the height estimation using barometer pressure, please go to Fig. 5. Each picking action was divided into frames of 12 samples (0.192 s, 16 ms/sample), from which statistical features as mean, standard deviation, maximum and minimum were calculated. In the case of the Warehouse-Box Experiment, the model was done using 1 min of static data from each compartment, and tested with five volunteers, in which the best case was 62,86% accuracy, and the worst case was 56.81% accuracy. The confusion matrix from the best case can be seen on the left side of Fig. 6. With regard to the body experiment, we tested 3 model scenarios, in the first scenario the model was based on

Level Distribution Training Data (Meters)

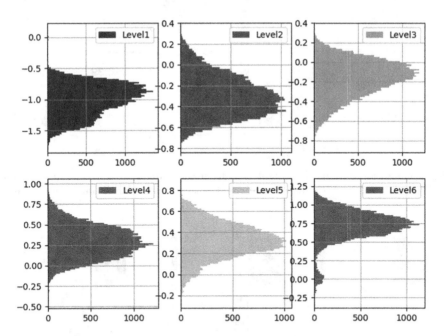

Fig. 5. Level distribution (vertical axis in meters) from the warehouse-box experiment.

the volunteer with the middle height, 177 cm(70% training), getting an accuracy scores of 82.03% (volunteer's height = 170 cm), 91.48% (volunteer's height = 177 cm) and 73.05% (volunteer's height = 190 cm). In the second scenario the model was based on the participant with a height = 170 cm (70% training), given accuracy results of 87.28%, 81.82% and 78.81% (In height increasing order). In the last scenario the model was based on the volunteer with height = 190 cm, with accuracy results of 86.39%, 85.23% and 84.25% (In height increasing order, the confusion matrices of the participants on the third scenario are shown in Fig. 7, this third scenario is the one with less variation on accuracy.

In order to compare our results, the same classifier with a model based on static data and an initial offset correction but without the RFID information was applied to the same data. The calculated height was directly the relative value between the RDevice and WDevice pressures, the resulted confusion matrix is shown on the right side of Fig. 6, in this case, only the drifting and the sudden changes on the pressure errors are considered. No paying attention to the offset dependency decreased the accuracy to 48.61%, and the identification of the middle levels are highly affected.

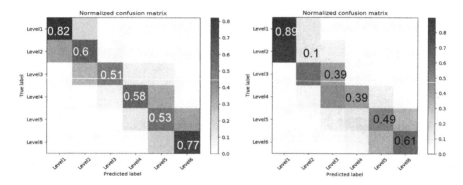

Fig. 6. Confusion matrix of the best case from the warehouse-box experiment using RFID-monitor error method(Left side), and without using RFID information(Right side)

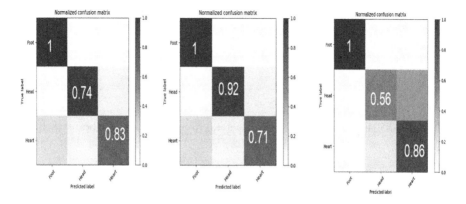

Fig. 7. Volunteer 1 (170 cm), Volunteer 2 (177 cm) and Volunteer 3 (190 cm) confusion matrices from the body-experiment

4   Results and Contributions

The use of relative height estimation by barometer pressure differences and the RFID as a monitor-error method improved the detection of the vertical position compared to using the barometer-height relationship without RFID, in which the dependency of the drifting, humidity and temperature were not taken into account. This goal was achieved by only using a simple linear model and an RFID chip to calculated the initial offset and to reduce the impact of the drifting and offset in the vertical position estimation, additionally to the reduction of the effects of sudden changes on pressure, due to the opening of windows or doors around the devices. This initial step could evolve into a fusion of sensor to obtain more accurate results. An important point to consider is that the prototyping hardware has a height of 11 cm, which means that the error will be on the measurement depending on the orientation of the wrist in the picking action.

Moreover, the linear fitting has a minimum mean-squared error of 4.27 Pa. For the simplicity and limitations of the system, this first step achieved relatively good results.

References

1. Koepp, R., Allen, T., Fassett, J., Teng, A.: Achieving high speed RFID die pick and place operation. In: 2008 33rd IEEE/CPMT International Electronics Manufacturing Technology Conference (IEMT), pp. 1–8 (2008)
2. Cho, W., Shin, M., Jang, J., Paik, J.: Robust pedestrian height estimation using principal component analysis and its application to automatic camera calibration. In: 2018 International Conference on Electronics, Information, and Communication, pp. 1–2 (2018)
3. Cola, G., Avvenuti, M., Piazza, P., Vecchio, A.: Fall Detection using a head-worn barometer. In: Perego, P., Andreoni, G., Rizzo, G. (eds.) MobiHealth 2016. LNICST, vol. 192, pp. 217–224. Springer, Cham (2017). https://doi.org/10.1007/978-3-319-58877-3_29
4. Ehrlich, C.R., Blankenbach, J.: Pedestrian localisation inside buildings based on multi-sensor smartphones. In: 2018 Ubiquitous Positioning, Indoor Navigation and Location-Based Services (UPINLBS), pp. 1–10 (2018)
5. Fishkin, K.P., Philipose, M., Rea, A.: Hands-on RFID: wireless wearables for detecting use of objects. In: Ninth IEEE International Symposium on Wearable Computers (ISWC 2005), pp. 38–41 (2005)
6. Hou, X., Arslan, T.: Monte carlo localization algorithm for indoor positioning using bluetooth low energy devices. In: 2017 International Conference on Localization and GNSS (ICL-GNSS), pp. 1–6 (2017)
7. Lee, D., Park, K.W., Park, C., Kang, I.: An efficient heave estimation using time-differenced gps carrier phase measurements and compensated barometer measurement applying error model. In: 2015 International Association of Institutes of Navigation World Congress, pp. 1–6 (2015)
8. Ogris, G., Stiefmeier, T., Junker, H., Lukowicz, P., Troster, G.: Using ultrasonic hand tracking to augment motion analysis based recognition of manipulative gestures. In: Ninth IEEE International Symposium on Wearable Computers, pp. 152–159 (2005)
9. Parviainen, J., Kantola, J., Collin, J.: Differential barometry in personal navigation. In: 2008 IEEE/ION Position, Location and Navigation Symposium, pp. 148–152 (2008)
10. Riyadi, M.A., Sudira, N., Hanif, M.H., Triwiyatno, A.: Design of pick and place robot with identification and classification object based on RFID using stm32vldiscovery. In: 2017 International Conference on Electrical Engineering and Computer Science (ICECOS), pp. 171–176 (2017)
11. Rodríguez-Martín, D., Samà, A., Pérez-López, C., Català, A.: Posture transitions identification based on a triaxial accelerometer and a barometer sensor. In: Rojas, I., Joya, G., Catala, A. (eds.) IWANN 2017. LNCS, vol. 10306, pp. 333–343. Springer, Cham (2017). https://doi.org/10.1007/978-3-319-59147-6_29
12. Wei, S., Dan, G., Chen, H.: Altitude data fusion utilising differential measurement and complementary filter. IET Sci. Measur. Technol. **10**(8), 874–879 (2016)
13. Woelfle, M., Guenthner, W.A.: Wearable RFID in order picking systems. In: RFID SysTech 2011 7th European Workshop on Smart Objects: Systems, Technologies and Applications, pp. 1–6 (2011)

Systems and Medical Applications

The Smart Insole: A Pilot Study of Fall Detection

Xiaoye Qian(iD), Haoyou Cheng(iD), Diliang Chen(iD), Quan Liu(iD), Huan Chen(iD),
Haotian Jiang(iD), and Ming-Chun Huang$^{(\boxtimes)}$(iD)

Case Western Reserve University, Cleveland, OH 44106, USA
{xxq82,hxc399,dxc494,qxl268,hxc556,hxj172,mxh602}@case.edu

Abstract. Falls are common events among human beings and raised a global health problem. Wearable sensors can provide quantitative assessments for fall-based movements. Automatic fall detection systems based on the wearable sensors are becoming popular in recent years. This paper proposes a new fall detection system based on the smart insole. Each smart insole contains pressure a pressure sensor array and can provide abundant pressure information during the daily activities. According to such information, the system can successfully distinguish the fall from other activities of daily livings (ADLs) using deep learning algorithms. To reduce the computational complexity through the classifiers, the raw data for each sensor in the time windows are utilized. Furthermore, the deep visualization approach is applied to provide an intuitive explanation of how the deep learning system works on distinguishing the fall events. Both quantitative and qualitative experiments are demonstrated in this paper to prove the feasibility and effectiveness of the proposed fall detection system.

Keywords: Pressure sensor array · Fall detection · Deep learning · Smart insole · Deep visualization

1 Introduction

Falls are the most common incident among human beings. It poses a global health problem. In the United States, more than 1.6 million adults receive treatment due to the fall-related accidents every year [7], and the financial costs associated with fall are rising in these years [10]. Approximately one-third of the aged population fall at least once a year, and the similar reports are also generated from other countries, such as Spain and Colombia [1]. With increasing age, the physical changes make people more prone to falls, and the fall injuries are exacerbated. Falls event leads to significant injuries including skin abrasions, upper limb and hip fractures, brain injuries and general connective tissue lesions [2, 11]. Falls not

We thank the Institute for Smart, Secure and Connected Systems (ISSACS) for support.

L. Mucchi et al. (Eds.): BODYNETS 2019, LNICST 297, pp. 37–49, 2019.
https://doi.org/10.1007/978-3-030-34833-5_4

only seriously threaten the health, but also cause the psychological problem like lowering the self-confidence and being afraid of independent life, which further weakens the quality of daily life [9]. In the past few decades, falls detection has attracted more attention from the public. Most of the time, the fallers might lose consciousness and are unable to call for help. Therefore, many automatic fall detection technologies have proposed in recent years [16].

It is generally known that the vision, sound, radar, and infrared sensors perform well to detect falls automatically [13]. However, these ambient sensor-based technologies have the problem of privacy and make the seniors face many constraints, for example, living in a restricted zone [12,14]. In the last decades, the development of the wearable sensor-device provides new chances for detecting fall-related accidents. The wearable sensor-based fall detection systems eliminate the space limitation compared with the systems based on the ambient technologies [12]. Due to the wearable accelerometers have the characters of small size and low price, many wearable fall detection systems are designed based on such sensors and place them on different positions on the subject of interest (SOI). However, in these ways, SOI have to wear many sensors during daily activities, which make them inconvenient. On the other hands, It is forgettable for the SOI to wear complicated wearable sensors, especially for seniors. Nowadays, smart insoles based on the wearable pressure sensors array placed in shoes can provide sufficient information for the gait analysis [8]. On the other hand, the characteristics of smart insole placed in the shoe are convenient and hard to be forgotten by the users.

In this article, we mainly focus on the fall detection based on the smart insole. To acquire the pressure information of an area, a high-spatial-resolution pressure sensor array has been developed over an individual pressure sensor. We extend smart insole with 48 pressure sensors array [8] to contain 96 pressure sensors for receiving more precise pressure information. The deep learning methods are applied to make the fall detection classifier. Besides, the comparison experiments of using the combinations of the smart insole with other wearable sensors including accelerometers and gyroscopes to perform the fall detection are also demonstrated. To further understand the deep learning model on distinguishing fall events, the saliency visualization [3] is introduced to present how the pressure information during the dynamic motion pattern contributes towards a fall classification.

2   Related Work

Most of the fall detection systems are designed by utilizing wearable devices [7,12,15,18]. The wearable devices are attached to clothes or part of the body of the SOI for detecting the falls [1,7,12]. The sensors as the main components of wearable devices measure the characteristics of the movements of SOI. The strategies of the fall detection system mainly monitor the variables of acceleration and speed primarily. The changes of the acceleration magnitude are utilized to detect the falls. When the value of accelerometers exceeds a specific threshold, the falls are recognized [15,19]. However, the threshold-based systems based on

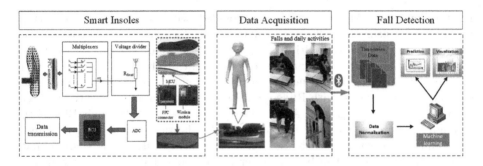

Fig. 1. The flowchart of the falls detection system. The data are collected from the pressure sensor array on the smart insoles that are attached to the SOI. The data are transmitted to the centralized data warehouse, and the machine learning algorithms are implemented for the falling recognition.

accelerometers are difficult to distinguish the falls from other activities that have similar characteristics in term of acceleration [1]. Some researchers enhance the system based on the accelerometers by applying more wearable sensors. The systems integrate the sensors that are placed on different positions such as the waist, ankle, and chest on the subject of SOI with data mining techniques [12,16–18]. Besides, the pressure sensor array designed on insole has been used in gait analysis and can provide sufficient information about the SOI movements [8]. In order to overcome the weakness of using a threshold, machine learning approaches are implemented including k-nearest neighbor (k-NN) [6], support vector machines (SVM) [7], decision tree [5] and artificial neural networks (ANNs) [1]. To understand the ANN-based classification models, several visualization techniques are used. Zeiler et al. [4] try to reconstruct the input of each layer from the output. Simonyan et al. [3] introduce a specific class saliency visualization approach to find the most influential part of a particular classification.

3   Methodology

The working flow of the proposed system is illustrated in Fig. 1. The smart insoles are applied in the proposed system to collect the data. The data are transmitted to a centralized data warehouse via Bluetooth. The fall detection movements are learned by the deep learning approaches and the deep learning visualization are applied for interpreting the deep learning classifier of the fall event.

3.1   Hardware Architecture of Smart Insole

The smart insole is applied in the proposed system for fall detection. Figure 1 shows the hardware architecture of smart insole utilized in the fall detection system. The smart insole is developed by integrating the circuit board and pressure sensor array through an insole shaped package. A high-performance Microcontroller Unit (MCU) is used for signal processing. Besides, twenty-four 12-bit

Digital Converter (ADC) channels are provided, which are used for measuring the pressure sensor array [8]. In this manuscript, each smart insole contains 96 pressure sensors. A Flexible Printed Circuit (FPC) connector connects the pressure sensor array with the signal processing circuit. Multiplexers are connected with all the pressure sensors and form a voltage divider circuit by connecting the selected pressure sensor with Rfixed, and the Analog could measure the voltage drop on the pressure sensor to ADC. The data can be transmitted via Bluetooth through the wireless module. The top layer is a fabric cover which guarantees the comfort of wearing and the pressure sensor array with insole shape is put into the middle layer. The bottom layer is an insole shaped package which is designed for settled battery and the circuit board.

3.2   Deep Learning Algorithms and Evaluation Metrics

To distinguish falls from other daily activities based on the data collected from smart insoles, Artificial neural networks (ANN) model is designed. Before the data are fed into the model, the data normalization is implemented. ANN has been proved to be efficient due to the promising results on the sensor data [1]. Hidden features are extracted from the input data through the Artificial neural networks, and more abstract features are calculated by deeper layers. Multi-Layer Perceptron (MLP) and convolutional neural network (CNN) are two primary subcategories of Artificial neural networks. To take advantage of the characteristic of time-series data dependency, the sliding window is employed in MLP and CNN for the falls detection. The performance can be validated by the following success criteria. *Sensitivity (Se)* represents the capacity of the automatic system on fall detection, $Se = TP/(TP + FN)$. *Precision (Pr)* is the precision of the system for detecting falls, $Pr = TP/(TP + FP)$. *Specificity(Sp)* measures the ability of the system for identifying ADLs, $Sp = TN/(TN + FP)$. Accuracy (Ac) clearly describe the correct differentiation between falls and non-falls, $Ac = (TP + TN)/(TP + FP + FN + TN)$. Here, TP (a fall occurs and the system recognizes it as a fall), TN (a fall does not occur and the system does not recognize it as a fall), FP (a fall does not happen but the system recognizes it as a fall), and FN (a fall happens but the system misses it) are used in the calculation of sensitivity, precision and accuracy.

3.3   Deep Learning Visualization

The deep neural network has made enormous progress over the last several decades and got tremendous attention from academia, industry, and health-care community. Many researchers have been considered about improvements in the knowledge of how to create high-performing architectures and learning algorithms. Historically, deep learning models have been thought of as "black boxes", meaning that the inner workings were different to understand or interpret. In order to shine the light into the "black boxes" to better understand exactly what the deep learning has learned, the deep learning visualization approach is applied.

In this section, the technique for the deep learning model visualization [3] is introduced. Saliency map is a quick way to tell which variation of the sensor data influenced the classification decision made by the network. Given a trained classification CNN, a specific activities class ac of interest, an sensor data I_s and the class score function $S_{ac}(I)$. The value of every single sensor I_s are sorted according to the influence on the score $S_{ac}(I_s)$. Take the linear score model as the example,

$$S_{ac}(I) = w_{ac}^T I + b_{ac} \tag{1}$$

where the I is the input sensor data, and w_{ac} and b_{ac} are the parameters in the model. The magnitude of elements w determines the importance though sensor I for the specific class. In CNN scenario, it is a highly non-linear problem. According to the first-order Taylor expansion, the $S_{ac}(I)$ can be approximated expressed with a linear function in the neighborhood of I_s.

$$S_{ac}(I) \approx w^T I + b, \; where \; w = \frac{\partial S_{ac}}{\partial I}|_{I_s} \tag{2}$$

Current deep learning Visualization is mostly focused on image-based system [4]. However, in the sensor-based system, it lacks efficient methods to know what the changes in movements make the models arrive at a certain classification decision. Here, exploring the deep learning visualization for the sensor-based system are mainly discussed. To acquire the saliency map from the time-series pressure sensor array, a two-dimension matrix should be utilized. The time is represented over one dimension while another dimension is expected to be related to the value of the pressure sensor array. The class saliency map $S \in R^{m \times n}$ can be calculated through the back-propagation process in the CNN and according to the derivative w. Researchers can elicit a particular interpretation using deep learning visualization for fall detection.

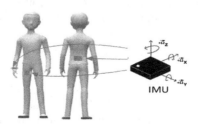

Fig. 2. The position where IMUs are attached.

4 Experiments

4.1 Dataset and Experimental Settings

It is commonly acknowledged that most of the falls occur with the directions of forwards, backward or sideways [20]. The experiments are designed with a

Table 1. The comparison experimental results of using smart insoles and wearable sensors placed on SOI for fall detection, W-waist, H-hand, T-thigh, I-smart insole, with k-nearest neighbor ($k$nn), support vector machines (svm), decision tree (dt), discriminant (dc), Multi-Layer Perceptron (mlp) and convolutional neural network (cnn).

	pr($k$nn)	se($k$nn)	sp($k$nn)	ac($k$nn)	pr(svm)	se(svm)	sp(svm)	ac(svm)
W	0.9385	0.9423	0.9896	0.9828	0.9458	0.9342	0.9910	0.9828
H	0.8566	0.8601	0.9758	0.9592	0.8477	0.8477	0.9744	0.9562
T	0.9336	0.9259	0,9889	0.9799	0.8943	0.9053	0.9820	0.9710
I	0.9555	0.9712	0.9924	0.9893	0.9874	0.9712	0.9979	0.9941
WI	0.9916	0.9753	0.9986	0.9953	0.9797	0.9918	0.9965	0.9959
HI	0.9872	0.9547	0.9979	0.9917	0.9917	0.9877	0.9986	0.9970
TI	0.9958	0.9794	0.9993	0.9964	0.9917	0.9877	0.9986	0.9970
WHTI	0.9958	0.9835	0.9993	0.9970	0.9918	0.9918	0.9986	0.9976
	pr(dt)	se(dt)	sp(dt)	ac(dt)	pr(dc)	se(dc)	sp(dc)	ac(dc)
W	0.9540	0.9383	0.9924	0.9846	0.9751	0.8066	0.9965	0.9692
H	0.8611	0.8930	0.9758	0.9639	0.8942	0.7253	0.9862	0.9503
T	0.9461	0.9383	0.9910	0.9834	0.9760	0.8354	0.9965	0.9734
I	0.9833	0.9712	0.9972	0.9935	0.9736	0.9095	0.9959	0.9834
W	0.9918	0.9877	0.9986	0.9970	0.9793	0.9753	0.9965	0.9935
HI	0.9833	0.9671	0.9972	0.9929	0.9706	0.9506	0.9952	0.9888
TI	0.9795	0.9835	0.9965	0.9947	0.9787	0.9465	0.9965	0.9835
WHTI	0.9836	0.9877	0.9972	0.9959	0.9756	0.9877	0.9959	0.9947
	pr(cnn)	se(cnn)	sp(cnn)	ac(cnn)	pr(mlp)	se(mlp)	sp(mlp)	ac(mlp)
W	0.9575	0.9783	0.9889	0.9911	0.9362	0.9565	0.9889	0.9852
H	0.9333	0.9130	0.9889	0.9793	0.8750	0.9130	0.9779	0.9704
T	0.9545	0.9348	0.9924	0.9852	0.8936	0.9130	0.9820	0.9734
I	0.9876	0.9794	0.9979	0.9953	0.9793	0.9660	0.9965	0.9921
WI	0.9959	0.9877	0.9993	0.9976	0.9862	0.9728	0.9976	0.9941
HI	0.9836	0.9877	0.9972	0.9959	0.9755	0.9835	0.9958	0.9941
TI	0.9916	0.9793	0.9986	0.9959	0.9714	0.9794	0.9952	0.9929
WHTI	0.9918	0.9918	0.9986	0.9976	0.9876	0.9835	0.9979	0.9959

group of falls containing backward falls, forward hard falls, forward soft falls, left falls and right falls. Note that, during the hard fall, SOI falls from vertical standing to the ground directly. A soft fall refers to the SOI fall to their knee before impacting on the ground. Regarding activities of daily livings (ADLs), activities can be divided into 9 groups with 12 most common activities: sit down, sitting (sitting on the chair and sitting on the sofa), walking (walking, walking upstairs and walking downstairs), bending, bend to pick up items, standing, squatting, squat to pick up items and laying. In this paper, the sample rate of the whole pressure sensor array is 30 Hz. Data obtained from the wearable devices accompanied with timestamps and videos which record the movements and provide a precise determination of each event (ground-truth). The counter is a kind of time stamp used for checking the synchronization and missed data. The fall detection system is validated on ten subjects with performing a set of movements including 12 ADLs and 5 falls. Each experiment trail is performed twice to ensure sufficient quantity and consistency. About 1.5 s sliding windows are utilized in the system to process the time-series sensor data. The time-series data which have inherent local dependency characteristics and can represent the activities such as gait, balance, and posture are collected by the smart insoles. In the system, the time-series data are collected from the smart insoles on two feet and are transmitted to a centralized data warehouse. For evaluating the performance of the machine learning algorithms, the 5-fold cross validation as the evaluation protocol is applied. As for the CNN architecture, it contains two convolutional layers, two max-pooling layers, and three fully-connected layers. six fully-connected layers build the MLP architecture in this paper.

Besides, the device that combines a 3-axis gyroscope, 3-axis accelerometer, 3-axis magnetometer is also applied through contrast experiments which are placed to thigh, waist, and hand as shown in Fig. 2. To acquire more precise information, the orientation is calculated by the raw sensor data from the accelerometer and the magnetometer. To further demonstrate the effectiveness of the system, four machine learning algorithms, the k-nearest neighbor, the support vector machines, the decision tree, and the discriminant are used for evaluating the system.

4.2   Results and Analysis

Both quantitative and qualitative experiments are demonstrated in this paper to prove the feasibility and effectiveness of the proposed fall detection system. As shown in Table 1, the comparisons of sensor combinations through six machine learning algorithm?s performances are illustrated. The input data are collected from the smart insoles and the predictions are 2 classes, fall or no fall. In the fall detection scenario, Using the Smart Insoles based on CNN achieve to the higher accuracy than using a single device (3-axis gyroscope, 3-axis accelerometer, 3-axis magnetometer) placed on the waist, right-hand or right-thigh with the widely-used machine learning algorithms. It is obvious that combining smart insoles with other sensors can achieve a better performance than using one single sensor units. The smart insoles can improve the performance of fall classification system. The smart insoles can acquire a higher precision than other single sensor units, which indicates that the system based on smart insoles guarantees a low risk regarding the daily activities as the fall.

This work proves that it is possible to achieve a high accuracy using smart insoles. Using only smart insoles can achieve to a high performance on fall detection (98.76% precision, 97.94% sensitivity, 99.79% specificity and 99.53% accuracy), which is better than using one single device placed on the waist, hand or thigh. Besides, for the combination scenarios, the best performance (99.59% precision, 98.77% sensitivity, 99.93% specificity and 99.76% accuracy) is achieved using the combination of smart insoles with the devices that placed at the waist. The waist sensor is close to the trunk. It has better performance than from the

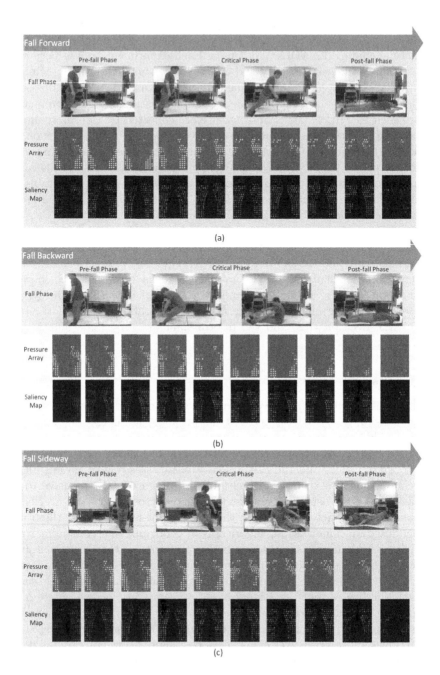

Fig. 3. The pressure changes and deep learning visualization for the time-series data of smart insole inside one window. For each fall events, the top is the fall in real life, the middle is the pressure changes of the smart insoles and the bottom is the corresponding saliency maps.

limbs because it is not easy to be affected by the interpersonal differences in the body movement during the daily activities. The smart insole can provide the pressure changes in various activities as shown in Fig. 3, the "pressure Array" reflects such changes when the fall forward, fall backward and fall sideways occurred.

As for the machine learning algorithms based on the input collected from the pressure insoles, the ANN algorithm is approved and satisfactory due to the high accuracy performance. The class of ANN covers several architectures including the CNN and the MLP. CNN can get the highest accuracy of 99.53% in all algorithms when using smart insoles. For the other machine learning algorithms, the k-NN algorithm produces 98.93% classification accuracy for the smart insoles and 98.28% accuracy with the single device that placed at the waist (the best performance of single device attached to SOI's waist, hand, and thigh). The SVM and Decision Tree have similar results as the k-NN. The best result of SVM can achieve to 99.41% when smart insoles units are used and Decision Tree can achieve to 99.35%. Discriminant gives 98.34% for using smart insoles to detect the fall. It is worthy to note that, CNN is more suitable for using only smart insoles on fall detection.

Fall Forward

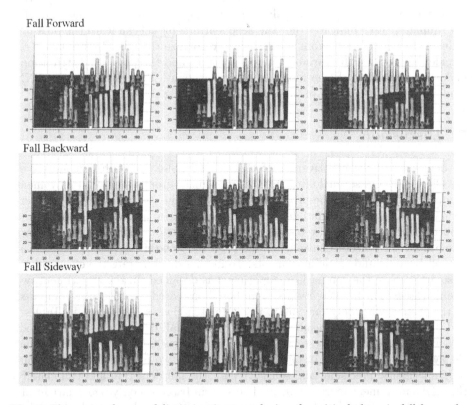

Fall Backward

Fall Sideway

Fig. 4. The major change of disciminative area during the critical phase in fall forward, fall backward and fall sideways.

To further explain how the system based on smart insoles with CNN algorithm works in fall detection, the deep learning visualization approach is applied. The saliency map gives the most discriminative part of the pressure array on the smart insole through the whole fall events. As shown in Fig. 3, in the fixed-length time-series data window, the "saliency map" is generated according to the input ("pressure array"). 10 frames in a window (total 40 frames) is selected to represent the variability in one fall incidents. Based on the results of combining the "pressure array" and "saliency map", the critical phase shows the most significant evidence among the entire falling process. During the critical phase, the discriminative area has changed. When the SOI falls forward, the discriminative area is changing roughly from the heel to the forefoot. As for the fall backward and fall sideways (e.g. right fall), the discriminative area is changing from the forefoot to the heel and from left to right. It is worthy to note that, "saliency map" shows the first few frames (Pre-fall phase) has less effect on the model to detect the falling incidents. The changes in the pressure array during the falls become an important part for the CNN models to recognize the falls. To make such changes more intuitive, the saliency map distribution for the critical phase with a wire-frame mesh in a foot-shaped 3-D map is illustrated as shown in Fig. 4. The deep learning visualization gives a good explanation of how the deep learning model recognizes fall during the fall detection. The change of the discriminative area indicates that the deep learning model can learn the pressure changes during the fall. From the result, to recognize the fall, CNN is based on the identification of the variability in the pattern and the pressure distributions under the foot through the foot-shaped sensor array. That is to say, the CNN model can learn the trend of pressure changes during the falling process.

5   Discussion

To demonstrate the effectiveness of the smart insole, the confusion matrix of the CNN of 13 classes including 9 ADLs-movement groups and a fall-movement group. We can see that the proposed system has achieved high recognition performance in the aspect of fall detection. Through entire movements, most of the movements have been well recognized. The fall detection system based on smart insole ensures the user's convenience and is proved to be effective in the classification of dynamic and static movements. To further demonstrate the effectiveness of smart insoles, the comparison experiment is designed. In the experiment, we mainly discuss the fall detection system based on paired smart insoles compared to the system with only one smart insole for ten classes. As shown in Tables 2 and 3, the experimental result based on CNN for fall detection is summarized. Generally speaking, the system with two insoles has better performance than the system with only one insole. The system with two insoles has better accuracy, specificity, precision, and sensitivity for the fall detection and can classify the ADLs movement more accurate. The system based on only one smart insole is more likely to classify the "confounding activities" such as suddenly sitting down into fall and identify the walk as fall, while two smart insoles mitigate this

Table 2. The confusion matrix using CNN with only **one** smart insole as inputs. CM-confusion matrix, Fa-Falling, SD-Sit Down, Wa-Walking, BP-Bend to Pick up, St-Standing, Be-Bending, Si-Sitting, Ly-Lying, Sq-Squatting and SP-Squat to pick up

Confusion matrix	Fa	SD	Wa	BP	St	Be	Si	Ly	Sq	SP
Falling	0.96	0.01	0.01	0.01	0	0	0	0.01	0	0
Sit Down	0.04	0.84	0.04	0.04	0.02	0.02	0	0	0	0
Walking	0.01	0	0.97	0.01	0.01	0	0	0	0	0
Bend to Pick	0	0	0	0.84	0.02	0.14	0	0	0	0
Standing	0	0	0	0.03	0.96	0.01	0	0	0	0
Bending	0	0	0	0.01	0	0.99	0	0	0	0
Sitting	0	0	0	0	0	0	0.99	0.01	0	0
Lying	0	0	0	0	0	0	0.10	0.90	0	0
Squatting	0	0	0	0	0	0	0	0	0.92	0.08
Squat to pick	0	0	0.04	0	0	0	0	0	0.17	0.79

Table 3. The confusion matrix using CNN with **two** smart insole as inputs.

Confusion Matrix	Fa	SD	Wa	BP	St	Be	Si	Ly	Sq	SP
Falling	0.98	0.01	0.01	0	0	0	0	0	0	0
Sit Down	0.04	0.88	0	0	0.04	0.04	0	0	0	0
Walking	0	0	0.99	0	0.01	0	0	0	0	0
Bend to Pick	0	0	0	0.72	0.08	0.2	0	0	0	0
Standing	0	0	0	0	0.99	0.01	0	0	0	0
Bending	0	0	0	0.01	0	0.99	0	0	0	0
Sitting	0	0	0	0	0	0	0.99	0.01	0	0
Lying	0	0	0	0	0	0	0	1	0	0
Squatting	0	0	0	0	0	0	0	0	0.88	0.12
Squat to pick	0	0	0	0	0	0	0	0	0.09	0.91

problem. The results show that using two paired smart insole for identifying fall and ADLs is more desirable.

6   Conclusion

In this paper, we evaluate the effectiveness and feasibility of using smart insole and ANN for fall detection. As expected, the experimental results show that the smart insoles with the pressure sensor array make good performance on fall detection. The advantage of capturing the pressure changes shows the huge potential for using smart insoles to recognize the fall. Besides, the deep learning visualization approach is applied to further demonstrate what model has learned and show the discriminative area as the fall event occurred. The results of deep learning visualization provide potential hints for the future application design not only the classification algorithm improvement but also the hardware upgrade.

Acknowledgement. The paper was carried out with support from the IoT Collaborative and the Cleveland Foundation and Ohio Bureau of Workers' Compensation: Ohio Occupational Safety and Health Research Program.

References

1. Vallejo, M., Isaza, C.V., Lopez, J.D.: Artificial neural networks as an alternative to traditional fall detection methods. In: 2013 35th Annual International Conference of the IEEE Engineering in Medicine and Biology Society (EMBC), pp. 1648–1651. IEEE (2013)
2. Abbate, S., Avvenuti, M., Bonatesta, F., Cola, G., Corsini, P., Vecchio, A.: A smartphone-based fall detection system. Pervasive Mobile Comput. **8**(6), 883–899 (2012)
3. Simonyan, K., Vedaldi, A., Zisserman, A.: Deep inside convolutional networks: visualising image classification models and saliency maps. arXiv preprint arXiv:1312.6034 (2013)
4. Zeiler, M.D., Fergus, R.: Visualizing and understanding convolutional networks. CoRR, abs/1311.2901v3 (2013)
5. Khawandi, S., Ballit, A., Daya, B.: Applying machine learning algorithm in fall detection monitoring system. In: 2013 5th International Conference on Computational Intelligence and Communication Networks (CICN), pp. 247–250. IEEE (2013)
6. Yu, M., Rhuma, A., Naqvi, S.M., et al.: A posture recognition-based fall detection system for monitoring an elderly person in a smart home environment. IEEE Trans. Inf. Technol. Biomed. **16**(6), 1274–1286 (2012)
7. Lara, O.D., Labrador, M.A., et al.: A survey on human activity recognition using wearable sensors. IEEE Commun. Surv. Tutor. **15**(3), 1192–1209 (2013)
8. Chen, D., Cai, Y., Huang, M.C.: Customizable pressure sensor array: design and evaluation. IEEE Sens. J. **18**(15), 6337–6344 (2018)
9. Cumming, R.G., Salkeld, G., Thomas, M., Szonyi, G.: Prospective study of the impact of fear of falling on activities of daily living, SF-36 scores, and nursing home admission. J. Gerontol. Ser. A: Biol. Sci. Med. Sci. **55**(5), M299–M305 (2000)
10. Costs of falls among older adults. https://www.cdc.gov/homeandrecreationalsafety/falls/fallcost.html
11. WHO global report on falls prevention in older age. https://www.who.int/ageing/projects/falls_prevention_older_age/en/
12. Delahoz, Y.S., Labrador, M.A.: Survey on fall detection and fall prevention using wearable and external sensors. Sensors **14**(10), 19806–19842 (2014)
13. Lapierre, N., Neubauer, N., Miguel-Cruz, A., Rincon, A.R., Liu, L., Rousseau, J.: The state of knowledge on technologies and their use for fall detection: a scoping review. Int. J. Med. Inform. **111**, 58–71 (2018)
14. Fortino, G., Gravina, R.: Fall-MobileGuard: a smart real-time fall detection system. In: Proceedings of the 10th EAI International Conference on Body Area Networks, pp. 44–50. ICST (Institute for Computer Sciences, Social-Informatics and Telecommunications Engineering) (2015)

15. Huynh, Q.T., Nguyen, U.D., Irazabal, L.B., Ghassemian, N., Tran, B.Q.: Optimization of an accelerometer and gyroscope-based fall detection algorithm. J. Sens. **2015**(1–8), 2015 (2015)
16. Gharghan, S., et al.: Accurate fall detection and localization for elderly people based on neural network and energy-efficient wireless sensor network. Energies **11**(11), 2866 (2018)
17. Taramasco, C., et al.: A novel monitoring system for fall detection in older people. IEEE Access **6**, 43563–43574 (2018)
18. Bourke, A.K., et al.: Evaluation of waist-mounted tri-axial accelerometer based fall-detection algorithms during scripted and continuous unscripted activities. J. Biomech. **43**(15), 3051–3057 (2010)
19. Kangas, M., Konttila, A., Lindgren, P., Winblad, I., Jämsä, T.: Comparison of low-complexity fall detection algorithms for body attached accelerometers. Gait Posture **28**(2), 285–291 (2008)
20. O'neill, T.W., et al.: Age and sex influences on fall characteristics. Ann. Rheum. Dis. **53**(11), 773–775 (1994)

Arrhythmia Detection with Antidictionary Coding and Its Application on Mobile Platforms

Gilson Frias[1]([⊠]), Hiroyoshi Morita[1][iD], and Takahiro Ota[2][iD]

[1] The University of Electro-Communications, Chofu, Tokyo 182-8585, Japan
`gilson.frias@mail.uec.jp, morita@uec.ac.jp`
[2] Nagano Prefectural Institute of Technology, Ueda, Nagano 386-1211, Japan
`ota@cse.pit-nagano.ac.jp`
`http://www.appnet.is.uec.ac.jp/`

Abstract. In response to the demand of memory efficient algorithms for electrocardiogram (ECG) signal processing and anomaly detection on wearable and mobile devices, an implementation of the antidictionary coding algorithm for memory constrained devices is presented. Pre-trained *finite-state* probabilistic models built from quantized ECG sequences were constructed in an offline fashion and their performance was evaluated on a set of test signals. The low complexity requirements of the models is confirmed with a port of a pre-trained model of the algorithm into a mobile device without incurring on excessive use of computational resources.

Keywords: ECG · Arrhythmia · Antidictionary · Werable · Mobile

1 Introduction

The Internet of things (IoT) revolution has driven the use of wearable devices for fitness tracking and health monitoring, empowering patients with the capability of doing self assessments about their health condition. The use of such technologies is expected to increment in the foreseeable future [1]. In that sense, the ambulatory monitoring of electrocardiogram (ECG) signals has proven to be of great importance for the early detection and treatment of a broad range of cardiac diseases. The small form factor and low power consumption characteristics of modern ECG monitors assure the necessity of efficient algorithms for the processing of the biosignals. Moreover, efficient lossless compression schemes are required in order to reduce the amounts of disk space for storage and bandwidth for wireless transmission.

The algorithm for Data Compression with Antidictionaries (DCA), first introduced by *Crochemore et al.* [2], makes use of the set of patterns that never appear

This work is supported by JSPS KAKENHI Grant Number JP17K00400.

on the source data set to effectively predict redundant symbols. The feasibility of the DCA for the compression of ECG signals has been previously studied, and it was also shown that the DCA method can be used for the detection of irregular heart beat patterns [3]. The algorithm constructs *finite-state* probabilistic models with the forbidden patterns obtained from the antidictionaries. The presence of expected patterns within the signals causes the algorithm to output a low and steady Compression Ratio, while the appearance of forbidden patterns such as those that occur on arrhythmias causes an increase on the Compression Ratio, thus enabling the DCA algorithm to be suitable for detection tasks.

It has been also shown that by translating the domain of the ECG distribution into a finite set of small integers it is possible to implement the detection algorithm with the use of less memory resources while maintaining an acceptable performance. This was done by the implementation of differentiation and a quantization stages on the signal processing chain that in effect redefines the signal in a restricted alphabet set [4].

In this paper, we present the results of porting the antidictionary coding algorithm into a mobile platform. Pre-trained models for the detection of Premature Ventricular Contractions (PVC) have been implemented on the IOS operating system, requiring relative small amounts of computational resources to process real time streams of ECG data transmitted through the Bluetooth Low Energy (LE) communication standard. Additionally, a new quantization method is introduced with the use of percentile statistical measurements from the ECG distribution.

Contents are presented in the following order: In Sect. 2 a brief overview on the characteristics of the ECG signal and the PVC arrhythmia will be presented. In Sect. 3 the theory behind Antidictionary Coding will be discussed. In Sect. 4, a description of the offline processing of the ECG is given, detailing the process involve in the construction of the probabilistic models and the selection criteria followed for picking the trained models used for a subsequent stage of online experimentation. Finally, in Sect. 5 the results of porting the offline-trained model into an IOS application for online processing of the ECG samples are shown.

2   The ECG Signal and Premature Ventricular Contractions

The Electrocardiogram (ECG) is a signal that represents the electrical activity of the heart. Usually measured directly on the body's surface, the ECG waveform is mainly composed of five characteristic components denoted by the letters P, Q, R, S and T. Each component marks the location of a specific peak or valley on the ECG signal that corresponds to a change in electrical activity in the heart and the consequent movement of the cardiac muscle. Sometimes an U component is also present following the T peak. The left part of Fig. 1 displays an overview of a typical ECG waveform. The P-peak on the waveform is generated with the activation of the upper chambers of the heart, the left and right atria, while the

QRS complex and the T-peak are generated with the activation process of the two lower chambers, the left and right ventricles [5].

The R-R interval is also pointed on the left side of Fig. 1, it is a measure of the time elapsed between consecutive heartbeats and is an important metric usually used for the calculation of the heart rate.

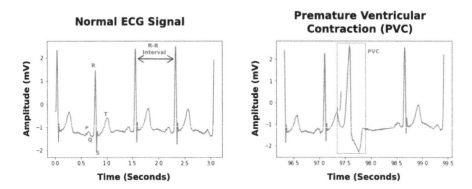

Fig. 1. Two ECG waveforms showing 4 heartbeats each. The second heartbeat on the left figure displays the location of main peaks and valleys that characterize the signal. The right figure shows an ECG waveform containing the occurrence of a PVC on the third heartbeat.

Premature Ventricular Contractions (PVC) are abnormal contractions that occur earlier than expected within the normal hearth cycle. The PVCs are generated on the ventricles, unlike the electrical impulses that drive the normal heart cycle, which are generated on the sinoatrial node [6]. The occurrence of PVCs can be an important indicator of the presence of an underlaying hearth disease, and they can be recognized on the ECG as abnormal and wide QRS complexes [7]. The right part of Fig. 1 shows an ECG waveform that contains one PVC. The occurrence of the premature heart beat disrupts the normal R-R interval and thus causing variability in the heart rate.

3   Finite State Machines (FSM) Probability Models with Antidictionaries

Let Σ_m be a finite set of integers $\{0, 1, \ldots, m-1\}$, called m-ary alphabet. For a string $\boldsymbol{x}^n = x_1 x_2 \ldots x_n$ of length n, we consider the set $\mathcal{D}(\boldsymbol{x}^n)$ called the dictionary of $\boldsymbol{x}^n$, as the set that contains all substrings of $\boldsymbol{x}^n$ including the null string $\boldsymbol{\lambda}$ of length zero. The antidictionary $\mathcal{A}(\boldsymbol{x}^n)$ of $\boldsymbol{x}^n$ is defined as the set of *minimal* strings that never appear in $\boldsymbol{x}^n$. An element $\boldsymbol{v} = v_1 v_2 \ldots v_k$ in $A(\boldsymbol{x}^n)$ is called Minimal Forbidden Word (MFW) which must satisfy the following three conditions:

1. $v \notin \mathcal{D}(x^n)$
2. A one-symbol shorter prefix of v, defined as $p(v) = v_1 v_2 ... v_{k-1}$, must be contained in $\mathcal{D}(x^n)$.
3. A one-symbol shorter suffix of v, defined as $s(v) = v_2 v_3 ... v_k$, must be also contained in $\mathcal{D}(x^n)$.

Data compression is achieved by the Data Compression using Antidictionary (DCA) algorithm [8]. From $\mathcal{A}(x^n)$, a proper set of MFWs is selected for the construction of a finite state machine, hereafter referred as FSM. The FSM can be utilized to build a probabilistic model that normally accepts substrings of x^n, but in the presence of an MFW it will lock itself in a terminal state. A simple example is introduced next to illustrate the concepts just established. Consider a string $w = 2210010$ over $\Sigma_3 = \{0, 1, 2\}$. As discussed previously, the antidictionary $\mathcal{A}(w)$ of w is given by the set of all MFWs of w, thus $\mathcal{A}(w) = \{02, 000, 11, 12, 101, 20, 222, 0100\}$. By taking a subset of $\mathcal{A}(w)$, say $\mathcal{A}_s(w) = \{02, 11, 20\}$, we construct a FSM probabilistic model, as shown in Fig. 2.

The FSM consists of seven states or nodes, with four states S_1, S_2, S_3 and S_4 being the internal states and the remaining three states R_1, R_2 and R_3 are the external states. Each internal state points to another state (or to itself) through an edge, in Fig. 2 an edge is defined by an arrow and the accompanying symbol that causes the transition to a new state.

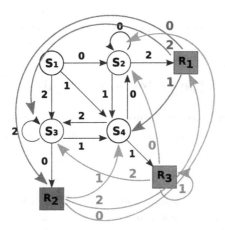

Fig. 2. An FSM model for MFWs 02, 11 and 20. Coloured edges denote the corresponding transitions after a forbidden state is reached. (Color figure online)

Now assume that the ith symbol of $x^n (1 \le i \le n)$ is being processed by the FSM, and we define the next state reached sequentially by x_i as s_i, where $1 \le i < n$ and s_0 denotes the initial state of the FSM. Moreover, we assume that the state sequence $s^m = s_0 s_1 ... s_m$ is uniquely determined by the input string $x^m = x_1 x_2 \ldots x_m (1 \leq m \leq n)$. The probability of transitioning to a state specified by the next symbol on the sequence, $P(x_{i+1}|s_i)$, is given by

$$P(x_{i+1}|s_i) = \frac{N(x_{i+1}|s_i)}{\sum_{c \in \Sigma} N(c|s_i)}, \quad 0 \leq i < n \tag{1}$$

where $N(c|s_i)$ denotes the number of times that a transition has happened from state s_i with symbol c.

The algorithm's output for a given symbol that is being encoded depends on whether the next transition leads to an internal state or to an external state. For a given integer sequence $1 \leq I_1 < I_2 < \cdots < I_{t+1} = n$, if the I_jth state $(1 \leq j \leq t)$ to be reached corresponds to an external state and the final state I_{t+1} does not necessary so, then it can be concluded that an MFW is present as a substring of the input sequence and the algorithm outputs the corresponding interval I_j of occurrence of the transition to the external state.

In the case of a transition to an external state s_i through symbol x_i, the algorithm would point next to the node that covers the sequence $v = x_{i-s} \ldots x_{i+1}$, where v coincides with the *Longest Common Prefix* with one MFW in $\mathcal{A}(w)$ and $(0 \leq s \leq i - 1)$.

In the case that the transition leads to an internal state, the algorithm's output depends on the total number of available edges, denoted by n_E, that lead to terminal states from the current node. If $n_E = 1$, then the next symbol can be predicted and the algorithm does not output anything. However, if $n_E > 1$, then the algorithm outputs the transition probability $P(x_{i+1}|s_i)$ associated with the next symbol x_{i+1} [3].

4   Description of the Detection System

Figure 3 shows the structure of the proposed detection system. The details concerning each stage in the processing pipeline will be discussed next.

4.1   Signal Differentiation

The shape of the probability distribution constructed from the ECG signals can be affected by the presence of noise and unwanted artifacts in the signals [9]. The presence of arrhythmia components within the signal can also cause asymmetry and flattening on the distribution [10]. The left part of Fig. 4 shows a histogram built from an ECG record consisting of 650,000 samples (with 11 bit resolution). The distribution clearly displays the asymmetry and flattening characteristics discussed earlier.

The detection algorithm proposed in this study relies in a quantization process aiming to convey the information contained in the ECG probability distribution into a new distribution defined over a smaller alphabet set. The irregularities in the shape of the ECG distribution can lead to uneven distribution of the samples in the new probability distribution created from the quantized signals.

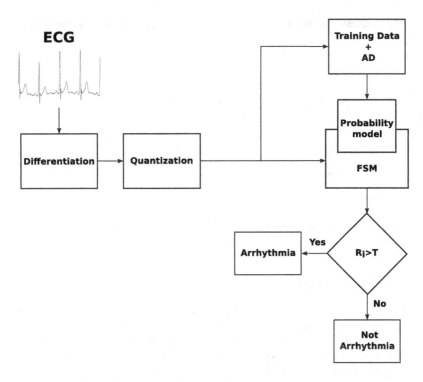

Fig. 3. Schematic diagram of the detection system.

To address this inconvenience, we introduce a differentiation step prior to the quantization process. In this context, we use the term *differentiation* to refer to the operation of subtraction of consecutive samples in the original signals.

For a sampled signal sequence denoted by $z^n = z_1 z_2 \ldots z_n$ where $z_i \in \Sigma_{2048}, 1 \leq i \leq n$, the differentiation process that yields the output sequence $y^n = y_1 y_2 \ldots y_n$ is stated as follows:

$$y_i = \begin{cases} z_i & i = 1 \\ z_i - z_{i-1} & 1 < i \leq n \end{cases} \tag{2}$$

where $|y_i| \leq 2047$ $(1 \leq i \leq n)$.

The histogram built from each component of y shows a shape that resembles the Laplace distribution although the former is a discrete distribution while the latter is a continuous one, with a considerable less amount of dispersion than the distribution of x. The right part of Fig. 4 displays the histogram of the distribution obtained after the application of the differentiation process on the ECG signal.

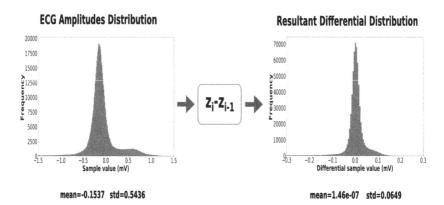

Fig. 4. Histograms for raw ECG signal distribution (left) and the resultant distribution after the differentiation process (right).

4.2   Signal Quantization

The next step in the signal processing pipeline aims to translate the information contained in the differential signals into a domain defined over a smaller alphabet set. Let's define Q as the odd number of quantization levels under which the quantization will take place. Any quantized symbol can be defined only on the set of integers $\{0, 1, \ldots, Q-1\}$. The quantization process is carried out with a simple ranking system that assigns each sample its corresponding quantized symbol depending on its differential amplitude value.

Hereafter, let us denote a sequence of quantized symbols of length n by a string x^n over Σ_Q where $m = Q$. The ith quantized symbol x_i on the sequence $x^n = x_1 x_2 \ldots x_n \in \Sigma_Q^n$ can be obtained from the differential sequence y^n and the set of quantization parameters $\{q_0, q_1, \ldots, q_{Q-2}\}$ where q_l's $(0 \leq l \leq Q-2)$ are reals and $q_i < q_j$ $(0 \leq i < j \leq Q-2)$.

Then, the quantization rule is given as follows:

$$x_i = \begin{cases} 0 & y_i \leq q_0, \\ l & q_{l-1} < y_i \leq q_l \\ Q-2 & y_i > q_{Q-2}. \end{cases} \tag{3}$$

The quantization procedure is illustrated on Fig. 5. Previous experiments with different quantization levels have shown that the algorithm perform at its best when $Q = 7$. Next, for the definition of the quantization parameters, lets consider the *percentile* P_r as the value on the ECG distribution below which a percentage $r(\%)$ of the samples is allocated. Then, the quantization parameters are given as:

$$q_0 = P_{1.5}, \quad q_1 = P_{10}, \quad q_2 = P_{25}, \quad q_3 = P_{75}, \quad q_4 = P_{90}, \quad q_5 = P_{98.5} \tag{4}$$

An example of the quantization operation over a differential distribution is presented on Fig. 5 for a value of $Q = 7$.

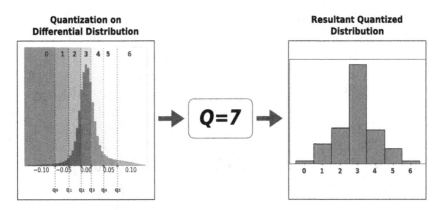

Fig. 5. Quantization operation on a differential ECG distribution (left) and the resultant quantized distribution (right). The location of the quantization parameters and the corresponding interval for each symbol are highlighted.

4.3   Training Data and Antidictinary AD Generation

The antidictionary set $\mathcal{A}$ to be used in the encoding process is generated from a segment of ECG data in a preprocessing stage as follows:

Step 1. First, let k be a certain positive integer denoting the total number of training files from which the antidictionary $\mathcal{A}$ will be constructed. Each training file $\boldsymbol{u}_i\,(1 \leq i \leq k)$ consists of 5 ECG waveforms (roughly between 3 and 5.5 seconds of ECG recording). Here, a waveform is defined as the portion of the signal covered by one R-R interval, as is described on the left waveform on Fig. 1. For each training file $\boldsymbol{u}_i$ an antidictionary set $\mathcal{A}(\boldsymbol{u}_i)$ is constructed and the process results in the family of antidictionaries

$$\mathcal{A}_K = \{\mathcal{A}(\boldsymbol{u}_1), \mathcal{A}(\boldsymbol{u}_2), \ldots, \mathcal{A}(\boldsymbol{u}_k)\}.$$

The process is described on Fig. 6.

Step 2. The antidictionary set $\mathcal{A}$ is conformed primarily by the set of MFWs that show a higher frequency of occurrence among all the generated antidictionaries $\mathcal{A}(\boldsymbol{u}_1), \mathcal{A}(\boldsymbol{u}_2), \ldots, \mathcal{A}(\boldsymbol{u}_k)$ in $\mathcal{A}_k$. Due to the periodic nature of the ECG signal, some MFWs are expected to appear constantly among the majority of the generated antidictionaries. However, the dynamic variations in the amplitude and periods of the training waveforms induce some variability on the frequency of occurrence of some MFWs. Given an MFW $\boldsymbol{w}$, the frequency of occurrence $f(\boldsymbol{w})$ on $\boldsymbol{w}$ is given by

$$f(\boldsymbol{w}) = |\{i\,|\,\boldsymbol{w} \in \mathcal{A}(\boldsymbol{u}_i), 1 \leq i \leq k\}|. \tag{5}$$

Step 3. Based on those f values, the MFWs are sorted and finally, the antidictionary set $\mathcal{A}$ can then be built with the MFWs that exhibit a relatively high frequency of occurrence. Experimental trials show that the MFWs with the higher frequency of occurrence are in general strings of length one or two. Those short strings usually perform poorly when implemented in the FSM model in the detection scheme. In that sense, for the construction of $\mathcal{A}$ the constraint of choosing MFWs of length greater than or equal to 3 is imposed in order to achieve better performance in the detection algorithm.

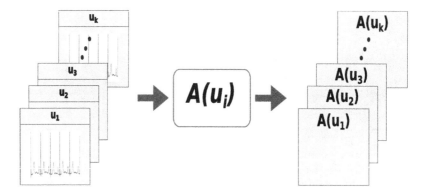

Fig. 6. Antidictionary set construction from the ECG training files set.

4.4 FSM Construction and Detection Criteria

With the appropriate set of MFWs picked from the antidictionary set $\mathcal{A}$, the FSM can be build alongside the accompanying probability model. Given a set of MFWs defined over an alphabet Σ_Q, in the implementation of the FSM each state is modeled with two memory registers for each outgoing edge associated with symbol $c \in \Sigma_Q$. The first register acts as a pointer to the next state reached through symbol c and the second register is implemented as a counter that holds the number of transitions to the next state though c. For the particular case of the FSM with $Q = 3$ on Fig. 2, there are seven states in total with three outgoing edges per state. Thus, the number of memory registers necessary for the implementation of the FSM would be equal to 42.

Once the FSM model is constructed, the transition probabilities are calculated by performing a second pass in the training data and updating the corresponding counter for each state transition.

Let $x^n = x_1 x_2 \ldots x_n$ be a string being processed with the detection algorithm by means of a FSM constructed with the appropriate probabilistic model. For $1 \leq i \leq n$ and a given number $d > 0$, the *instantaneous* compression ratio R_i defined on a sliding window w_i of size d is given by

$$
R_i =
\begin{cases}
\dfrac{1}{d} \displaystyle\sum_{k=i-d+2}^{i+1} \ln \dfrac{1}{P(x_k|s_{k-1})} & i - d > 0, \\[2.5em]
\dfrac{1}{i} \displaystyle\sum_{k=2}^{i+1} \ln \dfrac{1}{P(x_k|s_{k-1})} & i - d \leq 0.
\end{cases}
\tag{6}
$$

where $P(x_k|s_{k-1})$ is the transition probability defined in (1).

A threshold value T is chosen such as an instantaneous compression ratio R_i greater than T will signal the presence of an arrhythmia pattern in the input string. Figure 7 illustrates the case of a positive detection when the PCV located around 156 s time stamp causes an increase on the compression ratio, effectively surpassing the set threshold (2.5).

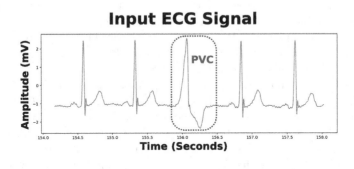

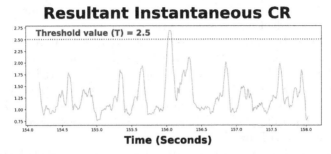

Fig. 7. Positive detection of a PVC heartbeat. The top figure displays an ECG sequence containing one PVC heartbeat while the bottom figure shows how the Instantaneous Compression Ratio goes above the set threshold value (T = 2.5), likely due to a forbidden pattern occurring within PVC.

5 Offline Preprocessing, Model Selection and Accuracy Assessment of FSM Models

In this section we describe the process involving the experimentation with the ECG records to obtain the best performance FSM models in an offline fashion. The test signals used for the experiments were taken from the MIT-BIH Arrhythmia Database, a library of ECG records commonly used for the evaluation of ECG arrhythmia detectors. It consists of 48 records, each one comprising 30 min of ECG recording on two channels digitized at 360 samples per second per channel at an 11-bit resolution spanning a 10 mV dynamic range. Each ECG record contains annotations given by two or more cardiologists, thus providing a medical grade benchmark for the assessment of the quality of arrhythmia detectors [11, 12].

In each experiment, training sets consisting of 50 training files (one training file containing 5 ECG waveforms, and one waveform consisting of the portion of ECG data covering the R-R segment) were used for the constructions of the antidictionaries. Only portions of the ECG signals from the MIT-BIH Arrhythmia Database annotated as "Normal" were employed for the construction of the training sets.

The MFWs from the antidictionary set where then sorted according to their f values, as described on Sect. 4.3. A common antidictionary set was then constructed from the top 20 MFWs on the sorted set. From the common antidictionary set, 190 different FSM models where then constructed taking into consideration all possible combinations of 2 MFWs.

The transition probabilities for each FSM model were calculated from the segment of training data previously used for the construction of the antidictionaries and then each FSM was tested with the whole ECG sequence. The accompanying annotations files from the MIT-BIH Arrhythmia Database where used for the posterior calculation of the detection evaluation metrics sensitivity and specificity. The sensitivity, or true positive rate, measures the ratio of true arrhythmia heartbeats detected while the specificity measures the ratio of normal heartbeats identified as such by the algorithm.

Table 1 shows the results obtained after processing 6 records from the database. The differentiation process resulted on distributions centered around zero with shapes similar to the distribution shown on the right part of Fig. 4. For the determination of the set of quantization parameters, the percentiles values where calculated from the distribution of ECG samples obtained within the first minute of recording (corresponding to 21,600 samples for records from the MIT-BIH Arrhythmia Database).

The results on Table 1 for records 105, 205 and 228 correspond to cases with FSM models of 2 MFWs, while in the cases of records 201, 215 and 221 slightly bigger models of 4 MFWs were employed to improve detection accuracy.

Table 2 contains the average metrics (sensitivity and specificity) obtained after processing the 6 aforementioned ECG records, where the metrics of other methods available on literature are given for comparison purposes.

While the proposed detection algorithm achieves high average values of Sensitivity, the average Specificity suffers in comparison with other methods, as described on Table 2. It is important to notice, however, that no prior treatment of the test signals was carried for conditioning or noise removal. It is very plausible that improvements on Specificity would follow with the use of appropriate methods for noise removal.

For the detection process, a sliding window size of $d = 25$ symbols was used for the calculation of the instantaneous compression ratio R_i and a dynamic range of threshold values T (in the range 1.8 to 3.2) was used to have an insight on how the variability on T can affect the detection process.

Table 3 shows a comparative description of the antidictionaries and FSM implementation characteristics for the proposed detection system and the detection system proposed in [3]. For the calculation of the antidictionary size values presented on Table 2, a byte has been assigned to describe every quantized symbol that conform an MFW.

Figure 8 displays the Receiver Operating Characteristics (ROC) curves for three different FSM built for record 228, evaluated on a range of threshold values T raging from 1.8 to 3.2 on increments of 0.01 units. The set of MFWs for FSM Model-1 is $AD_1 = \{656, 513\}$ while the antidictionary sets for the remaining two models (FSM Model-2 and FSM Model-3) are $AD_2 = \{656, 5351\}$ and $AD_2 = \{013, 514\}$, respectively.

A common MFW, 656, can be found on the antidictionary set of the two best performing FSM models (FSM Model-1 and FSM Model-2), thus suggesting that MFW very likely corresponds to a forbidden pattern within the PVCs morphology.

Table 1. Table of results (%) for the detection of PVC on 6 ECG records from the MIT-BIH database.

Record	Sen.	Spec.
105	100	94.77
201	98.98	98.40
205	97.18	99.57
215	93.29	79.74
221	97.97	94.43
228	97.79	96.44
Average	**97.53**	**93.89**

6   Implementation on a Mobile Platform

The second stage of experimentation consisted on the port of the detection algorithm into a mobile environment for the evaluation of performance at online operation. The experimental setup is described on Fig. 9. A pre-trained FSM model has been ported in addition to a quantization stage for the processing of a stream of ECG samples on real time. Continuing with the same methodology used on off-line experimentation, the records from the MIT-BIH Arrhythmia databased have been employed for testing the algorithm.

6.1   Wearable ECG Hardware Characteristics

A custom hardware configuration has been used to emulate the characteristics of a wearable ECG sensor handling the wireless transmissions of the ECG samples obtained from the annotated files on the MIT-BIH Arrhythmia database. The virtual wearable monitor is based around the ESP32-WROOM-32 Microcontroller Unint from Espressif Systems [16]. The ESP32-WROOM-32 contains the

Table 2. Comparison of the proposed method with other arrhythmia detectors.

Algorithm	Sensitivity	Specificity
Proposed method	**97.53**	**93.89**
Ota et al. [3]	97.9	98.6
Ittatinut et al. [13]	91.05	99.55
Adnane et al. [14]	97.21	98.67
Alajlan et al. [15]	100	93.71

Table 3. Antidictionaries and FSM implementation characteristics for quantized signals from six different ECG records. Results obtained previously in [3] are given for comparison purposes.

ECG record	105	201	205	215	221	228
Results obtained on Ota et al. [3]						
Number of MFWs	281	90	56	178	85	189
AD size (bits)	3,586	996	436	1,792	988	2,316
FSM size (kB)	24.2	6.5	2.6	11.5	6.5	15.4
Results obtained with the proposed method						
Number of MFWs	2	4	2	4	4	2
AD size (bits)	48	120	48	144	112	48
FSM size (kB)	**1.6**	**3.2**	**1.6**	**3.6**	**2.5**	**1.6**

ESP32 System on a Chip (SoC) device alongside flash memory and the hardware requirements to achieving low power Wi-Fi and Bluetooth Low Energy (LE) communication.

The Bluetooth LE standard enables low power communication between the ECG sensor and the mobile device and at the same time facilitates the easy implementation of the services both in the client and the server side, reducing the development time of the mobile application.

The ECG samples have been read from binary files stored on a SD card with the use of one of the multiple on-board Serial Peripheral Interface (SPI) buses available on the ESP32-WROOM-32 device. The ESP32 (SoC) device supports a broad range of open software initiatives, like the Arduino Open Software project. In our case, the whole configuration of the ESP32 core device was carried out on top of the SPI and Bluetooth libraries freely provided by Espressif Systems and the open source community [17].

In accordance to the Bluetooth LE specification, a custom Bluetooth Service and its corresponding Characteristic were implemented both in the wearable device and the mobile application [18]. Two randomly generated Universally Unique IDs (UUID) where used to identify both the Service and its Characteristic. ECG samples are treated as 16 bits unsigned numbers, and two samples are transmitted every 6 mS, for a rate of 333 ECG samples per second. The Blue-

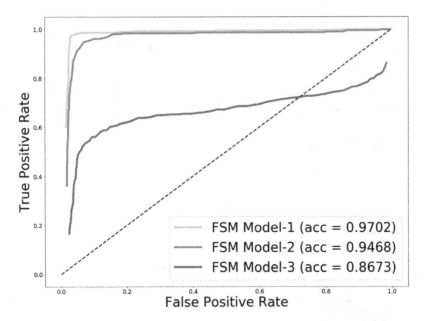

Fig. 8. Receiver Operating Characteristics curves for three different FSM trained to process record 228 under a wide range of threshold values (T). Maximum accuracy values and the corresponding threshold values for each model are given as follows: FSM Model-1 achieving 97.02% accuracy at $T = 2.56$, FSM Model-2 reaching 94.68 % at $T = 2.67$ and FSM Model-3 with 86.73% accuracy at $T = 2.63$.

tooth Characteristic is granted with the "Notify" property, and each time two samples are ready for transmission the notification alerts the mobile applications Bluetooth instance.

6.2 Mobile Application Deployment

The mobile application has been developed on the IOS mobile operating system. An object oriented approach has been adopted for the implementation of the quantization and FSM related data structures, to speed up development and facilitate code readability.

The deployed application was evaluated with Apple's Xcode development environment and tested on an Iphone 6s device. By using Xcode's memory profiler and benchmark tools, the performance of the application was evaluated with an average of 30MB of memory and 65% of CPU usage on one of the cores of the mobile device while processing the ECG samples in an on-line fashion. Figure 10 shows a screenshot of the running mobile application alongside the prototype of the ECG sensor. An USB connection is used to upload the firmware on the ESP32-WROOM-32 unit and to power it during operation.

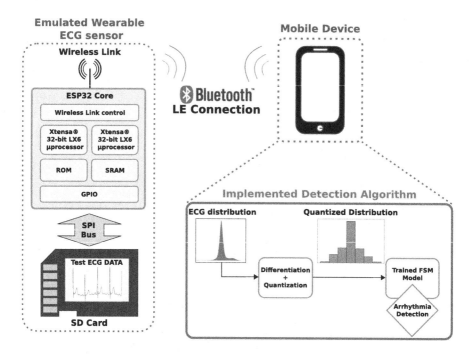

Fig. 9. Schematic digram of the experimental setup used for the evaluation of the detection algorithm on an mobile platform.

7   Discussion

In order to increase the sensitivity values on the measurements, further care should be taken for handling baseline wandering, mains interference and other sources of noise.

The offline processing of the records for the determination of the best set of antidictionaries and the construction of FSM models can prove to be a computationally intensive process, as each FSM model is evaluated with the entire ECG sequence over a range of threshold values. Next stages in our research efforts include the identification of specific MFWs patterns for PVCs and other types of arrhythmias to narrow down the pool of target MFWs and simplify the preprocessing stage.

The mobile application performed with a constant average usage of 30 MB of system memory while running a FSM of 9 nodes in the background and processing the ECG record 201 from the MIT-BIH database. The use of bigger FSM models for increasing accuracy should not lead to excessive increase on memory usage.

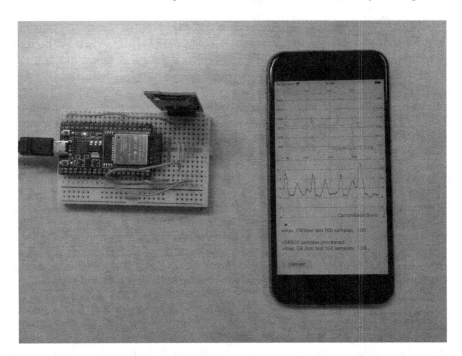

Fig. 10. The experimental setup for the online evaluation of the trained FSM models. The emulated ECG sensor (on the left) transmits the ECG samples through Bluetooth LE while in the mobile application the quantization and posterior processing in the FSM is effectuated to produce the output CR waveform displayed on the phone screen.

8 Conclusion

A system for the discrimination of irregular ECG patterns based on the scheme of antidictionary encoding applied to quantized signals has been presented, with a proof of concept port of a pre-trained FSM model into a mobile application.

The rescaling of the ECG distribution with the differentiation and quantization operations results on lower space complexity requirements for the implementation of the FSM probabilistic models. This is evidenced on Table 3, where an average size of 2.35 KB is calculated for the models constructed with the proposed approach while the models designed from binary ECG sequences require an average of 11.11 kB. This is further evidenced with the relatively low memory resources usage (30.5 MB) for online processing of ECG samples on the mobile application.

The achieved average metrics of sensitivity (97.53%) renders the proposed detection algorithm as a feasible alternative for PVC detection. Higher sensitivity values can be achieved with approaches such as the Gaussian Process Classifier (GPC) method suggested in [15], this at the expense of using bigger segments of training data and using a mix of time and frequency domain features to differentiate the pathological heartbeats.

Further research efforts aiming to increase the average specificity metrics could include the evaluation of additional time domain features, such as the R-R interval assessment made in [13] and band-limiting the ECG signal in a narrow frequency band to eliminate high frequency noise, as happens with the Discrete Wavelet Transform (DWT) method used on [14].

Besides, a deep dive in more specific details about the characteristic forbidden patterns that appear in each type of heartbeat could lead to the extension of the algorithm to a multi-class classification category.

References

1. Dias, D., Paulo Silva Cunha, J.: Wearable health devices—vital sign monitoring, systems and technologies. Sensors **18**(8), 2414 (2018)
2. Crochemore, M., Mignosi, F., Restivo, A., Salemi, S.: Text compression using antidictionaries. In: Wiedermann, J., van Emde Boas, P., Nielsen, M. (eds.) ICALP 1999. LNCS, vol. 1644, pp. 261–270. Springer, Heidelberg (1999). https://doi.org/10.1007/3-540-48523-6_23. https://hal-upec-upem.archives-ouvertes.fr/hal-006199 91/document
3. Ota, T., Morita, H., de Lind van Wijngaarden, A.J.: Real-time and memory-efficient arrhythmia detection in ECG monitors using antidictionary coding. IEICE Fundam. **E96–A**(12), 2343–2350 (2013)
4. Frias, G., Morita, H., Ota, T.: Anomaly detection on quantized ECG signals by the use of antidictionary coding. In: Proceedings of the 41st Symposium on Information Theory and its Applications, December 2018
5. Rajni, R., Kaur, I.: Electrocardiogram signal analysis - an overview. Int. J. Comput. Appl. **84**(7), 22–25 (2013)
6. Mayo Clinic: Premature ventricular contractions (PVCs), February 2018. https://www.mayoclinic.org/diseases-conditions/premature-ventricular-contractions/symptoms-causes/syc-20376757
7. ECGwaves.com: Premature Ventricular Contractions (premature ventricular complex, premature ventricular beats): ECG and clinical implications (2018). https://ecgwaves.com/premature-ventricular-contractions-complex-beats-ecg/
8. Ota, T., Morita, H.: On-line electrocardiogram lossless compression using antidictionary codes for a finite alphabet. IEICE Trans. Inf. Syst. **E93–D**(12), 3384–3391 (2010)
9. Zhao, Z., Zhang, Y.: SQI quality evaluation mechanism of single-lead ECG signal based on simple heuristic fusion and fuzzy comprehensive evaluation. Front. Physiol. **9**, 727 (2018)
10. Tziakouri, M., et al.: Classification of AF and other arrhythmias froma short segment of ECG using dynamic time warping. In: Computing in Cardiology, vol. 44, pp. 1–4 (2017)
11. Moody, G.B., Mark, R.G.: The impact of the MIT-BIH arrhythmia database. IEEE Eng. Med. Biol. Mag. **20**, 45–50 (2001)
12. Goldberger, A.L., Amaral, L., et al.: PhysioBank, PhysioToolkit, and PhysioNet: components of a new research resource for complex physiologic signals. AHA - Circulation **101**(23), E215–20 (2000)
13. Ittatirut, S., Lek-uthai, A., Teeramongkonrasmee, A.: Detection of premature ventricular contraction for real-time applications. In: 2013 10th International Conference on Electrical Engineering/Electronics, Computer, Telecommunications and

Information Technology, pp. 1–5, May 2013. https://doi.org/10.1109/ECTICon. 2013.6559531

14. Adnane, M., Belouchrani, A.: Premature ventricular contraction arrhythmia detection using wavelet coefficients. In: 2013 8th International Workshop on Systems, Signal Processing and their Applications (WoSSPA), pp. 170–173, May 2013. https://doi.org/10.1109/WoSSPA.2013.6602356

15. Alajlan, N., Bazi, Y., Melgani, F., Malek, S., Bencherif, M.A.: Detection of premature ventricular contraction arrhythmias in electrocardiogram signals with kernel methods. Sig. Image Video Process. **8**(5), 931–942 (2014). https://doi.org/10.1007/s11760-012-0339-8

16. Espressif Systems: Esp32-wroom-32 datasheet. https://www.espressif.com/sites/default/files/documentation/esp32-wroom-32_datasheet_en.pdf

17. Espressif Systems: Repository: Arduino core for esp32 wifi chip. https://github.com/espressif/arduino-esp32

18. The Bluetooth Special Interest Group (Bluetooth SIG): GATT services. https://www.bluetooth.com/specifications/gatt/services

Characterisation of Breathing and Physical Activity Patterns in the General Population Using the Wearable Respeck Monitor

D. K. Arvind[1(✉)], D. J. Fischer[1], C. A. Bates[1], and S. Kinra[2]

[1] Centre for Speckled Computing, School of Informatics,
University of Edinburgh, 10 Crichton Street,
Edinburgh EH8 9AB, Scotland, UK
dka@inf.ed.ac.uk
[2] London School of Hygiene and Tropical Medicine, Keppel Street,
London WC1E 7HT, England, UK

Abstract. Clinical trials employing manual processes for data collection and administering of questionnaires are time-consuming, expensive to run and result in noisy data. Wireless body-worn sensors coupled with mobile applications can be harnessed to automate the data collection process during clinical trials. This paper describes the use of the Respeck monitor, worn as a plaster on the chest, for characterising breathing and physical activity patterns in the general population during their normal everyday lives. Respeck data collected from 93 subjects for periods ranging between 24 to 72 h, amounting to a total of 106 days of continuous Respeck data. Analysis of the data revealed new insights, such as the respiratory rate levels dropped by 4.39 breaths per minute (BrPM) on average during sleeping periods, compared to the preceding day-time periods. This change is higher than typically reported levels when normally measured directly before the subjects fall asleep. Previous research in activity patterns in the general population were based on high-level activities logged using questionnaires. A method is presented for clustering simple, yet high-dimensional, activity patterns based on the Respeck data, by first extracting relevant features for each day. The results reveal four distinct groups in the cohort corresponding to different identifiable lifestyles: "Sedentary", "Moderately active", "Active walkers" and "Active movers".

Keywords: Wearable sensors · Respiratory rate · Physical activity

1 Introduction

Respiratory rate, pulse/heart rate, oxygen saturation, body temperature and blood pressure are vital signs to be monitored when assessing the state of health of a person. The measurement of respiratory rate is normally confined to clinical settings using nasal cannulae, masks, belts or similar devices. The Respeck [11] (Fig. 1) worn as a plaster on the chest monitors continuously the respiratory rate and respiratory effort/flow, by measuring the rotation of the chest wall using a triaxial accelerometer. Respeck data is communicated wirelessly to a mobile application on a phone for onward transmission to the server via WiFi or the cellular network [12]. The Respeck device is programmed to report "quiet breathing at rest", which is the metric used for comparing breathing rates in clinical pulmonary studies. The Respeck device detects physical activity [5] and filters those periods of rest to report respiratory rate and flow. The periods of physical activity are classified into different states, such as walking and other movement, and the periods of rest into sitting, standing and lying down. In summary, a single Respeck device provides respiratory data on breathing rate and flow, and information on the intensity of physical activity and its classification.

The paper reports on a study to investigate the respiratory rate profile and physical activity patterns in the general population during their everyday lives. The method uses the Respeck sensor which replaces the manual method of surveying the population using questionnaires, interviews and personal diary, which is expensive, time-consuming, and produces noisy data. The contributions of this paper are a novel method to monitor simultaneously the respiratory rate and flow and classification of physical activity using the wearable Respeck device, and the characterisation of 93 subjects aggregating to 106 days of continuous Respeck data. Breathing rate levels and variance are reported for day and night periods, together with results on clustering the activity data into four identifiable groups corresponding to different lifestyles.

Respiratory rate in the general population has traditionally been studied during the night-time, as wearing cumbersome recording equipment during day-time when people are going about their every-day lives was impractical. Respiratory rate levels are typically reported as being lower during sleep [10], although other studies [2] have reported higher levels during sleep compared to wake-time. One possible explanation for the disagreement in this regard is the ambiguous definition of the wake period. Respiratory rate will typically slow down during rest periods and if the wake levels of respiratory rate are only measured after the subject is already in lying position and preparing for sleep, the average levels will naturally be much lower than during the day-time.

There is a large body of research devoted to classifying activities such as walking, running, sitting, standing, lying down, cycling, and climbing stairs [1], using a single 3-axis accelerometer attached to different parts of the body, such as the wrist or the lower leg. In contrast, the Respeck is attached to the chest wall just below the last rib, in order to measure the breathing rate, and is unique in identifying these activities when attached to this part of the body. The recognition of these activities is helpful in providing contextual information to the subject [4], or in detecting abnormal behaviour [7], but it requires the combination of several activities into activity patterns to infer the lifestyle of the subject.

Clustering activity patterns to categorise subjects into groups is a well-known technique used in the field of social sciences. Questionnaires record high-level activities of the subjects, such as working, watching TV, or food shopping and one can infer levels of different types of activities and nutrition of sub-populations [6], or about typical work-habits and weekend activities [8]. In contrast to the questionnaire-based approaches, this paper presents the clustering of activities derived from the Respeck data recordings for the cohort of 93 subjects.

In the rest of this paper, Sect. 2 describes the methodology employed in this study and features selected for activity clustering, with Sects. 3 and 4 devoted to results and conclusions, respectively.

2 Methodology

The Respeck sensor (Fig. 1) developed at the Centre for Speckled Computing was validated in clinical trials at the Royal Infirmary Edinburgh against the nasal cannula as the reference monitor for measuring breathing rate/flow [3]. The Respeck also tracks continuously the activity of the wearer, such as sitting, standing and lying down based on the orientation of the device in relation to the direction of gravity, which is computationally inexpensive. Movement is detected based on the magnitude of the acceleration vector, and when it crosses a threshold level, fixed by analysing the training data, six times in succession regularly spaced with a tolerance of half-a-second, it is categorised as walking. The subjects in the cohort wore the device continuously for periods ranging between 24 to 72 h, only taking it off during their bath/shower. The dataset from the 93 subjects was analysed to offer cohort-level insights far more efficiently in terms of time and resources than the traditional manual approaches described in Sect. 1.

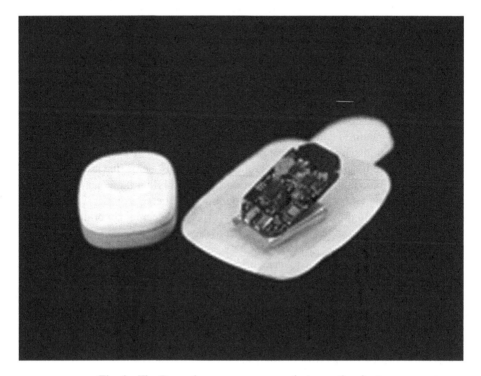

Fig. 1. The Respeck sensor worn as a plaster on the chest.

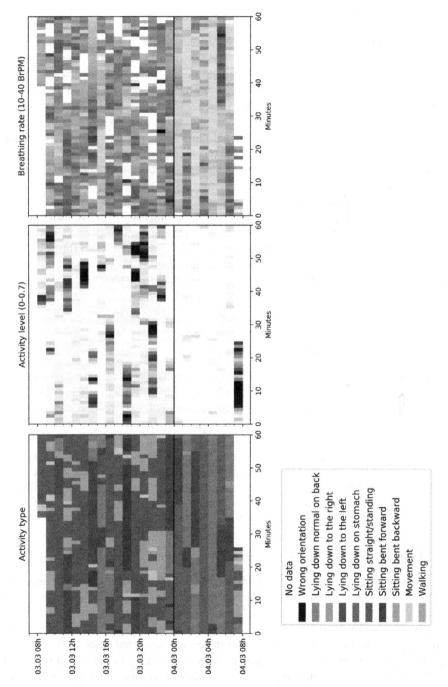

Fig. 2. "Pixelgram" for one valid day-night period. The darker shades represented higher values in Columns 2 and 3. (Color figure online)

2.1 Data Preparation

Of the-158 subjects recruited in a rural constituency, the data of 7 subjects were rejected as they were recorded incorrectly. The remaining 151 subjects were manually processed to remove records which were either too short (less than two hours during the day-night period), had too many interruptions, or the sensor was wrongly attached during the recording. The remaining 93 subjects (54 male and 39 female) had an average age of 42 ± 15 years. Figure 2 is an illustration of a Pixelgram representing three information channels, with each channel illustrating specific information for one subject over a day-night period. The sixty pixels along the x-axis in each information channel represents one minute-average recordings for one hour, and the 24 rows represent a day-long capture. In the first column on the left, activity types are colour-coded: blue - sitting/standing, orange/yellow - movement, and green - lying down. The other two columns display the activity levels, i.e., the intensity of movement [5], and the breathing rate, with darker shades representing higher values. The values in the brackets of the column titles show the minimum (white) and maximum (black) values of the grey scale. By scanning this plot, one can infer that this subject lay down approximately between 23:00 until 07:00 on the next day. The time of sleep onset can be inferred based on the following rules:

- The subject is lying down and stays that way for at least the next hour.
- The mean breathing rate level drops noticeably [10].
- The activity level is close to zero.

Conversely, waking up can be detected by a change in activity to sitting or movement, and a rise in activity level and breathing rate. Based on these rules, the subject in Fig. 2 slept from approximately 23:20 until 07:05 on the next day. The day period was then simply the start of the recording, or end of the previous sleeping period, until the start of the next day. Using this process for all 93 subjects, 84 subjects recorded one day and night period, five subjects recorded two valid periods and four subjects recorded three periods, resulting in a total of 106 day-night periods. As there are 2–3 recordings at most for any subject, and each day will be sufficiently different for the same subjects, it was decided to include all 106 periods for the following analysis, and treat them as 106 independent recordings.

2.2 Features for Activity Clustering

The activity patterns in the first column in Fig. 2 are prominently visible and the subjects can be clustered into groups, such as highly active groups and less active ones for those who take an afternoon nap. Jiang et al. [8] classify subjects into groups based on their work and leisure time-patterns, using nine activities logged with a questionnaire, such as at home, work, or school. The subjects are clustered based on this activity pattern, by first turning the 5-minute activity logs into a binary matrix (yes/no for each activity in the five-minute period), reducing the dimension using Principal Component Analysis, and applying K-means clustering on the resulting features. Their approach works well, but will not translate to the Respeck application for three principal reasons: the sample size is much smaller; the dimensionality is higher due to one-minute intervals as opposed to five-minute ones; and the activities are more abstract, and will therefore change more often.

Instead, a new set of features was chosen which best represented the patterns visible in the Pixelgrams during the day periods.

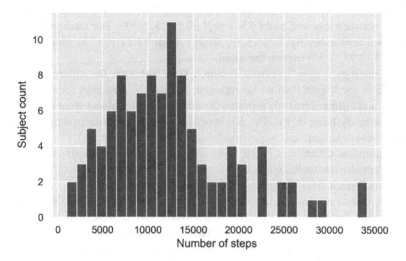

Fig. 3. Distribution of step counts for the cohort.

- **Step count:** The step count is recorded as part of the walking classification of the Respeck. A step is recorded when the mean length of the acceleration vector crosses a certain threshold several times in a row, regularly spaced. Figure 3 shows the distribution of step counts for all the 106-day periods.
- **Mean activity level:** The mean level of activity over the entire day [5].
- **Walking/Moving/Lying percentage:** The percentage of time spent walking, moving and lying down. Sitting/Standing is implicitly contained, as it is the absence of the other three.
- **Number of Walking/Movement/Lying/Sitting period:** The number of uninterrupted periods of that type.
- **Afternoon nap:** The number of instances of naps in the afternoon. A nap was registered when the subject lay down for at least 20 uninterrupted minutes and had a reduced breathing rate of at least two breaths per minute compared to the average.

The K-means module of the sklearn Python library [9] was employed to cluster the periods based on these features.

3   Results

3.1   Breathing Patterns

Taking the mean respiratory rate (RR) over day-night period for all 106 periods reveals the following pattern: The median (25th percentile, 75th percentile) RR during the day was 22.86 (21.67, 23.92), and during the night: 18.36 (17.02, 19.76). The median difference between day and night RR was 4.39 (3.29, 5.53). The median RR variance also dropped noticeably by 7.21 (3.39, 10.08), from 12.27 (10.13, 14.46) during the day to 4.84 (2.98, 7.33) during the night.

These findings support previous research [10], although the differences between day and night are bigger than so far reported. A likely explanation for this is that the RR during wake-time were only reported 20 min before the subject went to sleep, when they were already lying down. The RR would naturally be lower in that case and the difference between sleep and wake breathing would be smaller.

The significant differences in RR level also support the hypothesis that sleep onset may be detected with the RESpeck by a drop in RR level more accurately than by other accelerometer-based devices based on wrist movement, for instance.

This statement is valid even though one criteria for selecting the sleep periods in this study was the reduced RR itself, which would, by design, lead to a lower RR during that time. However, as this only affected the exact beginning of the night period, but not at other parts of the night, this intervention has a negligible effect on the statistics reported above.

3.2   Activity Patterns

Figure 4 shows the results using K-means clustering, by setting the number of clusters to four. Each plot corresponds to one cluster, with each line being the activity pattern for a subject over an entire day. The colour coding matches those in Fig. 2. The plots clearly show four different types of activity patterns:

- Sedentary (first graph): These are the least active subjects with few movement/walking periods during the day. Many subjects in this cluster take a nap in the afternoon. As this is a rural cohort, even the less active people show patterns more active than a typical urban office worker. This can also be seen in the step count histogram in Fig. 3, which shows a high level of step counts for the entire cohort.
- Moderately active (second graph): More active than the "Sedentary" cluster, with few subjects taking nap breaks.
- Active walkers (third graph): Subjects with an unusually high percentage of walking periods and a high step count.
- Active movers (fourth graph): Subjects with an unusually high percentage of non-walking movement, such as farmers and workers.

Six of the nine subjects with more than one day of recording were classified into more than one cluster. This is not surprising given the rural setting of the study, with less regular job activities than in an urban environment. In the future, recording data for

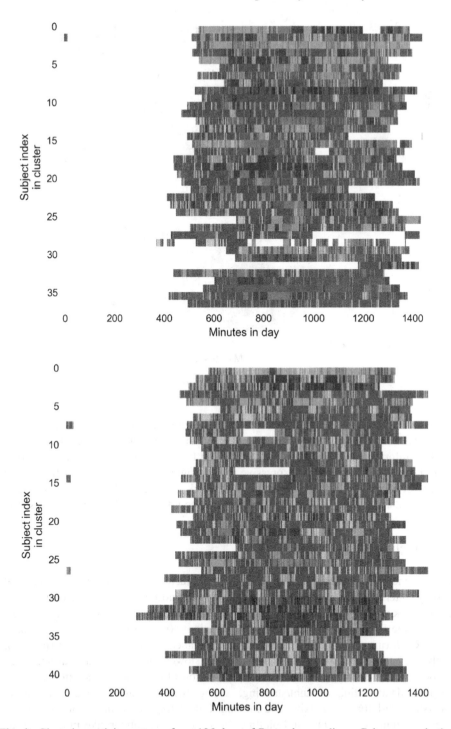

Fig. 4. Clustering activity patterns from 106 days of Respeck recordings. Colours encode the same activities as in Fig. 2. "Sedentary", first; "Moderately active", second; "Active walkers", third; "Active movers", fourth.

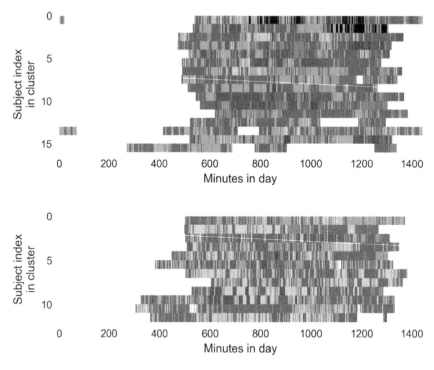

Fig. 4. (*continued*)

a full week, classifying each day into one of the clusters and taking the mode of all classifications as the predicted cluster will result in more accurate assignments.

This information about cluster affiliation can be used to estimate the lifestyle of a subject and is more stable and expressive than a single metric such as the activity level or number of walking periods alone. In future work, a sedentary lifestyle of subjects in the "Sedentary" cluster, coupled with a bad diet could be linked to health issues [6].

4   Conclusions

A novel methodology has been described for characterising respiratory and physical activity patterns in the general population during their normal every-day activities using the Respeck wearable sensor. Derived from 106 day-night recordings gathered from 93 subjects, the RR dropped by 4.39 breaths per minute (median) during sleep compared to the RR during day-time. The breathing rate variance also dropped by 7.21 (median), implying that the breathing is both considerably slower and more regular during sleep periods. Future work will validate the classification of other activities extracted from Respeck data: sitting straight/standing, sitting bent forward/backward, lying on back/stomach/left/right, walking and moving. Calculating the main activity performed in each minute of recording and plotting the values in a heatmap-like plot termed as *Pixelgram* revealed discernible activity patterns for each subject.

A selection of features extracted from this activity report enabled the clustering of all 106 day-night periods into four distinct groups, each containing visually similar records. The four groups corresponded to different lifestyles: "Sedentary", "Moderately active", "Active walkers" and "Active movers". Calculation of the most common label across several days of recording will lead to a relatively stable measure of lifestyle and will be a useful metric in assessing health parameters of subjects wearing the Respeck. Future studies are planned with patients with respiratory diseases such as asthma, emphysema, chronic bronchitis and upper airways obstruction to characterise causal relationships between physical activity and respiratory patterns. Other breathing rate patterns during the night, although not analysed in this report, could reveal information about the sleep quality in addition to its duration, once validated against reference polysomnography data.

Acknowledgements. This research was funded partially by the Centre for Speckled Computing, University of Edinburgh; the UK Medical Research Council, and the Natural Environment Research Council (NE/P016340/, project DAPHNE - Delhi Air Pollution: Health and Effects); and, the UK Medical Research Council and the Arts and Humanities Research Council (MC_PC_MR/R024405/1, project PHILAP - Public Health Initiative on LMIC Air Pollution). We wish to thank Ms. Santhi Bhogadi, Project Co-ordinator of APCAPS for managing the data collection and the volunteers who participated in the study.

References

1. Attal, F., Mohammed, S., Dedabrishvili, M., Chamroukhi, F., Oukhellou, L., Amirat, Y.: Physical human activity recognition using wearable sensors. Sensors **15**(12), 31314–31338 (2015). https://doi.org/10.3390/s151229858
2. Douglas, N.J., White, D.P., Pickett, C.K., Weil, J.V., Clifford, W.: Respiration during sleep in normal man. Thorax **37**(11), 840–844 (1982)
3. Drummond, G.B., Bates, A., Mann, J., Arvind, D.K.: Validation of a new non-invasive automatic monitor of respiratory rate for postoperative subjects. Br. J. Anaesth. **107**(3), 462–469 (2011). https://doi.org/10.1093/bja/aer153
4. Google: Activity Recognition API | Google Developers (2018). https://developers.google.com/location-context/activity-recognition/
5. Mann, J., Rabinovich, R., Bates, A., Giavedoni, S., MacNee, W., Arvind, D.K.: Simultaneous activity and respiratory monitoring using an accelerometer. In: 2011 International Conference on Body Sensor Networks, pp. 139–143 (2011). https://doi.org/10.1109/BSN.2011.26
6. Ottevaere, C., Huybrechts, I., Benser, J., et al.: Clustering patterns of physical activity, sedentary and dietary behavior among European adolescents: the HELENA study. BMC Public Health **11**(1), 328 (2011). https://doi.org/10.1186/1471-2458-11-328
7. Gayathri, K.S., Sukanya, P.: An unsupervised pattern clustering approach for identifying abnormal user behaviors in smart homes. IJCSN Int. J. Comput. Sci. Netw. **2**(3) (2013). ISSN 2277–5420
8. González, M.C., Jiang, S., Ferreira, J.: Clustering daily patterns of human activities in the city. Data Min. Knowl. Discov. **25**(3), 478–510 (2012)
9. Sklearn: sklearn.cluster.KMeans (2018). http://scikitlearn.org/stable/modules/generated/sklearn.cluster.KMeans.html

10. Snyder, F., Hobson, J., Morrison, D.F., Goldfrank, F.: Changes in respiration, heart rate, and systolic blood pressure in human sleep. J. Appl. Physiol. **19**, 417–422 (1964). https://doi.org/10.1097/00132586-196508000-0000. (Bethesda, Md.: 1985)

11. Bates, C.A., Ling, M., Mann, J., Arvind, D.K.: Respiratory rate and flow waveform estimation from tri-axial accelerometer data, In: Proceedings of 2010 International Conference on Body Sensor Networks, BSN 2010. IEEE, Singapore (2010)

12. Arvind, D.K., Bates, C.A., Fischer, D.J., Mann, J.: A sensor data collection environment for clinical trials investigating health effects of airborne pollution. In: Proceedings of 2018 IEEE International Conference on Biomedical and Health Informatics, 4–7 March 2018, USA (2018)

Medical Tele-Monitoring and Tele-Assistance for Diabetics Patients by Means of 5G Cellular Networks

S. Morosi[1(✉)], S. Jayousi[1], L. Mucchi[1], F. Peinetti[2],
L. Mastrantonio[2], G. Fioravanti[2], A. Giacomini[2], A. Fratini[3],
F. Padiglione[4], and F. De Lucia[5]

[1] Department of Information Engineering, University of Florence,
50139 Florence, Italy
{simone.morosi,sara.jayousi,lorenzo.mucchi}@unifi.it
[2] Enel X, Viale Tor Di Quinto 47, 00191 Rome, Italy
{federico.peinetti,luca.mastrantonio,
gabriele.fioravanti,andrea.giacomini}@enel.com
[3] OpEn Fiber, Rome, Italy
andrea.fratini@openfiber.it
[4] ADILIFE s.r.l, via Mosca 52, 00142 Rome, Italy
f.padiglione@adilife.net
[5] MENARINI DIAGNOSTICS, Bagno a Ripoli (FI), Italy
fdelucia@menarini.it

Abstract. This paper deals with the description of an effective solution for tele-monitoring and tele-assistance of diabetics patients which resorts to the use of the recently launched 5G cellular networks. The proposed solution allows the provision of a tele-monitoring service for chronic diabetic patients, which provides proactive remote interaction of the patient with a "Healthcare center". Moreover the paper shows the results of a recent experimentation which is based on the use of 5G network and has been realized in the town of Prato, Italy by presenting the results in terms of main performance indicators and describing the implemented e-health routines. Since these activities are achieved in the framework of one of the recent Italian pilot experimentations of the 5G networks, the presented e-Health services are one the first implementation that is based on this cellular system and take benefit of its outstanding performance.

Keywords: 5G cellular networks · E-health services · Tele-assistance · Telemonitoring

1 Introduction

Thanks to its remarkable performance the fifth Generation (5G) cellular networks will represent an enabling factor for different applications concerning the quality of life of the community of the territories by providing several advanced services. Focusing on the healthcare sector, the adoption of 5G networks will improve the citizen's health assistance system: e-health services, such as tele-assistance, tele-consultation and

© ICST Institute for Computer Sciences, Social Informatics and Telecommunications Engineering 2019
Published by Springer Nature Switzerland AG 2019. All Rights Reserved
L. Mucchi et al. (Eds.): BODYNETS 2019, LNICST 297, pp. 79–88, 2019.
https://doi.org/10.1007/978-3-030-34833-5_7

remote monitoring of patients and fragile subjects, will guarantee continuity of care and assistance and will push towards transition from the specialized hospital-based care models to patient-centered ones. These services and the introduction of the 5G networks will make the medical service more effective, reduce its costs and increase the quality of life of patients [1–3]: it is important to note that the Tele-Assistance/Tele-Consultation applications will take particular benefit from the distinctive features of the upcoming 5G networks, namely the ultra-low latency and very high bandwidth.

This new paradigm will allow the design and development of innovative solutions addressing some of the main problems related to the management of multiple patients in a care environment (hospital, rehabilitation structure, etc.) during all the different phases and to the remote assistance of convalescent or home patients (for diseases such as diabetes). The patient can be assisted "transparently" at any time through adaptive interactions among smart objects (sensors, drugs, doctors' terminals, patients, relatives, and pharmacies): the monitoring of some of the main parameters will afford immediate assistance in case of necessity. The transparency to the user, the flexibility, and the cooperation between the patient, the objects, and the network are of utmost importance in the disease context and can be specifically tailored to the assistance of patients affected by specific problems or pathologies [4, 5].

In this paper an effective solution for tele-monitoring and tele-assistance of diabetics patients is presented, which resorts to the use of the recently launched 5G cellular networks [6–8]: this solution allows the provision of a tele-monitoring service for chronic diabetic patients, which provides proactive remote interaction of the patient with a "Healthcare Center".

The proposed solution resorts to the adoption of an innovative 5G architecture that affords to experience the outstanding Key Performance Indicators (KPIs) of the upcoming cellular network. The interactions between the Patients, the Doctors and Healthcare Center are permitted by an original web app that has been specifically designed for the Use-Case experimentation: the application allows patients to monitor the status of their diabetes pathology and to be remotely monitored through frequent blood glucose and weight measurements. Measurements are performed by consumable and wearable devices and their results are automatically stored in the patient clinical records and made available and accessible at anytime and anywhere. Moreover, the connection to the H24 operating center permits medical monitoring of the measurements and the support in the decision-making process related to the management of their pathology. The adoption of the 5G network enables high quality tele-Assistance and represents a performance breakthrough with respect to current LTE/LTE-A (Long Tem Evolution/Long Term Evolution - Advanced) networks. Since the latency and the data-rate are both essential for this service, their values have been measured alongside the preliminary tests of the Use-Case: the measured values are also reported in the paper.

The article is organized as follows. The next paragraph presents an overview about the Diabetic Pathology with figures about number of patients and control routines. Then the main requirements of tele-monitoring services for diabetics patients are reported. In the successive paragraph the proposed solution for tele-monitoring and tele-assistance is introduced by describing the network architecture and the benefits that are due to the 5G exploitation. Then, the results of a recent experimentation which is based on the use of 5G network and has been realized in the town of Prato, Italy is presented by showing the results of the main performance indicators and describing the simulated e-health routines. Finally, conclusions and future developments are drawn in the final section.

2 An Overview of Diabetic Pathology: Some Figures About Number of Patients and Control Routines

The slow but inexorable increase in life expectancy of the world population and the equally significant decrease in some of the most widespread pathologies has made the growth of the incidence of diabetes in the world population evident. International Diabetes Foundation has recently revealed that while today one in 11 adults has diabetes, in 2040 the diabetics will be one in 10. This means that while today 415 million people have diabetes, this number will raise to 642 million in 2040. Moreover it is worth recalling that in 2015, around 5 million people died of diabetes-related causes (1 every 6 s) and that 193 million people live with undiagnosed diabetes, that is to say one in two adults [9].

The reasons for this diabetes epidemic are manifold and mainly attributable to a profound change in lifestyle, to increased life expectancy and ongoing social changes:

- the population of over-sixties is constantly growing;
- increased calorie intake and reduced physical activity led to the rapid increase in obesity and overweight.

Moreover, diabetes tends to be more common in the less well-off socio-economic groups and also in some specific ethnic groups. As a matter of facts, an ever-increasing number of people will have to live with diabetes and with the serious complications that it causes with a growing demand for assistance, social support, economic investments and reorganization of care. Therefore, the growth in health expenditure will risk to jeopardize the principle of equality of access to care with the consequent widening of poverty and fragility. Therefore, our societies will need a deeper attention and bigger resources to be dedicated to the prevention that, as it is known, tends to reduce the subsequent costs for the treatment of complications.

3 Monitoring Diabetic Patients: Main Requirements

The efficient management of diabetic patients requires a continuous monitoring of different parameters. The main ones are: glycaemia, weight, eating habits, physical activity, pre-scribed therapy adherence. By correlating the information coming from the monitoring of these parameters and analyzing the results that are achieved by taking also into account the history of the patients' health, the medical staff can evaluate the actual status of the patient and activate the adequate care path.

On the diabetic patient's side, the main identified needs:

- to increase the frequency of specialist visits;
- to easily store the glycaemia measurements and report them to the specialist (clinical history);
- to reduce the waiting times to schedule a visit;
- to be home-monitored due to both logistic difficulties in accessing public health facilities (e.g. long distances) and motor difficulties (e.g. complications of diabetes);
- to be motivated to improve his/her lifestyle (eating habits, physical activity);
- to be supported by qualified staff in the daily management of diabetes (e.g. lack of social and family support network);
- to be guided and motivated to improve adherence to therapy.

In this context, the adoption of ICT (Information and Communication Technologies) and of wireless and wearable medical devices affords the implementation of advanced tele-monitoring systems that are able to address most of the previous listed requirements. Although a large variety of services can be defined, the main components that should be considered in the design of such services are:

- Qualified tele-assistance for medical consultation or guidance;
- Tele-monitoring and information collection of the main critical parameters that are required for the assessment of a diabetic patient;
- Feedback mechanisms for motivating patients, improving patient's lifestyle, monitoring the adherence to therapy, activating corrective actions in case of anomalies, etc.

4   Proposed Solution

Starting from the main requirements for the monitoring of diabetic patients, the proposed solution relies on the usage of a simple app that allows patients to record and monitor their health parameters and receive qualified medical advice anywhere and anytime by phone or video call.

4.1   The Service: Integrating Tele-Monitoring and Tele-Assistance

The proposed service consists of two main components: tele-monitoring and tele-assistance.

Tele-Monitoring Component. It enables patients to monitor the status of their pathology and to be remotely monitored through:

- frequent blood glucose and weight measurements, which automatically are stored in the patient clinical record and are made available and accessible anytime and anywhere;
- a H24 operating center for proactive medical monitoring of the measurements performed by patients and for supporting them in the decision-making process related to the management of their pathology.

The patients will be equipped with a kit for measurements including a NFC (Near Field Communication) glucometer, a Bluetooth weight scale and a blood glucose lancing device.

Tele-Assistance Component. It enables patients to contact the Operating Assistance Center for:

- having a teleconsultation with medical staff;
- booking and having a tele-visit with a general practitioner or a specialist;
- being supported in coping with technical or administrative problems regarding the service itself.

In order to describe the proposed service a brief description of a use case integrating the two service components is provided in the following.

4.2   The Network Architecture

The objective of this section is to describe the network architecture that supports the proposed Service, highlighting the involved devices and communication technologies.

Figure 1 depicts the main components of the network architecture, showing the interactions among the three main players of the Service: the patient, a member of the medical staff and the Operating Assistance Service operator.

The data exchange among them are enabled by different communication access network technologies and by customized software applications (both as a mobile and a web versions) representing the interface with the Cloud Service Platform.

In the following the way each Platform user can access the Service is analyzed and the main functionalities of the Cloud Service Platform are presented.

Patient Side. The patient is equipped with a 5G smartphone running a customized App for accessing the tele-monitoring and tele-assistance Service and with a kit of smart devices for the measurements acquisition. In detail, the developed App is able to interface with the weight scale through a Bluetooth connection and with a glucometer with an NFC connection and to acquire automatically the results of the measurements. Once the measurement values are acquired by the smartphone, they are sent through a 5G link (eventually relayed by a 5G modem) to the Cloud service platform and stored in the patient health record.

Service Platform Side. The cloud platform allows the storage, processing and sharing of the uploaded measurements, which can be accessed and visualized (e.g. historical text or graphical output) by patients, medical staff members and Operating Assistance Service operators. In fact, all the patients' measurements are stored together with some additional diagnostic images and clinical reports (eventually integrated) in the Cloud Platform and they are always available and shared with the authorized people. More-over, Tele-assistance sessions (e.g. videoconference) between patient and medical staff or patient and Assistance Service operator are allowed for medical and technical assistance, respectively. In case of anomalous measurements (alert mechanism) the patient will be called by the Operating Assistance Service operator with the aim to further investigate on the patient's health status and, if needed, a tele-visit with a general practitioner or a specialist is booked.

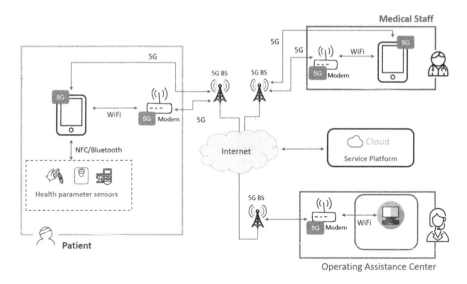

Fig. 1. Network architecture

All these interactions are enabled by the definition and development of a Platform web interface and a mobile interface, which allows patients, medical staff and operators to access the Service.

Medical Staff Side. Each member of the medical staff can run the customized Web App on his computer for remotely accessing patient health record and real time monitoring the patient's performed measurements. The historical health records and therefore the possibility of evaluating the trend of the patient's health status allow them to activate the proper countermeasures (e.g. tele-consultation, therapy calibration, etc.), if required.

Operating Assistance Service Side. The continuous monitoring of the uploaded data is guaranteed by the Operating Assistance Service operators, who access the Platform through a Personal Computer Wi-Fi connected to a 5G modem. In particular, the developed web interface allows an efficient patient management and monitoring.

4.3   The Benefits of 5G

Thanks to the flexibility that is guaranteed by new features such as the network slicing, the 5G networks will enable new business models in which operators, suppliers, end users, industry, companies, service providers, suppliers and other players in general will collaborate differently than today [6].

The evolution of business models will lead to the birth of new services or to the evolution of those that characterize the current telecommunications, which are mainly focused on personal communication (voice), on the interconnection of people between them (Instant Messaging and Social Networks) and on the use of multimedia content (Streaming and Internet browsing). These services will evolve both due to the increasing use of multimedia contents and to the interaction of "things" between them and the Web world. Moreover, unlike previous 3GPP mobile communication systems that are characterized by a single system configuration for all services, the 5G system will be able to provide differentiated and optimized support for a variety of deeply differentiated services, that are targeted for user communities with different needs. The 5G is therefore a multifunctional system capable of simultaneously supporting various combinations of performance characteristics, such as transmission speed, latency, positioning, reliability and availability.

As a consequence new and more stringent performance indicators such as: high data rate, very low latency, high reliability and availability, greater positioning accuracy, new minimum coverage requirements, connected device density and network capacity will have to be met.

As far as the e-Health use case is concerned, the use of 5G technology is especially required by tele-monitoring and tele-assistance services in order to guarantee the necessary network capacity (e.g. up to 200 Mbps per single stream, necessary for the transmission of HD video in case of videoconference between doctor and patient), and a reliability of at least 99% that is requested to ensure the correct continuity of the service.

More generally the considered services require the use of 5G technology to allow a more efficient realization than the ones that are possible with the current network technologies. Key features of 5G with a direct impact on the performance of the services developed in this eHealth trial are:

- the stability of the network to ensure continuity of service;
- the low latency required by monitoring and control applications;
- the high throughput required by video/teleconsultation applications.

Moreover it is worth recalling that 5G cellular networks will resort to the introduction of the Network Slicing, through which various eHealth services will be instantiated with isolation characteristics between different Customer traffic flows and performance guarantee in each slice.

5   Experimental Activities and Use Case

On March 16, 2017, the Ministry for Economic Development published a call for tenders for project proposals for pre-commercial testing of the 5G cellular network in the spectrum portion of 3.6–3.8 GHz. This call for proposals responds to the request of the European Commission for a 5G timely deployment as a strategic opportunity for Europe, with a coordinated approach and a common calendar among Member States.

This is the context of the joint initiative that has been promoted by the lead companies OpEn Fiber and Wind Tre, which combined their skills, infrastructures and investment capacity with the common goal of promoting a "5G City" project in which they are provided innovative services with a strong impact both in terms of social and economic utility. The initiative concerned the city of Prato while presenting characteristics of replicability and usability either on a National, an European and more generally, an International scenario. Therefore, a series of use cases were identified for which applications and services are intended with certain performance requirements, analyzing the strategic role of the 5G networks and the related economic and social impacts expected in the Prato area; among others, experimentation activities related to the improvement of the citizen's health care system have been launched.

As part of the activities planned for the Use Case 1 of the 5G Experimentation project promoted by the Italian Ministry of Economic Development (MISE), Enel is setting up a tele-monitoring service for chronic diabetic patients, which provides for proactive remote interaction of the patient with a "Healthcare center".

Enel aims to establish a Proof-of-Concept (PoC) test in Prato (which is the site selected for testing activities within Project 5G), to simultaneously determine the values of the main KPIs and perform tests on the integrated service. In order to provide further details on the KPI measurement link, Fig. 2 shows the protocol architecture of the segment of interest of the 5G network; the entities that are represented in this figure are the Customer Premise Equipment (CPE), the Evolved Radio Access Network (E-UTRAN), the Serving Gateway (SGW) and the Packet Data Network Gateway (PDN GW) that is also the point of connection with the Internet. The layers of the protocol stack and the interfaces are depicted for all the involved entities.

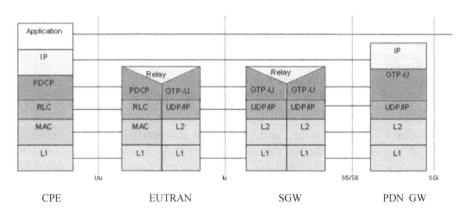

Fig. 2. 5G network architecture: network segment subject to measurement for KPI verification.

As for the KPIs, the following Tables 1 and 2 give a summary of the results that have been achieved in the preliminary tests: the entities that are mentioned in these tables are the CPE, the Base Station, the Evolved Packet Core (EPC) Network and the PDN. Multiple tests have been performed for all the considered parameters: particularly the bandwidth has been measured both for the UDP (User Datagram Protocol) and the TCP (Transmit Control Protocol) cases.

Table 1. Results of latency tests.

Latency (CPE - Base Station - EPC Core - PDN)					
	Measured values [ms]			Requirements [ms]	Test result
	Min	Mean	Max	Range	
Round trip time	9	10	12	20–100	Passed
One way delay	4.5	5	6	10–50	Passed

Table 2. Results of bandwidth tests.

Bandwidth (CPE - Base Station - EPC Core - PDN)					
	Measured values [Mbit/s]		Requirements [Mbit/s]		Test result
	DOWN	UP	DOWN	UP	
UDP	170	60	100	50	Passed
TCP	155	55	100	50	Passed

As regards the measured values, it has to be noticed that both the latency and the bandwidth satisfy the requirements that have been identified for the monitoring service of diabetic patients, namely the high data transmission speed (50 ÷ 100 Mb/s) and the moderately low latency (10 ÷ 50 ms, one way).

As for the service, Enel X and A. Menarini Diagnostic have developed an innovative solution that allows to record and monitor health parameters and to receive qualified medical advice anywhere, anytime, by either phone or video call. This solution is based on the implementation of the previously described network architecture, the use of suitable medical devices and the design of a simple app. Particularly, the parameters telemonitoring protocol allows to synchronize glycemic and weight results directly from the smartphone. The patient can view the measurements and get a graphical and organized view of the trend over time, with notifications in the event of values out of range. On the other hand the telephone and video-consultation assistance with a Diabetologist permits to request, 24 h a day, telephone assistance with doctors of the Operational Center and book a video-consultation with a Diabetologist, by simply clicking on mobile, comfortably at home.

As depicted in Fig. 3, a diabetic patient will program the daily measurement routines with the considered devices. During one of these probes, the glucometer will detect high/low glycaemia values. This condition will trigger the emission of an alert towards the smartphone with a callback request; on the same time, a Doctor in

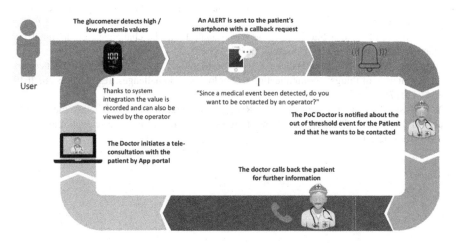

Fig. 3. The proposed tele-monitoring and tele-assistance routine.

Healthcare Center will be notified with the report and pre-alerted for a possible call by a patient. If the patient will proceed with the call, the Doctor will contact him to clarify the situation by means of a specific Teleconsultation through the app portal.

6 Conclusions and Further Works

An effective solution for tele-monitoring and tele-assistance of diabetics patients which resorts to the use of the recently launched 5G cellular networks has been presented. The results of a recent experimentation, which is based on the use of 5G network and has been realized in the town of Prato, Italy have been also shown by presenting the results of the main performance indicator and describing the simulated e-health routines. Future activities encompass further tests for the validation of the application and evaluation of the User Experience over a restricted set of real patients.

References

1. Brito, J.C.M.: Trends in wireless communications towards 5G networks—the influence of e-health and IoT applications. In: Proceedings on IEEE 2016 International Multidisciplinary Conference on Computer and Energy Science (SpliTech) (2016)
2. Lal, K.N., Kumar, A.: E-health application over 5G using content-centric networking (CCN). In: Proceedings on IEEE 2017 International Conference on IoT and Application (ICIOT) (2017)
3. Baker, S.B., Xiang, W., Atkinson, I.: Internet of things for smart healthcare: technologies, challenges, and opportunities. IEEE Access 5, 26521–26544 (2017)
4. Del Re, E., Morosi, S., Ronga, L.S., Jayousi, S., Martinelli, A.: Flexible heterogeneous satellite-based architecture for enhanced quality of life applications. IEEE Commun. Mag. 53(5), 186–193 (2015)
5. Del Re, E., Morosi, S., Mucchi, L., Ronga, L.S., Jayousi, S.: Future wireless systems for human bond communications. Wirel. Pers. Commun. 88(1), 39–52 (2016)
6. Marabissi, D., et al.: A real case of implementation of the future 5G city. Future Internet 11(4), 1–16 (2019)
7. Shafi, M., et al.: 5G: a tutorial overview of standards, trials, challenges, deployment, and practice. IEEE J. Sel. Areas Commun. 35(6), 1201–1221 (2017)
8. Akpakwu, G.A., Silva, B.J., Hancke, G.P., Abu-Mahfouz, A.M.: A survey on 5G networks for the internet of things: communication technologies and challenges. IEEE Access 6, 3619–3647 (2017)
9. NCD Risk Factor Collaboration (NCD-RisC): Worldwide trends in diabetes since 1980: a pooled analysis of 751 population-based studies with 4.4 million participant. Lancet 387, 1513–1530 (2016)

Physical Activity Monitoring

Group Walking Recognition Based on Smartphone Sensors

Qimeng Li[1], Raffaele Gravina[1(✉)], Sen Qiu[2], Zhelong Wang[2],
Weilin Zang[3], and Ye Li[3]

[1] Department of Informatics, Modeling, Electronics and Systems,
University of Calabria, 87036 Rende, Italy
`qimeng.li@unical.com`, `r.gravina@dimes.unical.it`
[2] School of Control Science and Engineering, Dalian University of Technology,
Dalian 116024, China
{`qiu,wangzl`}`@dlut.edu.cn`
[3] Key Laboratory for Health Informatics,
Shenzhen Institutes of Advanced Technology, Chinese Academy of Sciences,
Shenzhen, China
{`wl.zang,ye.li`}`@siat.ac.cn`

Abstract. Human group activity represents a potentially valuable contextually relevant source of information, which can be analyzed to support diverse human-centric applications. In recent year, more and more sensors are being pervasively spread in daily living environments, so giving excellent opportunities for using ubiquitous sensing to recognize group activities. In this paper, we used smartphone-based data and edge computing technologies to address group activity recognition, with particular focus on group walking. The data is provided by two groups of participants using a smartphone with embedded 9-DoF inertial sensors; several features are generated to identify group membership of each subject. Our results showed that the accelerometer rarely can be used alone to identify the group motion; in most situations, multiple sensor sources are required to determine group membership. Moreover, the use of 9-DoF sensors to identify group affiliation is still challenging, because, in a multi-user scenario, individual behaviors often have mutual contingency; therefore, the concept of proximity is also introduced to improve the classification algorithm.

Keywords: Multi-user activity · Group membership · Walking group clustering · Wearable sensors

1 Introduction

In recent years, thanks to ubiquitous sensing and Internet of things (IoT), more and more human-centric data has been captured, analyzed, and used to support or improve human's life. Human activity recognition (HAR) [1–3], in this

Published by Springer Nature Switzerland AG 2019. All Rights Reserved
L. Mucchi et al. (Eds.): BODYNETS 2019, LNICST 297, pp. 91–102, 2019.
https://doi.org/10.1007/978-3-030-34833-5_8

situation, becomes a relevant building block to address several problems in diversified application areas such as public safety, transportation, healthcare, wellness, manufacturing.

HAR, which is distinguished by the number of people involved in a given task, can be roughly divided in individual activity and group (multi-user) activity. From decades, most of studies were focused on recognizing individual activities, while research on group activity detection is much less developed. With the advent of technologies such as cloud computing, many researchers began to use computer-vision [4,5] to identify group activities because still images and video streams are very information-rich signals. Even though the recognition performance can be excellent, computer-vision have non trivial drawbacks and limitation, such as the raising privacy concern, deployment location selection of a fixed camera or battery capacity and energy consumption of a mobile camera. The recent continuous development of microelectronics and Internet of Things (IoT) technology, which have capability to provide massive amount of data from the more and more sensors being pervasively spread in daily living environments, has given an excellent opportunity for using ubiquitous sensing to recognize group activities.

In this paper, we propose a preliminary research on group membership identification in different walking groups. We used a smartphone to collect the 9-DoF (degree of freedom) data and generate features to recognize individual activity; then, all features with recognition results will be sent to the Edge or the Cloud layer to determine the walking group membership.

The remainder of the paper is organized as follows. Section 2 discusses some the state-of-art works on group activity recognition. Section 3 describes the proposed group activity detection architecture. Section 4 reveals the building blocks of the programming model for group activity detection. Finally, Sect. 5 concludes the paper and outlines planned future work.

2   Related Work

There is an established literature on group activities, involving group identification, group membership affiliation selection, group activity recognition. Most studies focuses specifically on the recognition of specific group activities. In this particular case, most researches focused on detecting individual activities/behaviors from each group member, and used such meta-knowledge to recognize the group activities.

Computer-vision approaches have been often applied. Ibrahim et al. [3] adopted a long short-term memory (LSTM) algorithm to build up a deep model for recognize group activity recognition. In their model, 2-stage LSTM (i.e., person dynamics and group dynamics) was used and experimental results demonstrate that the model has a good performance for group activity recognition. Deng et al. [4] proposed a framework which combined graphical models with deep neural networks, and their results showed the model could handle highly structured learning tasks on group activity recognition.

Another recent emerging approach, called *channel state information*, proposes the analysis of Wi-Fi signals to recognize human activities. Feng et al. [5]proposed a scheme termed Multiple Activity Identification System (MAIS) to identify multiple activities of different subjects in a group. However, all of the approaches above could not properly address requirements such as privacy, low portability, low power consumption, and mobility.

Thanks to the technical improvements of microelectronics, the wearable sensors are becoming more lightweight, less energy demanding, and often embedded in daily life wearable accessories (glasses, watches, rings) and garments (t-shirts, shoes, gloves). Abkenar et al. [6] proposed a modeling language (i.e., GroupSense-L) and a distributed middleware (i.e., GroupSense) for mobile group activity recognition (GAR). Experimental analysis showed excellent results in recognizing group activities such as playing table tennis, eating together, and picking cherry in an orchard. Gordon et al. [7] presented a method using mobile phone sensor data to recognize group affiliations in multi-group environments. The experimental results showed the approach can correctly detect 93% of group affiliations. Bourbia et al. [8] presented a generic framework, which is based on the concept of *patterns* for mining interval-based relationships between users' temporally overlapped actions, for group activity recognition using simple non-obtrusive sensors. Yu et al. [9] also proposed a framework with a two-stage process (i.e., sensing modality selection and multimodal clustering) to identify subgroups in a homogeneous group activity using smartphone embedded sensors.

In contrast with previous literature, with the aim of accurately recognizing group activities and group membership, we propose a framework that uses smartphone sensors to identify walking group membership and the group activities which generated by different groups. In this framework, we take into account additional information (i.e. proximity) to support the group activity recognition step.

3   Methodology

In this paper, we propose a framework (see in Fig. 1) to identify walking groups. It is composed of three different layers:

- *Sensing layer* - to collect and analyze all sensor data for further recognition;
- *Edge layer* - if the area is covered with Edge devices, this layer will receive the generated features and classified individual activities to recognize the group activity and identify group membership;
- *Cloud layer* - if the area is not covered by edge devices, the smartphone will connect to Cloud backend which will support the group activity recognition.

Figure 2 depicts the processing workflow of the proposed method. It is composed of three main tasks:

- *Data collection* - to acquire and store raw sensor data;
- *Pre-processing* - the pre-processing step reduces noise from the raw signals;

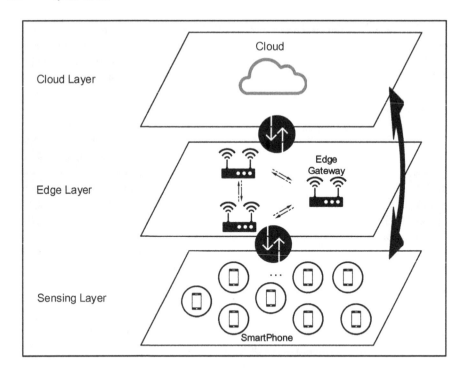

Fig. 1. Framework of the proposed method.

- *Data segmentation and feature generation* - data is segmented into fixed length windows; the segmented data will generate the feature sets;
- *Individual activity classification* - feature sets are sent to a local classifier running on the smartphone and results will be sent to the Edge (or Cloud) layer for group activity recognition;
- *Walking group recognition* - the Edge (or Cloud) layer executes a group recognition classifier that considers only feature sets from potential groups (i.e. cluster of users that are in mutual proximity).

3.1   Data Collection

Data is directly generated by embedded 9-DoF inertial sensor. Collected data is stored in a file which is structured into CSV format. The Edge and Cloud layers will calculate the distance from each user's smartphone.

3.2   Pre-processing

To reduce the noise present in the raw signals, a Finite Impulse Response (FIR) filter is adopted to inertial sensor streams to smooth the data. After de-noising, the raw smartphone sensor (accelerometer, gyroscope, magnetometer) data is normalized in the range $[0, 1]$.

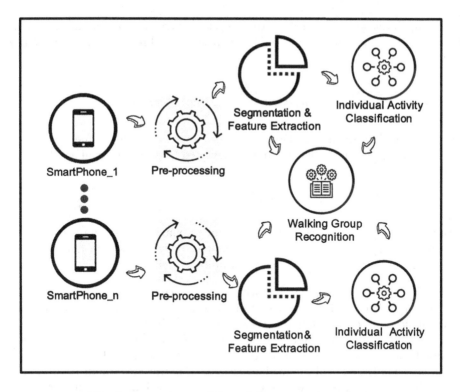

Fig. 2. Processing workflow of the proposed method.

3.3   Data Segmentation and Feature Generation

For the accelerometer data, we fixed the time length for the sliding windows as $l = 1$ s. Similarly, the gyroscope and magnetometer data can be divided into windows corresponding to the segmentation of acceleration data.

Feature extraction and selection are crucial in a machine learning process; in this paper, we extracted the following features: direction, signal magnitude vector (SMV), mean, root mean square (RMS), standard derivation (STD), and proximity. The most important features are defined and described in the next subsections.

Direction. Magnetometer and acceleration signals can be fused to estimate the angle between Magnetic North and the user heading. Equation 1 and Eq. 2 calculate respectively the pitch angle θ and the roll angle γ of the user. The g, g_x, g_y, g_z represent the components on three axes of the gravity acceleration vector.

$$\theta = \arcsin\left(-\frac{g_x}{g}\right) \tag{1}$$

$$\gamma = \arctan\left(\frac{g_y}{g_z}\right) \tag{2}$$

Then, the heading angle ψ (with respect to magnetic north) can be calculate using Eq. 3, which $m_x, m_y, and\, m_z$ represent the three axes elements of the magnetic field.

$$\psi = \arctan\left(-\frac{m_y \cos\gamma - m_z \sin\gamma)}{m_x \cos\theta + m_y \sin\theta \sin\gamma + m_z \sin\theta \cos\gamma}\right) \qquad (3)$$

Signal Magnitude Vector. Signal magnitude vector provides a measure of the degree of movement intensity; it can be calculated from the tri-axial acceleration values using Eq. 4.

$$a = \sqrt{a_x^2 + a_y^2 + a_z^2} \qquad (4)$$

Proximity. In our scenario, the concept of proximity represents a feature to measure the distance among different users and between the user and the edge device. In the framework, we consider two different situations:

– *in-door* - if the area is covered with edge devices, the Edge layer will calculate the distance from each surrounding user's smartphone; this allows to construct and keep updated a (user-to-user) proximity map;
– *out-door* - if the area is not covered by edge devices, the GPS module is activated and all the data (feature sets and individual activity class) transmitted to the Cloud layer will be geo-localized. In this way the Cloud layer is able to construct and keep updated a (user-to-user) proximity map similar to the one constructed by the Edge layer.

3.4 Individual Activity Classification

In this step, a previously proposed HMM-based algorithm [10] is used to classify individual user activity. In this work, we specifically focus on two activities: walking and standing. In our HMM, a continuous activity can be represented by a finite number of states. Each state consists of transition probabilities to other states as well as observation probabilities of all the discrete symbols from every state. In this model, each kind of activity represents a trained HMM. Thus, when we obtain a discrete observations sequence $\{O_1, O_2, \ldots, O_n\}$, the appropriate HMM can be found through the maximum likelihood and the recognition had been carried out by the Eq. 5.

$$c = \arg\max_{\mu} P(O_{1:n}, S_{1:n} \mid \lambda_\mu)P(\lambda_\mu) \qquad (5)$$

3.5 Walking Group Recognition

When individual activities are classified, the classification results and previous generated features will be sent to an Edge node or Cloud (see Fig. 1) to recognize the group activities. First of all, Algorithm 1 will calculate the size of the group and make a list of possible group members.

Algorithm 1. Member list for classification.

Input: Proximity (P_n) The sets of previous classification result for current batch, $S = \{S_1, S_2, \ldots, S_n\}$; Previous group member list, L_{t-1}; Previous potential member list, R_{t-1};

Output: Group member list, L_t; Removed member list, R_t;
 1: initial list: Calculate proximity and make member list;
 2: **function** UPDATE GROUP MEMBER LIST(L_t, R_t)
 3:     Calculate the number of the no walking state occurrences (N) for group member list, in period t
 4:     **if** $N > Threshold$ **then**
 5:         Remove the User for the group member list, add to potential member list;
 6:     **else**
 7:         Keep;
 8:     **end if**
 9: **end function**
10: **function** UPDATE POTENTIAL MEMBER LIST(L_t, R_t)
11:     Calculate the number of the no walking state occurrences (N) for potential member list, in period t
12:     **if** $N < Threshold$ **then**
13:         Remove the User for the potential member list, add to group member list;
14:     **else**
15:         Keep;
16:     **end if**
17: **end function**
18: **return** Group member list, L_t; potential member list, R_t;

In this step, we used a k-NN algorithm to determine the group. Assuming that the sample set $D = \{x_1, x_2, \ldots, x_n\}$ contains n unlabeled samples, each of $x_i = \{x_{i1}, x_{i2}, \ldots, x_{im}\}$ is a m-dimension feature vector (including direction, signal magnitude vector (SMV), mean, etc.); the clustering algorithm divides the sample set D into k disjoint clusters $\{C_l | l = 1, 2, \ldots, k\}$. The output recognition result can be described as in Eq. 6.

$$\lambda = \lambda_1, \lambda2, \ldots, \lambda_n \tag{6}$$

4   Experiment and Results

4.1   Experiment Description

The data has been collected during an experiment carried out in a previous research [11]. In this experiment, ten volunteers used the same smartphone model (i.e., Samsung Galaxy sIII) to collect data in a real-world environment. Each participant held the mobile phone in the hand during walking sessions. Along other information, accelerometer, gyroscope, magnetometer data were also collected although not used nor further analyzed in that work. The ten participants were

---

Algorithm 2. Walking group classification.

Input: The sets of features and previous classification result for current batch, $D = \{x_1, x_2, \ldots, x_n\}$; Cluster number, k;

Output: Cluster division on the current batch, C;

1: initial vector: randomly select k samples from set D: $\{\mu_1, \mu_2, \ldots, \mu_k\}$;

2: **repeat**

3:      Let $C_i = \emptyset (1 \leq i \leq k)$;

4:      **for** $j = 1, 2, \ldots, n$ **do**

5:          Calculate distance: $d_{ji} = \|x_j - \mu_i\|_2$;

6:          Determine cluster tag: $C_{\lambda_j} = C_{\lambda_j} \cup \{x_j\}, \lambda_j \in \{1, 2, \ldots, k\}$;

7:      **end for**

8:      **for** $i = 1, 2, \ldots, k$ **do**

9:          Calculate new mean vector: $\mu_i^{'} = \frac{1}{|C_i|} \sum_{x \in C_i} x$;

10:          **if** $\mu_i^{'} \neq \mu_i$ **then**

11:              Update the current mean vector μ_i to $\mu_i^{'}$;

12:          **else**

13:              Keep the current mean vector μ_i;

14:          **end if**

15:      **end for**

16: **until** No updates;

17: **return** Cluster division, C;

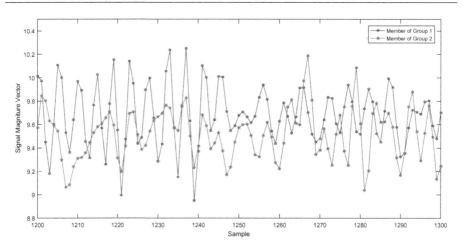

Fig. 3. Filtered acceleration data from different groups.

equally divided into two groups. The protocol of the experiment consisted of the two groups crossing each other, walking in opposite but parallel directions. The two groups were staggered for a short period, then they re-aggregated and continue walking forward altogether.

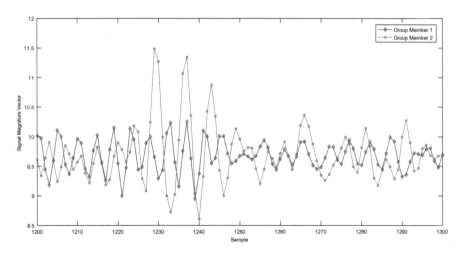

Fig. 4. Filtered acceleration data from same group.

4.2 Heading Direction Detection

In Fig. 5, the red and black lines indicate that there are two participants standing back to back, and the angle between their smartphones is almost 180°. The blue line represents the walking participant direction, and it is nearly the same direction of the standing participant which is marked in red line. This means that the walking participant is facing magnetic north. Obviously, when the participant changes direction, the indication of the magnetic field will change accordingly.

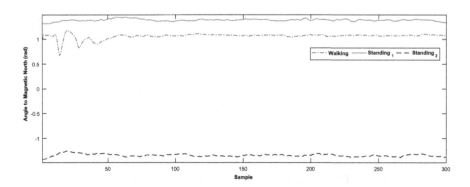

Fig. 5. Group member direction detection. (Color figure online)

4.3 Acceleration Data Analysis

As shown in Fig. 3, users from the same group often accelerated or decelerated in the same pattern; and in Fig. 4, the pattern in some areas is different, due to the

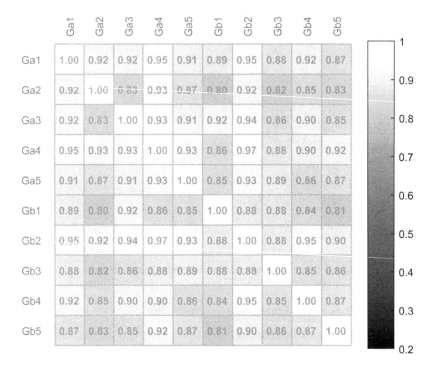

Fig. 6. Cosine similarity between each member.

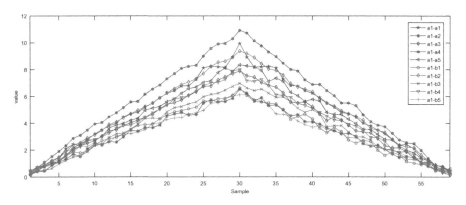

Fig. 7. Cross-correlation of each member (30 samples).

participants are in a different accelerative situation. Still, all of the above can not indicate that users have a similar pattern just from the same group; their motion pattern also could have a similarity between different groups. Human motion patterns are usually random, and different groups of people may have the same motion pattern at the same time. Besides, human activities are usually very subjective, and individual consciousness may lead to inconsistent actions at the same time, and it will result in different motion patterns for people in the same group.

Figures 6 and 7 show the cosine similarity and the cross-correlation between each member; these indicators show that there is no very strong relation by the acceleration changes between each member, even if the participants are in similar patten. Thus, the acceleration data only can be used in recognize the motion state (e.g., waling, standing) of the participant.

5   Conclusion

In this paper, we proposed a framework for the recolonization of group activity and walking group membership. The work is based on mobile, edge, and cloud computing which are selected to support the recognition in different scenarios. Data is generated by several smartphones from each participant, and it is used to identify individual activities. Then, the classified data and features are send to a Raspberry PI edge node or cloud to mining the group activity and the membership.

Results showed that the accelerometer can be used to recognize individual activities such as walking and standing but it has important limitations in mining the pattern of group activities. Therefore, we are planning to apply information fusion methods to combine accelerometer data with heading direction and proximity indicators, so to support a more accurately recognition of the group membership.

References

1. Gravina, R., Li, Q.: Emotion-relevant activity recognition based on smart cushion using multi-sensor fusion. Inform. Fusion **48**, 1–10 (2018)
2. Lara, O.D., Labrador, M.A.: A survey on human activity recognition using wearable sensors. IEEE Commun. Surv. Tutor. **15**(3), 1192–1209 (2013)
3. Ibrahim, M.S., Muralidharan, S., Deng, Z., Vahdat, A., Mori, G.: A hierarchical deep temporal model for group activity recognition. In: Proceedings of the IEEE Conference on Computer Vision and Pattern Recognition, pp. 1971–1980 (2016)
4. Deng, Z., Vahdat, A., Hu, H., Mori, G.: Structure inference machines: Recurrent neural networks for analyzing relations in group activity recognition. In: Proceedings of the IEEE Conference on Computer Vision and Pattern Recognition, pp. 4772–4781 (2016)
5. Feng, C., Arshad, S., Liu, Y.: MAIS: multiple activity identification system using channel state information of WiFi signals. In: Ma, L., Khreishah, A., Zhang, Y., Yan, M. (eds.) WASA 2017. LNCS, vol. 10251, pp. 419–432. Springer, Cham (2017). https://doi.org/10.1007/978-3-319-60033-8_37
6. Abkenar, A.B., Loke, S.W., Zaslavsky, A., Rahayu, W.: GroupSense: recognizing and understanding group physical activities using multi-device embedded sensing. ACM Trans. Embed. Comput. Syst. (TECS) **17**(6), 98 (2019)
7. Gordon, D., Wirz, M., Roggen, D., Tröster, G., Beigl, M.: Group affiliation detection using model divergence for wearable devices. In: Proceedings of the 2014 ACM International Symposium on Wearable Computers, pp. 19–26, September 2014

8. Bourbia, A.L., Son, H., Shin, B., Kim, T., Lee, D., Hyun, S.J.: Temporal dependency rule learning based group activity recognition in smart spaces. In: 2016 IEEE 40th Annual Computer Software and Applications Conference (COMPSAC), Vol. 1, pp. 658–663, June 2016

9. Yu, N., Zhao, Y., Han, Q., Zhu, W., Wu, H.: Identification of partitions in a homogeneous activity group using mobile devices. Mob. Inform. Syst. **2016**, Article ID 3545327, 14 p. (2016)

10. Ma, C., Li, Q., Li, W., Gravina, R., Zhang, Y., Fortino, G.: Activity recognition of wheelchair users based on sequence feature in time-series. In: Proceedings of the 2017 IEEE International Conference on Systems, Man, and Cybernetics (SMC), pp. 3659–3664, October 2017

11. Álvarez Lacasia, J., Leppänen, T., Iwai, M., Kobayashi, H., Sezaki, K.: A method for grouping smartphone users based on Wi-Fi signal strength. In: Forum on Information Technology, vol. 32, pp. 450–452 (2013)

Towards Body Sensor Network Based Gait Abnormality Evaluation for Stroke Survivors

Sen Qiu[1,2(✉)], Xiangyang Guo[2], Hongyu Zhao[1,2], Zhelong Wang[1,2], Qimeng Li[3], and Raffaele Gravina[3]

[1] Key Laboratory of Intelligent Control and Optimization for Industrial Equipment of Ministry of Education, Dalian University of Technology, Dalian 116024, China
{qiu,zhaohy,wangzl}@dlut.edu.cn
[2] School of Control Science and Engineering,
Dalian University of Technology, Dalian 116024, China
[3] Department of Informatics, Modeling, Electronics and Systems,
University of Calabria, Via P. Bucci, 87036 Rende, CS, Italy

Abstract. Due to the technological advances of micro-electro-mechanical sensor and wireless sensor network, gait analysis has been widely adopted as an significant indicator of mobility impairment for stroke survivors. This paper aims to propose an wearable computing based gait impairment evaluation method with distribute inertial sensor unit (IMU) mounted on human lower limbs. Temporal-spacial gait metrics were evaluated on more than twenty post stroke patients and ten healthy control subjects in the 10-meters-walk-test. Experimental results shown that significant differences exist between stroke patients and healthy subject in terms of various gait metrics. The extracted gait metrics are consistent with clinical observations, and the position estimation accuracy has been validated by optical device. The proposed method has the potential to serve as an objective and cost-efficient tool for rehabilitation-assisting therapy for post stroke survivors in clinical practice.

Keywords: Body sensor network · Human gait analysis · Information fusion · Rehabilitation · Micro-electro-mechanical sensor

1 Introduction

As a fundamental human need, people's health needs are constantly increasing with the development of social economy. Especially in the reality of accelerated aging of the population all over the world. One fifth people will be over the age of 60 by 2050 according to the statistics of United Nations. This means that the need for devices with health monitoring and managing functions will continue to grow. The health crisis is likely to become more and more severe, especially

© ICST Institute for Computer Sciences, Social Informatics and Telecommunications Engineering 2019
Published by Springer Nature Switzerland AG 2019. All Rights Reserved
L. Mucchi et al. (Eds.): BODYNETS 2019, LNICST 297, pp. 103–113, 2019.
https://doi.org/10.1007/978-3-030-34833-5_9

for some chronic diseases. For example, stroke is a leading cause of death all around the world as population ages. Nearly four fifths of stroke survivors are suffering from hemiparesis which tends to severely deteriorate limbs mobility due to muscle weakness and Joint degeneration. Walking dysfunction is one of the main problems in the rehabilitation of stroke patients. A typical symptom manifest as gait disorder, characterized by asymmetry between dual feet, insufficient foot elevation, deviant gait phase distribution and reduced range of joint motion (ROM) such as ankle joint. Note that ankle joint is an essential clinical concern, i.e., the plantarflexion and dorsalflexion come from ankle joint are used as an evaluation factor by clinic in post stroke rehabilitation programs [1–5]. Gait assessment has thus become a useful tool to study the effect of gait retraining in stroke patients.

Gait is the external manifestation of human body structure and movement, motor regulation system, behavior and mental activity during walking. Any nerve, muscle and joint disease can lead to walking dysfunction [6–9]. Pathological gait refers to the abnormal state of uncoordinated walking. It is actually caused by diseases of the nervous and motor systems of the human body, skewness of the pelvis, trunk lateral flexion and other reasons. Gait analysis system is based on wearable motion capture system, which captures the movement data of lower limbs and then analyzes and evaluates the walking state of people. Traditional optical device based human gait tracking approach and pressure sensor based methods universally suffer from high cost and rigorous requirements of testing setup, hence limited the larger scale application in the field [10,11]. Regardless of the approach, gait parameters derived from wearable inertial sensors have showed significant differeces between post stroke patients with walking aids and healthy subjects able to walk normally without auxiliary facilities [12–15].

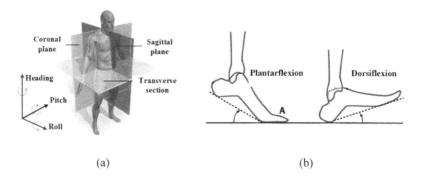

(a)   (b)

Fig. 1. Three-dimensional anatomical structure and foot movement schematic (a) three planes of the human body (b) foot plantarflexion and dorsiflexion

The three-dimensional anatomical structure is the reference from which all other orientation description are based [16–19], where the subjects' faces are directed forward, while the toes facing forward, as shown in Fig. 1(a). In this case, three anatomical planes can be defined: the sagittal plane, the transverse plane and the coronal plane, respectively. The coronal plane divides the body into anterior (front) and posterior (rear) sections. The transverse plane divides the body into superior (upper) and inferior (lower) sections. The sagittal plane divides the body into left and right halves. With regards to gait analysis, the majority of movements occur within the sagittal plane. Note that the ankle movement to point the toes is called plantarflexion while the movement to bring the toes closer to the body is called dorsiflexion, as shown in Fig. 1(b).

2 Methodology and Materials

2.1 Hardware Platform Based on Wearable IMU

The self-made sensor module weights less than 20 g, the maximum size is not more than 60 mm. The total power consumption does not exceed 200 mW. The lightweight design of sensor module is for the demand of gait analysis and intended to have minimal effect on natural gait of the subjects. The inertial sensor array specification is shown in Table 1. We have designed a bandage that binds the sensor tightly on lower limbs, avoiding direct contact with the skin and allowing the sensor nodes to be adapted to different types of shoes without compromising the reliability of the sensor installation. In the gait assessment scenario, the subject wear multiple sensor nodes on both lower limbs, and their daily activities will not be affected. Movement data from wearable sensors were recorded when the subjects walked at an preferred speed for 10 m along straight line path. The embedded operating system μCOS is adopted to collect the raw sensor data and transmit the data to the host through 2.4 Ghz wireless communication with the data transmission rate of 100 Hz. In addition to real-time wireless transmission, the system can rely on the memory card for offline recording, which supporting more than 10 h of continuous monitoring. This performance enhances its portability and is very helpful in outdoor testing scenario, where subjects are not restricted to stay in the settled wireless communication coverage area. Figure 2 illustrate the raw motion data of dual foot during normal walking.

Table 1. Inertial sensor array specification

Unit	Accelerometer	Gyroscope	Magnetometer
Dimensions	3 axes	3 axes	3 axes
Dynamic scope	$\pm 50\,\mathrm{m/s^2}$	$\pm 1200°/s$	$\pm 750\,\mathrm{mGauss}$
Bandwidth	30 Hz	40 Hz	20 Hz
Nonlinearity	0.2%	0.1%	0.25%
Axis misalignment	0.1°	0.1°	0.1°

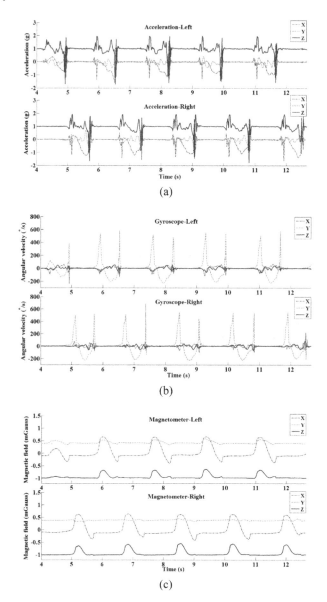

Fig. 2. Raw data collected from IMU (a) Acceleration measurement (b) Gyroscope measurement (c) Magnetometer measurement

The data from the wearable inertial sensors are compared with measurements obtained from an optical motion tracking system. On account of the misalignment error, the accelerometer is accurately calibrated with a linear least squares method. Note that the magnetometer performance is easily distracted by other magnetic source [14,20–23]. Therefore, it is necessary to estimate the magnetic

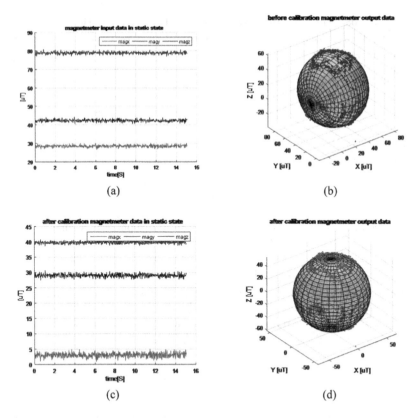

Fig. 3. Fitting results of ellipsoid before and after calibration (a) raw magnetometer measurement (b) ellipsoid fitting before calibration (c) magnetometer measurement after calibration (d) ellipsoid fitting after calibration

interference when using the observation data of the magnetometer to estimate the heading. Set $\boldsymbol{m^s} = [m_x^s, m_y^s, m_z^s]|$ as the measured magnetic field for ground reference, when meet the following criterion, can be directly used magnetic measurement. The threshold λ is set to 0.2 after several tries and errors. Figure 3(a) (b) and (c) (d) are fitting results of ellipsoid before and after calibration respectively. One rotation of the magnetometer is enough to ensure the accuracy of the magnetometer calibration.

$$| \frac{arctan(m_x^s/m_z^s) - arctan(m_x^g/m_z^g)}{arctan(m_x^g/m_z^g)} | \geq \lambda \tag{1}$$

2.2 Gait Metrics Definition

Gait metrics definition are described in Table 2. The statistics of gait metrics may varied greatly between normal and pathological status. For example, under normal circumstances, the swing phase accounts for 40% of a gait cycle, and the stance phase takes the remaining 60% [24–27]. For stroke patients, in order to alleviate the pain caused by dystonia, they tend to adopt a relatively comfortable posture, which leads to the increase of stance phase, along with lower foot elevation and gait asymmetry.

Table 2. Typical spatio-temporal gait metrics

Gait metrics	Description
Stride length (m)	Distance between two consecutive footprint of the same foot
Walking speed (m/s)	Stride length divided by walking cycle
Stance ratio (s)	The proportion of the stance phase in a single walking cycle
Foot elevation (m)	Foot elevation in swing phase, which reflects the muscular strength
Gait symmetry	Symmetry of walking motion between left and right side of lower limbs
Ankle ROM (°)	Range of ankle flexion during a single stride

$$q = q_0 + q_1\mathbf{i} + q_2\mathbf{j} + q_3\mathbf{k} \tag{2}$$

This research adopts quaternion to represent rigid body rotation, as illustrated in Eq. 2. Note that the rotation from body frame to reference frame can be represented by a rotation angle α around a phasor axis. It is widely acknowledged that the rotation matrix C can describe a rotation of rigid body as follows:

$$C = \begin{bmatrix} q_0^2 + q_1^2 - q_2^2 - q_3^2 & 2(q_1q_2 + q_0q_3) & 2(q_1q_3 - q_0q_2) \\ 2(q_1q_2 - q_0q_3) & q_0^2 - q_1^2 + q_2^2 - q_3^2 & 2(q_2q_3 + q_0q_1) \\ 2(q_1q_3 + q_0q_2) & 2(q_2q_3 - q_0q_1) & q_0^2 - q_1^2 - q_2^2 + q_3^2 \end{bmatrix} \tag{3}$$

where

$$\psi = -\arctan(\frac{2(q_1q_2 - q_0q_3)}{q_0^2 + q_1^2 - q_2^2 - q_3^2}) \tag{4}$$

$$\theta = \arcsin(2(q_2q_3 + q_0q_1)) \tag{5}$$

$$\varphi = -\arctan(\frac{2(q_1q_3 - q_0q_2)}{q_0^2 - q_1^2 - q_2^2 + q_3^2}) \tag{6}$$

The combination of roll angle φ, pitch angle θ and yaw angle ψ determine the three-dimensional orientation, which lay a solid foundation for position estimation.

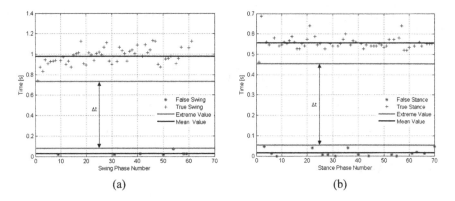

(a)   (b)

Fig. 4. Gait phase detection by k-mean clustering algorithm (a) swing phases detection (b) stance phases detection

As illustrated in Fig. 4, the k-mean clustering algorithm efficiently classifies the detected swing phases and stance phases into true and false clusters based on time durations, respectively. Meanwhile, the extreme values of each cluster are illustrated by red lines. Results shown that time constraint parameters were determined adaptively for different data sets using the k-mean algorithm, in this case, false gait phases detection due to sensor data fluctuation could be properly eliminated (Fig. 4).

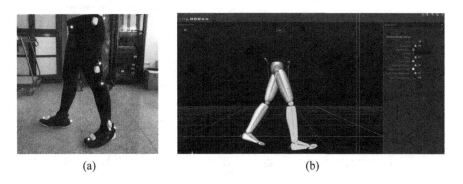

(a)   (b)

Fig. 5. Experimental scene and optical system validation (a) Inertial sensor installation and high reflection marker for optical motion tracking (b) 3D orientation and position ground truth provided by optical apparatus

2.3   Experimental Results and Discussions

In this research, the subjects included the patients group and the control group. The patients group consists of twenty stroke survivors (ten females and ten

Table 3. Gait parameters comparison for healthy subjects and patients. Results are presented as mean (±SD)

Gait metrics	Healthy subjects	Stroke survivors
Stride length (m)	1.17 ± 0.15	0.72 ± 0.48
Walking speed (m/s)	0.96 ± 0.15	0.64 ± 0.37
Stance ratio (%)	59 ± 4	70 ± 16
Foot elevation (m)	0.22 ± 0.05	0.011 ± 0.09
Gait symmetry	0.93 ± 0.07	0.74 ± 0.26
Ankle ROM (°)	66 ± 9	39 ± 18

Table 4. 3D position estimation error

Position error	X-axis (m)	Y-axis (m)	Z-axis (m)
Trial 1	0.017 ± 0.005	0.023 ± 0.004	0.008 ± 0.003
Trial 2	0.014 ± 0.003	0.019 ± 0.005	0.006 ± 0.004

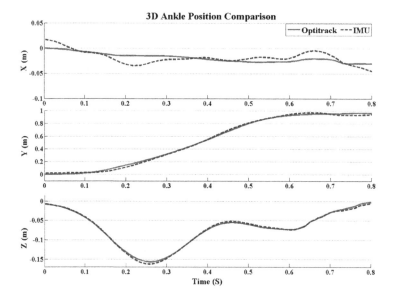

Fig. 6. Results of comparative experiments using Optitrack device

males age from 38 to 67) with varying degrees of gait abnormality. The control group includes ten healthy subjects (five females and five males age from 22 to 46) who participated in the control tests. The tests consist of multiple walking trials along the specific straight line path for each subject at their comfortable pace. The experiment took place in the corridor of first affiliated hospital of Dalian Medical University. The extracted gait metrics are presented in Table 3, the stride lengths, walking speed, foot elevation, gait symmetry and ankle range of motion (ROM) are relatively low in stroke survivors, which are consistent with clinical observation. The mean value of stride length of healthy subjects are 1.12 ± 0.18, with the minimum being 0.98 m. The system validation scenario is shown in Fig. 5, and the results of comparative experiments using Optitrack device are shown in Table 4 and Fig. 6.

3   Conclusions

In this work, an IMU based system for ambulatory gait monitoring was presented. The physical interface is connected to the computer by a Bluetooth link, and provides feedback to the medical staff and patients while performing walking trials. The system allows for in-home rehabilitation at an affordable cost.

The essential aspect of wearables sensors in healthcare applications is monitoring the health of users. Body sensors network provides the foundation of numerous medical applications by measuring and processing physiological information upon which medical staff can make intelligent decisions and inform the subjects with quantitative data. Particularly, IMU sensors consist of accelerometers and gyroscopes are readily available on contemporary smartphones and wearable devices. They have been widely adopted in the area of limb movement disorder recognition, fall detection and step counting applications being prominent examples in this field. In the long run, only the combination of hospital, data and equipment can fully reflect the advantages of big data and wearable computing. The battery life, data processing, data collection, transmission and the ability of computers to analyze the data independently are the key to the ultimate solution of gait analysis in the big data era.

Acknowledgments. This research was funded by National Natural Science Foundation of China (61803072, 61873044 and 61903062), China Postdoctoral Science Foundation (2017M621131 and 2017M621132), Liaoning Natural Science Foundation Key Project no. 20180540011, Dalian Science and Technology Innovation fund (2019J13SN99 and 2018J12SN077), Fundamental Research Funds for the Central Universities no. DUT18RC(4)034, and National Defence Pre-research Foundation no. 614250607011708.

References

1. Gravina, R., Alinia, P., Ghasemzadeh, H., Fortino, G.: Multi-sensor fusion in body sensor networks: state-of-the-art and research challenges. Inf. Fusion **35**, 68–80 (2016)
2. Fortino, G., Galzarano, S., Gravina, R., Li, W.: A framework for collaborative computing and multi-sensor data fusion in body sensor networks. Inf. Fusion **22**, 50–70 (2015)
3. Horak, F.B., King, L., Mancini, M.: Role of body-worn movement monitor technology for balance and gait rehabilitation. Phys. Ther. **95**(3), 461–70 (2015)

4. Gravina, R., et al.: Cloud-based activity-aaservice cyber-physical framework for human activity monitoring in mobility. Future Gener. Comput. Syst. **75**, 158–171 (2017)
5. Qiu, S., Wang, Z., Zhao, H., Liu, L., Jiang, Y., Li, J.: Body sensor network based robust gait analysis: toward clinical and at home use. IEEE Sens. J. **19**, 1–9 (2019)
6. Al-Amri, M., Nicholas, K., Button, K., Sparkes, V., Sheeran, L., Davies, J.L.: Inertial measurement units for clinical movement analysis: reliability and concurrent validity. Sens. (Switz.) **18**(3), 1–29 (2018)
7. Kumar, P., Mukherjee, S., Saini, R., Kaushik, P., Roy, P.P., Dogra, D.P.: Multimodal gait recognition with inertial sensor data and video using evolutionary algorithm. IEEE Trans. Fuzzy Syst. **27**(5), 956–965 (2019)
8. Qiu, S., Wang, Z., Zhao, H., Liu, L., Jiang, Y.: Using body-worn sensors for preliminary rehabilitation assessment in stroke victims with gait impairment. IEEE Access **6**, 31249–31258 (2018)
9. Wang, Q., Markopoulos, P., Yu, B., Chen, W., Timmermans, A.: Interactive wearable systems for upper body rehabilitation: a systematic review. J. NeuroEngineering Rehabil. **14**, 1–21 (2017)
10. Baghdadi, A., Cavuoto, L.A., Crassidis, J.L.: Hip and trunk kinematics estimation in gait through Kalman Filter using IMU data at the Ankle. IEEE Sens. J. **18**(10), 4253–4260 (2018)
11. Leal-Junior, A.G., Frizera, A., Avellar, L.M., Marques, C., Pontes, M.J.: Polymer optical fiber for in-shoe monitoring of ground reaction forces during the gait. IEEE Sens. J. **18**(6), 2362–2368 (2018)
12. Lu, R., Lin, X., Liang, X., Shen, X.: A secure handshake scheme with symptoms-matching for mHealthcare social network. Mob. Netw. Appl. **16**(6), 683–694 (2011)
13. Qiu, S., Liu, L., Zhao, H., Wang, Z., Jiang, Y.: MEMS inertial sensors based gait analysis for rehabilitation assessment via multi-sensor fusion. Micromachines **9**(9), 442 (2018)
14. Wang, Z., et al.: Using wearable sensors to capture posture of the human lumbar spine in competitive swimming. IEEE Trans. Hum.-Mach. Syst. **49**(2), 194–205 (2019)
15. Majumder, S., Mondal, T., Deen, M.J.: A simple, low-cost and efficient gait analyzer for wearable healthcare applications. IEEE Sens. J. **19**(6), 2320–2329 (2019)
16. Favre, J., Jolles, B., Siegrist, O., Aminian, K.: Quaternion-based fusion of gyroscopes and accelerometers to improve 3D angle measurement. Electron. Lett. **42**(11), 3–4 (2006)
17. Zhao, H., Wang, Z., Qiu, S., Shen, Y., Zhang, L., Tang, K.: Heading drift reduction for foot-mounted inertial navigation system via multi-sensor fusion and dual-gait analysis. IEEE Sens. J. **19**(19), 8514–8521 (2019)
18. Gouwanda, D., Gopalai, A.A., Khoo, B.H.: A low cost alternative to monitor human gait temporal parameters-wearable wireless gyroscope. IEEE Sens. J. **16**(24), 9029–9035 (2016)
19. Ahmed, M., Naude, J., Birkholtz, F., Glatt, V., Tetsworth, K.: Gait & Posture the relationship between gait and functional outcomes in patients treated with circular external fi xation for malunited tibial fractures. Gait Posture **68**, 569–574 (2019)
20. Qiu, S., Wang, Z., Zhao, H., Qin, K., Li, Z., Hu, H.: Inertial/magnetic sensors based pedestrian dead reckoning by means of multi-sensor fusion. Inf. Fusion **39**, 108–119 (2018)
21. Huang, H., et al.: Attitude estimation fusing quasi-newton and cubature Kalman filtering for inertial navigation system aided with magnetic sensors. IEEE Access **6**, 28755–28767 (2018)

22. Gheorghe, M.V., Member, S., Bodea, M.C., Member, L.S.: Calibration optimization study for tilt-compensated compasses. IEEE Trans. Instrum. Meas. **67**(6), 1486–1494 (2018)
23. Choe, N., Zhao, H., Qiu, S., So, Y.: A sensor-to-segment calibration method for motion capture system based on low cost MIMU. Measurement **131**, 490–500 (2018)
24. Zhao, H., Wang, Z., Qiu, S.: Adaptive gait detection based on foot-mounted inertial sensors and multi-sensor fusion. Inf. Fusion **52**, 157–166 (2019)
25. Qiu, S., Wang, Z., Zhao, H., Hu, H.: Using distributed wearable sensors to measure and evaluate human lower limb motions. IEEE Trans. Instrum. Meas. **65**(4), 939–950 (2016)
26. Wang, Z., et al.: Inertial sensor-based analysis of equestrian sports between beginner and professional riders under. IEEE Trans. Instrum. Meas. **67**(11), 2692–2704 (2018)
27. An, W.W., et al.: Neurophysiological correlates of gait retraining with real-time visual and auditory feedback. IEEE Trans. Neural Syst. Rehabil. Eng. **27**(6), 1341–1349 (2019)

Motion Recognition for Smart Sports Based on Wearable Inertial Sensors

Huihui Wang[1(✉)], Lianfu Li[1], Hao Chen[1], Yi Li[1], Sen Qiu[2],
and Raffaele Gravina[3]

[1] School of Fundamental Education, Dalian Neusoft University of Information,
Dalian 116023, China
{wanghuihui,lilianfu,chenhao}@neusoft.edu.cn
[2] School of Control Science and Engineering, Dalian University of Technology,
Dalian 116024, China
[3] Department of Informatics, Modeling, Electronics and Systems,
University of Calabria, Via P. Bucci, 87036 Rende, CS, Italy

Abstract. With the development of wearable technology and inertial sensor technology, the application of wearable sensors in the field of sports is becoming more extensive. The notion of Body Sensor Network (BSN) brings unique human-computer interaction mode and gives users a brand new experience. In terms of smart sports, BSN can be applied to table tennis training by detecting individual stroke motion and recognizing different technical movements, which provide a training evaluation for the players to improve their sport skills. A portable six-degree-of-freedom inertial sensor system was adopted to collect data in this research. After data pre-processing, triaxial angular velocity and triaxial acceleration data were used for table tennis stroke motion recognition. The classification and recognition of stroke action were achieved based on Support Vector Machine (SVM) algorithm after Principal Component Analysis (PCA) dimension reduction, and the recognition rate of five typical strokes can reach up to 96% using the trained classification model. It can be assumed that BSN has practical significance and broad application prospects.

Keywords: Body sensor network · Information fusion · Motion recognition · Wearable computing · Micro-electro-mechanical sensor

1 Introduction

As the earliest innovative Technology in MIT media lab in 1960 s, wearable computing technology is one of the most promising advanced technologies in modern human-machine interaction domain. The technology combines sensors, wireless communication, multimedia, signal process technologies, et al., and is mainly used to provide data monitoring support and auxiliary decision-making for users [1–4]. Traditional optical device based human motion tracking approach and pressure sensor based methods universally suffer from high cost and

© ICST Institute for Computer Sciences, Social Informatics and Telecommunications Engineering 2019
Published by Springer Nature Switzerland AG 2019. All Rights Reserved
L. Mucchi et al. (Eds.): BODYNETS 2019, LNICST 297, pp. 114–124, 2019.
https://doi.org/10.1007/978-3-030-34833-5_10

rigorous requirements of testing setup, hence limited the larger scale application in the field [5,6]. Wearable sensors not only have small volume and light weight, but also have the characteristics of low power consumption, simple operation and wireless data transmission, which have been attracting a large number of researchers' attention. In the context of intelligence and big data era, the ultra-miniaturization of electronic devices as well as the continuous progress of forward-looking computing models have boosted microelectronics technology and communication technology. At present, wearable technology is increasingly widely used in intelligent sports, mainly in physical physiological information detection, physical rehabilitation, physical education and research. Initial applications of wearable devices mainly include a simple pedometer, a heart-rate device or other devices to collect various physiological parameters of the exerciser [7,8]. With the continuous development and improvement of inertial sensor technology, inertial sensors have been widely used in smart watches, smart bracelets and other popular personal belongings, which can accurately obtain the inertial data generated by the user's daily activities and provide data for identification and motion analysis [9–16].

As China's "national sport", table tennis is one of the most common sports in Chinese society. According to the survey, there are tens of millions of Chinese people who love playing table tennis, especially among teenagers. It is possible for table tennis enthusiasts to apply wearable sensors during table tennis training to detect and evaluate individual stroke movements, so as to improve their sport skills. In this paper, a wearable sensor system is applied to table tennis training, and the wearer's inertial sensor is used to collect table tennis players' motion throughout the process. Angular velocity and acceleration signals are used to generate the corresponding strokes classifier to complete the recognition of various types of strokes. Recognition algorithm is introduced to classify and recognize the typical stroke action of the players.

As for classification models, researchers have proposed many research methods, such as Decision Trees [17], K Nearest neighbor (KNN) [18], Bayes method [18,19], Hidden Markov Models (HMM) [20], Support Vector Machine (SVM) [21–23] and so on. In literature, various methods for dimension reduction of high-dimensional features of samples in classification and recognition tasks are proposed [24–29]. Current stroke action recognition researches based on wearable sensors is still at an initial stage due to the actual environment variable and the diversity of stroke category, and there are still many problems need to be solved.

2   Methodology and Materials

2.1   Hardware Platform Based on Wearable Inertial Sensors

In this paper, the wearable sensor system is used to collect the stroke movement data in table tennis sport. This system consists of low cost six-axis inertial sensor, which can obtain high-precision motion data and well meet the design needs. The research focus on data preprocessing, sample feature extraction, classifier recognition process. Through the reasonable processing of data and classification model training, it is expected to obtain high-precision recognition performance at reasonable processing speed.

Table 1. Inertial sensor array specification

Unit	Accelerometer	Gyroscope
Dimensions	3 axes	3 axes
Dynamic range	$\pm 18\,g$	$\pm 2000°/s$
Bandwidth (Hz)	50	40
Bias stability (unit 1σ)	0.02	1
Noise density ($units/\sqrt{Hz}$)	0.05	0.05
Alignment error (deg)	0.2	0.2

Figure 1(a) is a the portable motion tracking system developed by Manlyn Ltd (Dalian, China). The lightweight design of sensor module is for the demand of ambulatory and long time monitoring. Sensor array specification is shown in Table 1. Figure 1(b) shows the table tennis stroke assessment scenario, in which the subject may wear sensor nodes on each upper limbs, and their sport activities will not be affected. Movement data from wearable sensors was recorded when the subjects played table tennis. The embedded operating system collect the raw sensor data and transmit the data to the host wirelessly. The 3D human upper limbs model in Fig. 1(c) indicates the ground truth of motion tracking provided by optical device (Made by Optitrack Ltd).

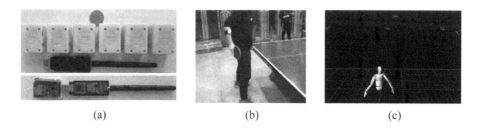

(a) (b) (c)

Fig. 1. Raw data collected from IMU (a) Inertial measurement Unit (b) Sensor installation (c) Ground truth provided by optical device (Made by Optitrack Ltd.)

2.2 Feature Extraction and Selection

After simple extraction, triaxial angular velocity and triaxial acceleration data were used for actual motion recognition. Five typical table tennis stroke movements including forehand stroke, flat push, forehand chop, backhand chop and smash, which are classified and identified respectively based on KNN algorithm and SVM algorithm. The collected raw data needs to be converted into a numerical matrix for subsequent recognition processing. Feature extraction is carried out then and for each data sample we can get a 48-dimensional feature vector, that is to calculate the mean value, variance, kurtosis, covariance, skewness, correlation coefficient, entropy and energy for the angular velocity data and acceleration data in the direction of X, Y and Z axes, as shown in Table 2.

Table 2. Eight features extracted from inertial data

Type of features	Statistical characteristics	Computational formula
Time-domain	Mean value	$\bar{X} = \frac{1}{n} \sum_{i=1}^{n} X_i$
	Variance	$s^2 = \frac{\sum_{i=1}^{n}(X_i - \bar{X})^2}{n}$
	Kurtosis	$K = \frac{\sum_{i=1}^{n}(X_i - \bar{X})^4 f_i}{n\,s^4}$
	Covariance	$\mathrm{cov}(X,Y) = \frac{\sum_{i=1}^{n}(X_i - \bar{X})(Y_i - \bar{Y})}{n-1}$
	Skewness	$SK = \frac{n\sum_{i=1}^{n}(X_i - \bar{X})^3}{(n-1)(n-2)\,s^3}$
	Correlation coefficient	$i_{xy} = \dfrac{\sum_{i=1}^{n}(X_i - \bar{X})(Y_i - \bar{Y})}{\sqrt{\sum_{i=1}^{n}(X_i - \bar{X})^2}\,\sqrt{\sum_{i=1}^{n}(Y_i - \bar{Y})^2}}$
Frequency-domain	Entropy	$H(X) = - \sum_{k=1}^{N} X_i(k) \log X_i(k)$
	Energy	$E = \dfrac{\sum_{k=1}^{N} X_i(k)^2}{N}$ $(X_i(k) = \sum_{n=1}^{N} x_i\, e^{-j2\pi kn/N}, k = 1,2,3,...,N)$

Feature normalization is normally necessary. Common methods of feature normalization include linear normalization and zero mean normalization as follows:

$$\overset{*}{X}_{linear} = \frac{x - x_{\min}}{x_{\max} - x_{\min}} \tag{1}$$

$$\overset{*}{X}_{zero} = \frac{x - \bar{x}}{\sigma}. \tag{2}$$

Compare the two normalization method, the linear normalization rely too much on minimum and maximum values, while zero mean normalization can get better recognition performance in the preliminary study. The characteristics of the original sample differ greatly in numerical value. After the normalization and dimensionality reduction, the characteristic values are limited to a certain range with little numerical difference, and the characteristics of the sample data represented by each feature are not changed.

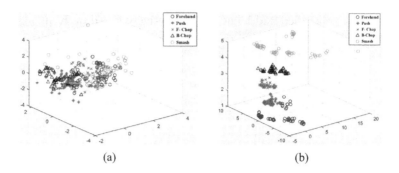

Fig. 2. Sample characteristic scatter plot (a) before PCA dimension reduction (b) after PCA dimension reduction

The main advantage of PCA (Principal Component Analysis) is that the principal components are orthogonal to each other after dimensionality reduction, which can eliminate the interaction between the components of the original data. In addition, PCA is an unsupervised learning of information measured by variance, which is not subject to sample label limit. Furthermore, its calculation process is simple and easy to realize. Figure 2 shows the effect of PCA dimensionality reduction. Figure 2(b) is the characteristic scatter diagram after dimensionality reduction of PCA. The aggregation number of the same type of stroke data can be seen in the figure, and the degree of differentiation of different actions is large, which lays a good foundation for the subsequent classification by SVM.

Table 3. Recognition rate of classifier using KNN method

K value	1	2	3	4	5	6	7	8	9	10	11	12
Recognition accuracy (%)	93	92	94	92	91	90	89	88	86	84	82	82

When using KNN method, it can be clearly seen from Table 3 that the recognition rate of classifier corresponding to different values of K (from 1 to 12 in this study). the recognition rate of the corresponding classifier is obtained by 10-fold cross validation. It can be concluded that when K = 3, the corresponding classifier model has the highest recognition rate. Therefore, in the task of classifying and recognizing the table tennis stroke action of players in this research, K = 3 is selected as the optimal value of K when using KNN method. Since the best performance is still less than 94%, SVM method is hence adopted to complete optimize recognition.

SVM based machine learning toolbox Libsvm (Matlab) is adopted in this study. Parameters train were completed through experimental tests. After several experimental tests, parameters and types with better recognition performance were finally selected, it turned out that C-svm was selected as SVM type

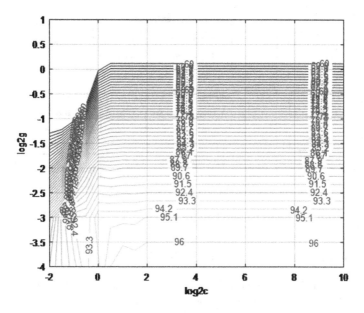

Fig. 3. Contour map of SVM corresponding matrix with different c and g parameters

and Gaussian kernel (as shown in the following formula) was selected as kernel function to achieve optimal recognition performance. Optimal punish coefficient c and kernel function radius g were selected through actual tests where the parameter c and g increasing gradually within a certain range. The test results are expressed in matrix contour plot, as shown in Fig. 3. The horizontal and longitudinal axiss show the parameter c and g taking logarithm of 2, respectively. The red numbers in the figure are recognition rates corresponding to different parameter values of c and g. During actual tests, c and g were increased sharply in the beginning, and the incremental amplitude range were gradually reduced according to the test results. The final result can be seen in the figure. In the end, the optimal output parameters are as follows: c = 2, g = 0.0625.

$$k(x_i, x_j) = \exp(-\frac{||x - y||^2}{\sigma^2}) \tag{3}$$

When training the classification model, the method of 10-fold cross validation is adopted to randomly divide the sample feature data into ten parts, one part of which is taken as the test set and the other nine parts as the training set. During training, the training set is divided into two parts: feature and label, and the classifier is trained by the classification algorithm. When testing, input the test set to output the recognition result and recognition rate. The flowchart of the proposed recognition process is shown in Fig. 4.

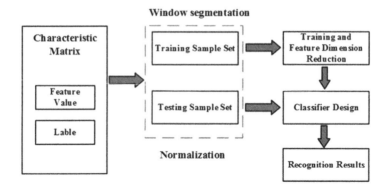

Fig. 4. The flowchart of proposed stroke motion recognition process

2.3   Experimental Results and Analysis

In the experimental stage, five different stroke actions of fifteen subjects were collected with 10 times for each stroke. A total of 750 strokes were collected and analyzed afterwards. The built-in low cost inertial sensor unit can measure the x, y and z axes of acceleration and angular velocity of the player at the same time, as shown in Fig. 5. The synchronization signal can be sent to each acquisition nodes to realize the synchronous measurement of multiple nodes. The data acquisition software can control the acquisition instructions and process the data.

In this paper, the Confusion matrix is used to display the precision of the classification results in a Confusion matrix by comparing the classification results with the actual type. Each column of the obfuscation matrix represents the prediction category, and the total number of each column represents the number of data in that category. Each row represents the true category to which the data belongs, and the total number of data instances for each row represents the number of data instances for that class. The values in each column represent the number of classes that the actual data is expected to be of. The correct classification is located on the diagonal of the confusion matrix, while the wrong classification is located outside the diagonal (Fig. 6 and Table 4).

It can be seen from the above mentioned recognition results that the KNN classification algorithm can not meet the actual application accuracy requirements due to the lower recognition rate (94%). KNN directly compares test samples with training samples without training the model, which is time-consuming and inefficient. In addition, the KNN method is largely dependent on the training sample size and has great limitations in practical application. Therefore, it can be seen from the above that the KNN algorithm can not meet the practical application requirements for the classification and recognition of table tennis stroke actions. With regard to SVM algorithm, satisfactory classification and recognition of stroke actions can be achieved. After the above processing of sample data, the recognition rate of the trained classification model can reach up to

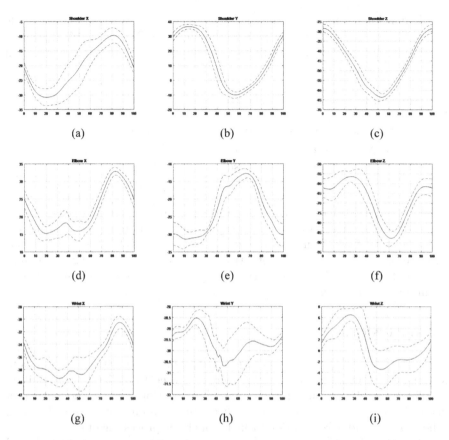

Fig. 5. Raw accelerometer data collected from IMU when a typical subject performs forehand stroke (a) shoulder X axis (b) shoulder Y axis (c) shoulder Z axis (d) elbow X axis (e) elbow Y axis (f) elbow Z axis (g) wrist X axis (h) wrist Y axis (i) wrist Z axis

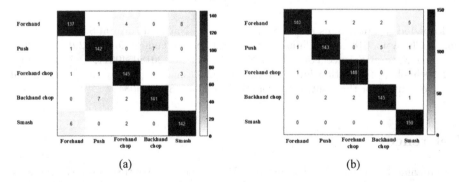

Fig. 6. Table tennis skilled movement recognition results (a) Confusion matrix of five different strokes using KNN classifier (b) Confusion matrix of five different strokes using SVM classifier

96.86%. It is known that KNN method relies too much on the training sample size and has great limitations in practical application. Therefore, SVM is more suitable for the practical application of classification and recognition tasks in the proposed research.

Table 4. Recognition rate of classifier using different feature dimension

Classifier	24 dimensions	48 dimensions	Mean accuracy (%)
KNN	90.86%	94.12%	92.49%
SVM	92.28%	96.86%	94.57%

We can conclued that when using acceleration data and angular velocity data for motion recognition, both algorithms have better performance than merely using acceleration data, and the recognition rate is basically $4\% \sim 5\%$ higher. Therefore, this study adopted both triaxial acceleration and triaxial angular velocity data to identify different strokes of table tennis sport, ensuring better recognition performance.

3   Conclusions

In this paper, wearable sensors are applied to table tennis stroke recognition, and the data collected by the wearable sensor is used to realize the recognition of 5 different stroke actions. In the design of recognition process, the method of machine learning is introduced, which reflects the advantage of machine learning method to this kind of recognition task. Through the processing of angular velocity and acceleration data of various kinds of stroke motions collected by inertial sensors, the recognition methods based on KNN and SVM are presented. In the future, various machine learning methods would be studied. Meanwhile, other features can be extracted to explore whether other features can better improve the identification accuracy of the whole system.

Acknowledgments. This research was funded by National Natural Science Foundation of China no. 61803072, China Postdoctoral Science Foundation no. 2017M621132, Liaoning Natural Science Foundation Key Project no. 20180540011, Dalian Science and Technology Innovation Fund no. 2019J13SN99, and in part by the Fundamental Research Funds for the Central Universities no. DUT18RC(4)034.

References

1. Gravina, R., Alinia, P., Ghasemzadeh, H., Fortino, G.: Multi-sensor fusion in body sensor networks: state-of-the-art and research challenges. Inf. Fusion **35**, 68–80 (2016)
2. Fortino, G., Galzarano, S., Gravina, R., Li, W.: A framework for collaborative computing and multi-sensor data fusion in body sensor networks. Inf. Fusion **22**, 50–70 (2015)

3. Horak, F.B., King, L., Mancini, M.: Role of body-worn movement monitor technology for balance and gait rehabilitation. Phys. Ther. **95**(3), 461–70 (2015)
4. Gravina, R., et al.: Cloud-based Activity-aaService cyber-physical framework for human activity monitoring in mobility. Futur. Gener. Comput. Syst. **75**, 158–171 (2017)
5. Qiu, S., Wang, Z., Zhao, H., Qin, K., Li, Z., Hu, H.: Inertial/magnetic sensors based pedestrian dead reckoning by means of multi-sensor fusion. Inf. Fusion **39**, 108–119 (2018)
6. Huang, H., et al.: Attitude estimation fusing quasi-newton and cubature Kalman filtering for inertial navigation system aided with magnetic sensors. IEEE Access **6**, 28755–28767 (2018)
7. Qiu, S., Wang, Z., Zhao, H., Liu, L., Jiang, Y.: Using body-worn sensors for preliminary rehabilitation assessment in stroke victims with gait impairment. IEEE Access **6**, 31249–31258 (2018)
8. Martinez-Hernandez, U., Mahmood, I., Dehghani-Sanij, A.A.: Simultaneous Bayesian recognition of locomotion and gait phases with wearable sensors. IEEE Sens. J. **18**(3), 1282–1290 (2018)
9. Seshadri, D.R., Drummond, C., Craker, J., Rowbottom, J.R., Voos, J.E.: Wearable devices for sports: new integrated technologies allow coaches, physicians, and trainers to better understand the physical demands of athletes in real time. IEEE Pulse **8**(1), 38–43 (2017)
10. Al-Amri, M., Nicholas, K., Button, K., Sparkes, V., Sheeran, L., Davies, J.L.: Inertial measurement units for clinical movement analysis: reliability and concurrent validity. Sens. (Switz.) **18**(3), 1–29 (2018)
11. Qiu, S., Wang, Z., Zhao, H., Liu, L., Jiang, Y., Li, J.: Body sensor network based robust gait analysis: toward clinical and at home use. IEEE Sens. J. 1–9 (2019)
12. Wang, Z., Qiu, S., Cao, Z., Jiang, M.: Quantitative assessment of dual gait analysis based on inertial sensors with body sensor network. Sens. Rev. **33**(1), 48–56 (2013)
13. Baghdadi, A., Cavuoto, L.A., Crassidis, J.L.: Hip and trunk kinematics estimation in gait through Kalman filter using IMU data at the Ankle. IEEE Sens. J. **18**(10), 4253–4260 (2018)
14. Albert, M.V., Azeze, Y., Courtois, M., Jayaraman, A.: In-lab versus at-home activity recognition in ambulatory subjects with incomplete spinal cord injury. J. NeuroEngineering Rehabil. **14**(1), 1–6 (2017)
15. Qiu, S., Liu, L., Zhao, H., Wang, Z., Jiang, Y.: MEMS inertial sensors based gait analysis for rehabilitation assessment via multi-sensor fusion. Micromachines **9**(9), 442 (2018)
16. Foxlin, E.: Pedestrian tracking with shoe-mounted inertial sensors. IEEE Comput. Graph. Appl. 38–46 (2005)
17. Wang, Z., et al.: Using wearable sensors to capture posture of the human lumbar spine in competitive swimming. IEEE Trans. Hum.-Mach. Syst. **49**(2), 194–205 (2019)
18. Mandery, C., Terlemez, Ö., Do, M., Vahrenkamp, N., Asfour, T.: Unifying representations and large-scale whole-body motion databases for studying human motion. IEEE Trans. Robot. **32**(4), 796–809 (2016)
19. Albert, M.V., Kording, K., Herrmann, M., Jayaraman, A.: Fall classification by machine learning using mobile phones. PLoS ONE **7**(5), 3–8 (2012)
20. Qiu, S., et al.: Body sensor network based gait quality assessment for clinical decision-support via multi-sensor fusion. IEEE Access **7**, 59884–59894 (2019)

21. Liu, Z., Wang, L., Zhang, Y., Chen, C.P.: A SVM controller for the stable walking of biped robots based on small sample sizes. Appl. Soft Comput. **38**(1), 738–753 (2016)
22. Teichmann, D., Kuhn, A., Leonhardt, S., Walter, M.: Human motion classification based on a textile integrated and wearable sensor array. Physiol. Meas. **34**(9), 963–75 (2013)
23. Choe, N., Zhao, H., Qiu, S., So, Y.: A sensor-to-segment calibration method for motion capture system based on low cost MIMU. Measurement **131**, 490–500 (2018)
24. Qiu, S., Wang, Z., Zhao, H., Hu, H.: Using distributed wearable sensors to measure and evaluate human lower limb motions. IEEE Trans. Instrum. Meas. **65**(4), 939–950 (2016)
25. Wang, Z., et al.: Inertial sensor-based analysis of equestrian sports between beginner and professional riders under. IEEE Trans. Instrum. Meas. **67**(11), 2692–2704 (2018)
26. Brzostowski, K.: Toward the unaided estimation of human walking speed based on sparse modeling. IEEE Trans. Instrum. Meas. **67**(6), 1389–1398 (2018)
27. Zhao, H., Wang, Z., Qiu, S.: Adaptive gait detection based on foot-mounted inertial sensors and multi-sensor fusion. Inf. Fusion **52**, 157–166 (2019)
28. Miezal, M., Taetz, B., Bleser, G.: On inertial body tracking in the presence of model calibration errors. Sens. (Switz.) **16**(7), 1132 (2016)
29. Mario, M.O.: Human activity recognition based on single sensor square HV acceleration images and convolutional neural networks. IEEE Sens. J. **19**(4), 1487–1498 (2019)

Pulse Wave Characteristics Based on Age and Body Mass Index (BMI) During Sitting Posture

Fatemeh Heydari, Malikeh P. Ebrahim, Jean-Michel Redoute, and Mehmet R. Yuce[✉]

Department of Electrical and Computer Systems Engineering, Monash University, Melbourne, Australia
mehmet.yuce@monash.edu

Abstract. Measurement technologies of arterial parameters are mostly based on processing blood pulse wave which is an important representation of cardiac activity. The pulse wave is structured with forward and reflected waves which are affected by individual physiological parameters such as the blood intensity, the elasticity of the aorta, artery elasticity and the reflection location. The pulse wave is also an important parameter in invasive cuff-less blood pressure measurement methods. However, different physiological circumstances can lead to pulse waveforms with different characteristics including the curve factors, amplitude and time landmarks. In this study, the pulse wave signal is obtained by bio-impedance (BImp) via shoulder and photoplethysmography (PPG) from the left ear. Four age groups, as well as three (body mass index) BMI groups, are considered as physiological circumstances and the effect of them on five characteristics factors of the pulse wave, are compared. Overall, the results displayed a significant effect of the aging and BMI on the pulse wave's characteristics.

1 Introduction

Cardiovascular diseases (CVDs) and strokes are the main reasons for death worldwide with causing 15.2 million death in 2016 [1]. There has been an enormous interest in extracting computerized arterial parameters using cardiovascular signals as an initial symptom of the CVDs. These parameters can be utilized to estimate the operative and anatomic variations of the arterial wall. Arterial parameters measurement technologies have been focused on methods that capture a pulse of blood travels from the heart to the other organs (blood pulse wave) which is a significant representation of cardiac activity. The pulse wave can illustrate the heart and arteries activities and peripheral resistance [2,3].

Forward and reflected waves are produced in the pulse wave structure. The forward wave is generated with the start of the blood ejection from heart (systolic phase) and rises until the peak pressure (the crest of forward wave or systolic

© ICST Institute for Computer Sciences, Social Informatics and Telecommunications Engineering 2019
Published by Springer Nature Switzerland AG 2019. All Rights Reserved
L. Mucchi et al. (Eds.): BODYNETS 2019, LNICST 297, pp. 125–132, 2019.
https://doi.org/10.1007/978-3-030-34833-5_11

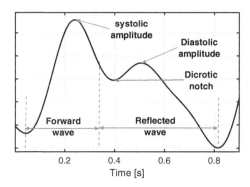

Fig. 1. Forward and reflected waves of pulse waveform.

amplitude). Then, until the ventricular ejection turning point, the pressure waveform starts to drop. At the turning point, the diastolic heart activity begins and the reflected wave is produced. During the reflected wave, the pressure decreases until the dicrotic notch, then with reflected wave passing through the ventricle, the pressure increases to the highest point (diastolic amplitude) of the reflected pressure wave [4]. Then pressure decreases waiting for the next cardiac period (Fig. 1). Forward wave is mostly affected by the blood intensity and the elasticity of the aorta while the reflected wave is associated with the artery elasticity and the reflection location [5,6]. TThis changes the pulse waveform characteristics between different subjects [7].

The pulse wave is also an important parameter in invasive cuff-less blood pressure measurement methods. These methods require different steps of data processing where feature extraction is the most important step and directly changes the results of the blood pressure estimations. To calculate the blood pressure using the pulse wave, first, the signal waveform is recorded from on-body sensors and then, features are extracted by measuring the time difference of the ECG's R-peak and characteristic landmarks on the pulse wave [8]. Since, different physiological circumstances can lead to producing different pulse waveform with different characteristics including the curve factors, amplitude and time landmarks, blood pressure measurement will be affected significantly.

Different types of biotic indicators can be selected as a pulse wave representative such as photoplethysmography (PPG) [9,10], electrical bio-impedance (BImp) [11,12], ballistocardiogram (BCG) [13] and seismocardiogram (SCG) [14,15]. These methods require on-body sensor attachment to neck, ear or arm. In [11,12], pulse wave is extracted from the carotid and subclavian arteries with placing BImp sensors across the shoulder of the patient. In this way, instead of the peripheral arteries, the pulse wave is measured over the central elastic arteries, which reduced the changes caused by vasomotion.

In this study, the pulse wave signal is obtained by both BImp and PPG signals. The BImp is captured using 4-lead sensors placed on the subjects' shoulder and the PPG is recorded from left ear sensor. Signals were collected on human

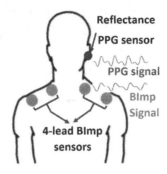

Fig. 2. Sensors placement on the body.

subjects, preliminarily recorded for a blood pressure monitoring project [12], during sitting position for 6 min. Five different characteristics of the pulse wave are extracted for both signals' pulse waveform. Four age groups as well as three (body mass index) BMI groups are considered as physiological circumstances and the effect of them on extracted characteristics are compared.

2   Methods and Implementation

2.1   Subjects and Experimental Details

Subject selected are 52% male, aged 40 ± 15 years, height 168 ± 10 cm and weighted 60 ± 16 kg. Signals were recorded with six minutes sitting position. The placements of the BImp and PPG sensors on body is shown in Fig. 2.

2.2   Signal Processing

The block diagram of signal processing is described in Fig. 3. Both raw sensors' recorded signals (BImp and PPG) are passed through a Chebyshev type II band-pass filter (BPF) modified using Matlab filter design. The heart rate frequency and signals total frequency ranges defined the cutoff frequencies of the filter. To extract the heart rate frequency, the fast Fourier transform (FFT) of the PPG

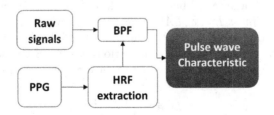

Fig. 3. Signal processing block diagram.

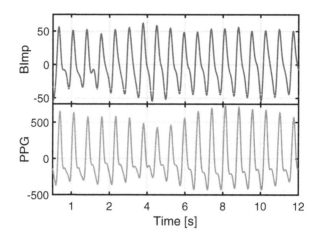

Fig. 4. Filtered BImp and PPG signals samples.

signal is extracted, (the biggest harmonic in the FFT domain of PPG is approximately equal to HRF). This was due to fewer effects of motion and respiration on BImp compared to that of on BImp. A sample of the signal processing output for both BImp and PPG signals is presented in Fig. 4.

2.3   Characteristics Selection

There are various parameters extraction methods that measure amplitude and time information of the pulse wave [16]. In this paper the following characteristics of pulse wave are extracted to be investigated based on age and BMI:

1. *Maximum slope*, the value of the of pulse wave where the first derivative is maximum.
2. *Maximum value (systolic peak)*, the maximum value of the pulse wave.
3. *Augmentation (AI)*, the ratio of the systolic peak to the inflection point which determines the arteries wave reflection.

$$AI = \frac{x}{y}. \tag{1}$$

4. *Crest time*, the time interval between the foot and the systolic peak.
5. *Large Artery Stiffness Index (LASI)*, the time interval between systolic peak and inflection point which indicates the stiffness of the artery.
6. *Inflection Point Area Ratio (IPA)*, the ratio of the S_1, S_2, S_3 and S_4 selected areas under the pulse waveform which indicates the total resistance of the peripheral.

$$IPA = \frac{S_1 + S_2}{S_3 + S_4}. \tag{2}$$

The definition of above characteristics has been illustrated in Fig. 5.

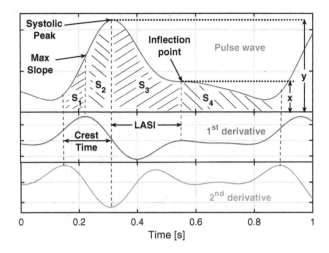

Fig. 5. Pulse waveform characteristic selection.

3   Results and Discussion

To extracted the features, the foot to foot of pulse waves within each recorded signal are extracted. Then, by applying minimum and maximum thresholds, the outlying values are omitted. The results are averaged and final pulse wave is calculated. The characteristics described in Sect. 2.3 are extracted from average pulse wave by using zero-crossing detection of the first and second derivatives. In Fig. 6 samples of all extracted and average pulse waves for both BImp and PPG are presented obtained from three different subjects.

The following four age groups are provided based on the baseline of the subjects:

1: $30 <$ age ≤ 40 2: $41 <$ age ≤ 50 3: $51 <$ age ≤ 60 4: age ≤ 60.

The BMI is calculated using the following equation:

$$BMI = \frac{Weight[Kg]}{Height^2[m]}, \tag{3}$$

and based on the distribution of the extracted BMI for subjects, the next three groups are defined:

1: BMI ≤ 30 2: $30 <$ BMI ≤ 40 3: BMI ≤ 50.

In Fig. 7, the bar charts of the extracted pulse wave (for both BImp and PPG) characteristics based on different age groups is presented. As can be seen, with age increase, the systolic peak, crest time, Max slope and AI values raise while LASI reduces. The IPA values increase from age group 30–40 to 51–60 and then fall in age older than 60. The AI values increasing rate for BImp is almost stable, while for PPG there is a significant rise in age groups over 60. From the figure, it can be seen that, overall aging increases amplitude and timing terms of the pulse wave, while it decreases the stiffness of the artery and peripheral resistance.

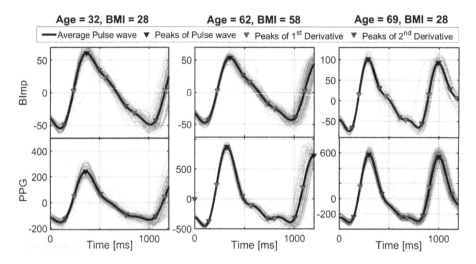

Fig. 6. Samples of extracted average pulse waves of the BImp and PPG for three different subjects: subject1: age = 32, BMI = 28, subject2: age = 62, BMI = 58 and subject3: age 69 and BMI = 28.

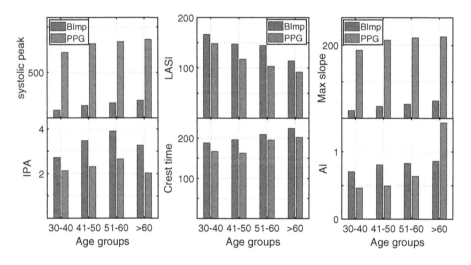

Fig. 7. Pulse wave characteristics based on age groups.

Figure 8, shows the charts of the measured parameters based on BMI groups. The systolic peak, LASI, Max slope, and IPA values reduce due to BMI growth, when in the opposite the crest time and AI increase. There are noteworthy reductions in both systolic peak and max slope values from under 30 to over 30 BMI. The AI increasing and the LASI reduction show that extra weight increases the arteries reflection and decreases its stiffness.

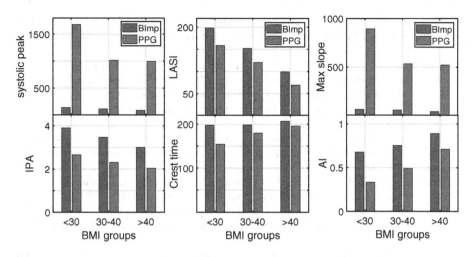

Fig. 8. Pulse wave characteristics based on BMI groups.

4 Conclusion

In this paper, we investigated age and BMI effects on the pulse wave characteristics. Two pulse wave signals from BImp and PPG are analyzed. Data is collected from 43 adult participants in sitting position for the duration of six minutes. We extracted pulse waves from each signal and calculated an average pulse wave for each subject. Five pulse wave characteristics are extracted from average pulse waves and their changes are presented based on four age and three BMI groups. From the obtained results in this paper, the pulse wave information varies due to both age and BMI change. Aging overall increases amplitude and timing terms of the pulse wave and decreases the stiffness of the artery and peripheral resistance and BMI growth increases the arteries reflection and decreases its stiffness. Hence, there is a considerable merit to include age and BMI factors into pulse wave based methods especially blood pressure measurements algorithms. For our future work, we suggest to study data with several conditions and age groups and investigate different physical situations.

Acknowledgments. M. R. Yuces work is supported by Australian Research Council Future Fellowships Grant FT130100430.

References

1. Top 10 causes of death. Global Health Observatory (GHO) data, World Health Organization, Geneva, 24 May 2018
2. Dutt, D.N., Shruthi, S.: Digital processing of ECG and PPG signals for study of arterial parameters for cardiovascular risk assessment. In: 2015 International Conference on Communications and Signal Processing (ICCSP), pp. 1506–1510, April 2015

3. Saito, M., Matsukawa, M., Asada, T., Watanabe, Y.: Noninvasive assessment of arterial stiffness by pulse wave analysis. IEEE Trans. Ultrason. Ferroelectr. Freq. Control **59**(11), 2411–2419 (2012)
4. Xing-Yun, D., Qing, C., Chao, S.: Study on the extract method of time domain characteristic parameters of pluse wave. In: 2016 IEEE International Conference on Signal and Image Processing (ICSIP), pp. 432–436, August 2016
5. Elgendi, M.: On the analysis of fingertip photoplethysmogram signals. Curr. Cardiol. Rev. **8**(1), 14–25 (2012)
6. Avolio, A.P., Butlin, M., Walsh, A.: Arterial blood pressure measurement and pulse wave analysis their role in enhancing cardiovascular assessment. Physiol. Meas. **31**(1), R1 (2009)
7. Kelly, R., Hayward, C., Avolio, A., O'rourke, M.: Noninvasive determination of age-related changes in the human arterial pulse. Circulation **80**(6), 1652–1659 (1989)
8. Buxi, D., Redouté, J.-M., Yuce, M.R.: A survey on signals and systems in ambulatory blood pressure monitoring using pulse transit time. Physiol. Meas. **36**(3), R1 (2015)
9. Ding, X., Zhang, Y., Liu, J., Dai, W., Tsang, H.K.: Continuous cuffless blood pressure estimation using pulse transit time and photoplethysmogram intensity ratio. IEEE Trans. Biomed. Eng. **63**(5), 964–972 (2016)
10. Tamura, T., Maeda, Y., Sekine, M., Yoshida, M.: Wearable photoplethysmographic sensors-past and present. Electronics **3**(2), 282–302 (2014)
11. Buxi, D., Redouté, J.M., Yuce, M.R.: Blood pressure estimation using pulse transit time from bioimpedance and continuous wave radar. IEEE Trans. Biomed. Eng. **64**(4), 917–927 (2017)
12. Heydari, F., et al.: Continuous cuffless blood pressure measurement using body sensors. In: 2018 IEEE SENSORS, pp. 1–4, October 2018
13. Fierro, G., Silveira, F., Armentano, R.: Central blood pressure monitoring method oriented to wearable devices. Health Technol. **6**(3), 197–204 (2016)
14. Yang, C., Tavassolian, N.: Pulse transit time measurement using seismocardiogram, photoplethysmogram, and acoustic recordings: evaluation and comparison. IEEE J. Biomed. Health Inform. **22**, 733–740 (2017)
15. Verma, A.K., Fazel-Rezai, R., Blaber, A., Tavakolian, K.: Pulse transit time extraction from seismocardiogram and its relationship with pulse pressure. Comput. Cardiol. **42**, 37–40 (2015)
16. Sharma, M., et al.: Cuff-less and continuous blood pressure monitoring: a methodological review. Technologies **5**(2), 21 (2017)

In-Body Communications

A Novel Galvanic Coupling Testbed Based on PC Sound Card for Intra-body Communication Links

Anna Vizziello$^{(\boxtimes)}$ ⓘ, Pietro Savazzi ⓘ, Farzana Kulsoom ⓘ,
Giovanni Magenes ⓘ, and Paolo Gamba ⓘ

Department of Electrical, Computer and Biomedical Engineering,
University of Pavia, 27100 Pavia, Italy
{anna.vizziello,pietro.savazzi,giovanni.magenes,paolo.gamba}@unipv.it,
farzana.kulsoom01@universitadipavia.it

Abstract. Intra-Body Communication (IBC) is an emerging research area that will transform the personalized medicine by allowing real time and in situ monitoring in daily life. A galvanic coupling (GC) technology is used in this work to send data through weak currents for intra-body links, as an energy efficient alternative to the current radio frequency (RF) solutions. A sound card based GC testbed is here designed and implemented, whose main features are: (i) low equipment requirements since it only employs two ordinary PCs and Matlab software, (ii) high flexibility because all the parameters setting may be modified through Matlab programs, and (iii) real time physiological data set transmissions. Experimental evaluation with a real chicken tissue are conducted in terms of bit error rate (BER) proving the feasibility of the proposed solution. The developed GC testbed may be easily replicated by the interested research community to carry out simulation-based experiments, thus fostering new research in this field.

Keywords: Intra-body networks · Intra-body communication · Galvanic coupling technology · Sensor networks

1 Introduction

Implanted sensors will enable the next generation of healthcare by in situ testing of abnormal physiological conditions, personalized medicine and proactive drug delivery. The paradigm of interconnecting the implants is known as intra-body network (IBN) and allows implants to transmit measurements to an external processing center for real time monitoring, to receive updates on drug delivery volumes, and to directly start actions by embedded actuators. All these examples require energy efficient data communication between implants through body tissues.

However, the state of the art (SoA) for intra-body communication (IBC) relies on high frequency radio (RF) signals. Short-range RF communication

Published by Springer Nature Switzerland AG 2019. All Rights Reserved
L. Mucchi et al. (Eds.): BODYNETS 2019, LNICST 297, pp. 135–149, 2019.
https://doi.org/10.1007/978-3-030-34833-5_12

techniques, such as Bluetooth, ANT, and Zigbee [1] are useless for intra-body communication as they are affected by severe attenuation within the human tissues, which are composed of 40–60% water, high power consumption, and limited battery lifetime. Moreover, emitted RF signals propagates also around the body, creating privacy risks.

Non-RF IBC Techniques. Non-RF techniques that use the human body as a medium for data communication include ultrasound (US) technology, which consists of mechanical vibrations and works well in mediums with high water content such as the body [2]. The main US drawbacks are severe multi-path fading and the high delay caused by slow propagation speeds. Another alternative to RF is inductive coupling (IC) [3]: coils wrapped around anatomy are used to generate and receive magnetic energy and the efficiency of the data transfer is directly proportional to the coupling efficiency (i.e. correct resonance frequency matching between the transmitter and the receiver), which is not always easy to achieve. Capacitive coupling (CC) [1] uses electrical signals with a couple of electrodes at the transmitter and receiver, respectively. Only one of the electrodes at each side is attached to the body while the other electrode is floating (ground electrode needs only to be in proximity) and the signal is generated through the body channel transceiver by making a current loop through the external ground. Thus, unfortunately, the path loss has high variability based on environmental conditions.

We use an alternative cable-less architecture for IBNs using galvanic coupling (GC) technology for communications among implants. GC utilizes low or medium frequency (1 kHz–100 MHz) and weak (<1 mW) electrical currents, which are modulated with data and coupled directly to the tissue [4]. Differently from SoA RF solutions, GC IBNs does not show privacy risks since the signals do not propagate outside the body, and consumes two orders of magnitude less energy than RF method [5,6].

Related Works. Existing GC efforts focused on signal strength changes in tissues [1,4,7] and the characterization of human tissues [1,5,8], which are a valuable base to explore the feasibility of communication schemes that are difficult to be performed directly on the human body.

Some works have been conducted in developing GC testbeds. For example, a test system has been designed and implemented, which considers a complex programmable logic device (CPLD) containing all the digital signal processing blocks of the transmitter, and, besides the analog units, a field-programmable gate array (FPGA) at the receiver to provide the digital demodulation and interfaces [7]. More recently, a baseband transmission has been implemented in a FPGA board based on impulse radio (IR) employing a pulse position modulation (PPM) [9]. In [10] design a testbed using two USRP software defined radios (SDRs), one at the transmitter and the other at the receiver side, supporting low frequency daughterboards. Anyhow, an effective and repeatable GC platform to carry out experiments is still a challenge.

Proposed Sound Card Based GC Testbed. We here design and implement a GC testbed that is based on PC sound card and Matlab environment, hence easily replicable for the interested research community. The main advantages of the proposed testbed architecture are that: (i) such scheme requires limited equipment since only ordinary PCs and Matlab software are needed; (ii) allows high flexibility since all parameters, including carrier frequency, bandwidth and modulation order, may be varied directly in the TX/RX Matlab programs allowing a quick evaluation of the resulting effects; (iii) real time option for the receiver by including a Data Acquisition Toolbox (Daq Tbx) in Matlab that exploits the real time data logging feature of the toolbox [11], so that real time transmission and evaluation of physiological data sets are possible; (iv) BER evaluation of the experimental setup.

2   Background on GC Communication Technology

An alternative ultra-low power solution that uses the human body as a communication medium is GC technology. In GC, a pair of electrodes is used to directly couple a weak electric current into the human body, so that the electrical signal is applied differentially between the two electrodes of the transmitter and secondary paths of propagation are used for potential difference detection at the electrodes of the receiver [1]. Recommendation from ICNIRP [12] suggests to limit the signal within the safe bound of 1 mA, which is easily matched from GC technology, usually injecting currents in the order of 0.5 mA [13].

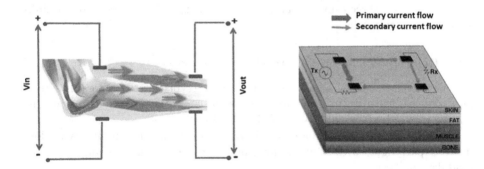

Fig. 1. GC setup on skin surface with detail on multiple tissues

Figure 1 represents the conceptual illustration of GC: the transmitter is composed of a pair of electrodes with typical distance of 5 cm (on-skin case is depicted in Fig. 1, although the electrodes could be places in any tissue) to inject low intensity electrical currents as data signals. While the primary current flows through the two transmitter electrodes, weak secondary electrical currents carry the information to a distant pair of receiver electrodes using layered tissues conduction. Experiments prove that a weak secondary current can be detected at the receiver with a transmission range of 20–30 cm. GC may use any type of electrode, whose usual size is approximately 10 mm [14], and consumes only 0.24 nJ per received bit compared to 106 nJ/b of Zigbee [1]. Indeed, due to its frequency range, the GC signal is restricted to the body so that GC communication is highly energy efficient, resulting in a long lifetime for battery-powered implants. The tissue heating is low due to the limited attenuation at the frequencies used, and communication is interference-free and secure from external fields. The operative frequency range of GC is a tradeoff among tissue attenuation, interference with other natural signals (e.g., ECG and EEG signals), and other impairments. Experiments show that the usable frequency range is 1 kHz–100 MHz [4], so that other natural signals are not impaired.

2.1   Channel Model for the Human Body

The main approaches modeling the electrical behavior of human tissues include wave numerical techniques, for instance, finite element analysis (FEA) and finite difference time domain method (FDTD) [15,16], quasi-static approximations, [17,18], and equivalent circuit analysis (ECA) models.

Field analysis with FEA and FDTD are accurate but expensive for the required time computation. The quasi-static approximations of field distribution are less computationally complex but only model low frequency Maxwell's equations, so that they are not valid for high frequency applications.

The ECA model gives an easy transfer function with accurate gain calculation, and is valid for a wide range of frequency. Several ECA methods focus on single tissue layer, such as [8], while a recent analytical model has been proposed that considers a three dimensional multi-layered tissue, validated through finite element simulations [5].

2.2   Related Works on GC Testbed

Some works have been conducted to develop GC testbeds with different hardware and software features, in order to validate the aforementioned channel models and/or prove the GC viability as IBC technology.

A low power single chip biomedical system is designed in [19], firstly exploiting GC paradigm, with a continuous phase frequency shift keying (CPFSK) modulation scheme.

The test system in [15] includes battery powered transceiver and an FPGA as interface between analog front-end and digital communication link. Two modulation schemes have been used, frequency shift keying (FSK) and binary phase shift keying (BPSK), with a 128 and 255 kbps, respectively.

In [20], the authors build up a transceiver to communicate with both on-body and implanted sensors with a frequency range in the order of tens to hundred MHz and a data rate up to 5 Mbps.

Baseband transmissions are developed in a FPGA board based on impulse radio (IR) with a PPM, and the corresponding BER performance is evaluated [9].

A GC testbed has been proposed recently based on off-the-shelf SDR platforms with low frequency daughterboards and Matlab environment, which presents BER performance for differential BPSK (DBPSK) modulation for different level of transmitted power in case of one transmitter and one receiver implant [10], and BER QPSK performance in case of two transmitters and one receiver [12].

Finally, given the heterogeneity of experimental setups and conditions, and some discrepancies observed between results in literature, some studies have been conducted to evaluate the influence of different experimental settings on GC measurements [21]. On that purpose, different experimental setups have been considered to analyze specific key issues such as load resistance, grounding, effect of cables, and type of measurement device [21].

Anyhow, all the developed systems require specific hardware and software and show low flexibility, resulting in GC platforms difficult to replicate for carrying out experiments.

3   GC Testbed Architecture

Since the common sound cards support signals whose frequency range is included in the GC frequency range (1 kHz–100 MHz), we develop and implement a GC

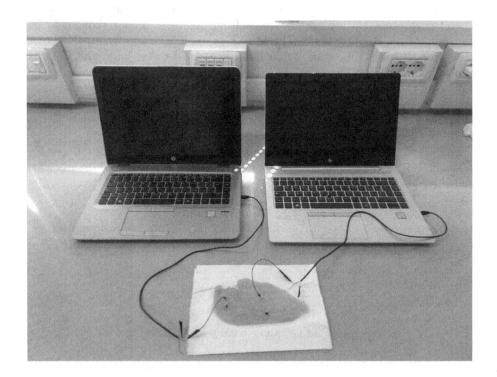

Fig. 2. Experimental setup of the GC testbed

testbed for intra-body communication links employing only ordinary PCs with sound card support and Matlab software, resulting in a simple platform to emulate a single implanted sensor transmission/reception.

The developed system may be easily reproduced and is flexible since all the parameters may easily changed in the TX/RX Matlab programs, while allowing real time transmission of physiological data sets. The developed testbed manages all aspects of communication, including, among the others, bit generation, preamble insertion and raised cosine filtering.

3.1   Blocks Design of the GC System Architecture

The main advantage of the proposed GC system architecture is its limited equipment requirement, consisting of two common PCs with sound card and the basic Matlab package for transmitter and receiver development, as shown in Fig. 2 and in the block diagram in Fig. 3. Bridging the channel and the two PCs, we ensure to use battery powered PCs without connection to the grid, in order to isolate the common ground return paths of the transmitter and the receiver, as required from GC technology [12].

Figure 3 illustrates that only two Matlab sessions are required, one per PC, to implement the transmitter and receiver respectively, and the sound cards are used to support real signal transmission/reception in a subset frequency range of GC technology [4]. On that purpose, Fig. 3 shows that the transmitted data generated through Matlab are converted from digital to analog domain to be sent over the sound card of the transmitter. A cable is connected to the *LINE OUT* jack to carry the signal outside the PC. As detailed later, the cable is attached to two electrodes that represent the GC transmitter, which send the signal over the tissue through GC communication technology. At the other side, the two receiver's electrodes bring the received signal to the other PC through the cable connected to the *LINE IN* jack. The data are thus processed in the Matlab session II where the receiver program is running.

In the following, the blocks diagram of the proposed audio-band GC system are described, including the functional blocks of the transmitter and the receiver, shown in Figs. 4 and 5, respectively.

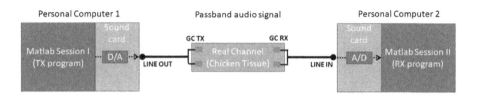

Fig. 3. Setup of the GC audio-band testbed using two PCs

3.2 Functional Blocks of the GC Transmitter

Before detailing each block of the transmitter shown in Fig. 4, we summarize in the following Table 1 the main parameters values of the system. Note that both transmitter and receiver parameters are included for completeness.

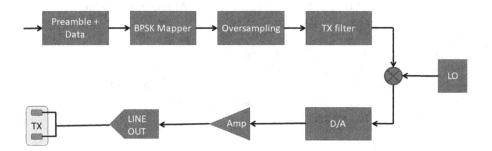

Fig. 4. Block diagram of the GC transmitter

Table 1. Parameters setting

Parameter	Value
Carrier frequency f_c (KHz)	15
Waveform sampling frequency f_{s_a} (KHz)	48
Oversampling frequency f_s in number of samples	4
Sampling time T_s (ms)	0.16
RX oversampling frequency $f_{s_{rx}}$ in number of samples	2
Roll-off of TRX filters R	0.2
Delay of TRX filters D in number of samples	8
QAM modulation order M	2
RX Wiener filter length N_f in number of samples	11
Modulated sequence N in number of symbols	1000
Preamble length N_{pre} in number of symbols	192

Figure 4 shows that after bit generation, a preamble is inserted and the data are modulated in BPSK. The sequence is oversampled by 4, as specified in Table 1, and passes through a squared-root-raised-cosine (SRRC) filter. The corresponding baseband samples $x(nT_s)$ are thus generated, with $n = 0, 1, ..., f_s N - 1$ and sampling time T_s.

The resulting sequence is then upconverted to the carrier frequency by multiplying it by the *cos* signal, which represents the local oscillator (LO) obtained via software-define radio in Matlab program. This yields an audio passband transmitted signal s_{tx}:

$$s_{tx}(nT_{s_a}) = x(nT_{s_a})\cos(2\pi f_c nT_{s_a}) \tag{1}$$

where $T_{s_a} = 1/f_{s_a}$ with $f_{s_a} = 48000\,\text{Hz}$, whose value is chosen according to the standard sample frequency of PC sound card, and f_c is the carrier frequency. According to the parameters setting in Table 1, $T_s = 8\,T_{s_a}$ with a net data rate $R = 6\,\text{kbs}$, in line with several biomedical applications showing sparse and low rate traffic generated by implanted sensors [6, 13]. Anyhow, the achievable data rate may be increased by appropriately choosing the value of f_s, f_{s_a}, f_c shown in Table 1.

Figure 4 illustrates that the obtained audible signal s_{tx} passes through the sound card's internal amplifier, which may be replaced with an external amplifier circuit using Arduino. Then, the signal is sent out to the *LINE OUT* jack by using the following simple Matlab statements in Table 2, which play the software-generated transmitted signal:

Table 2. Matlab audio playing statements

sObj = audioplayer(s_{tx},48000); % To create an audioplayer object for signal s_{tx},	
	using sample frequency at 48000 Hz
playblocking(sObj);	% To play from beginning till playback completes

Through a wire, the output signal is then connected to two electrodes, that represent the GC transmitter.

3.3 Functional Blocks of the GC Receiver

The main blocks of the receiver developed in Matlab are shown in Fig. 5 and may be split in the following two macro-blocks: (i) signal recording and digital down-conversion and (ii) burst detection and symbol timing estimation.

Signal Recording and Digital Down-Conversion. A Matlab session must to be open in the PC connected with the GC receiver for running the receiver program, which includes the following Matlab statements in Table 3 to record the received signal and store the data in the array s_{rx}.

As shown in Fig. 5, after recording the signal s_{rx} in digital format, which passes through the sound card amplifier, a digital down-conversion is performed by multiplying the received sampled signal by $\cos(2\pi f_c nT_{s_a})$, where f_c is the carrier frequency at the receiver. The sequence then is sent to an SRRC filter, resulting in a baseband received signal $y(nT_{s_a})$ with $n = 0, 1, ..., f_s N - 1$.

The output signal is then decimated by two so that the next blocks, described below, work at two samples per symbol ($f_{s_{rx}} = 2$ as specified in Table 1). The obtained sampled signal may be expressed as

$$y(nT_s) = s_{tx}(nT_s)e^{j\theta} + v(nT_s) \tag{2}$$

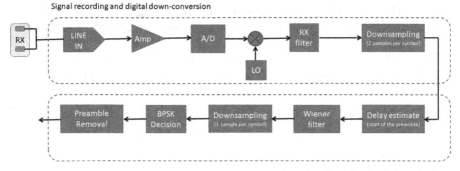

Fig. 5. Block diagram of the GC receiver

Table 3. Matlab recording statements

recObj=audiorecorder(48000,16,1);	% To create a 48000 Hz, 16-bit, 1 channel recorder object;
Tsamp=1/48000;	% Sampling time;
Trecord=$N * f_s * T_{s_a}$;	% Recording time, where:
	N is the modulated sequence lenght,
	fs is the oversampling freq equal to 4;
recordblocking(recObj,Trecord+3);	% To record for length of time, Trecord+3, expressed in seconds;
s_{rx} = getaudiodata(recObj);	% To return the recorded audio data as a double array.

where $n = 0, 1, ..., f_{s_{rx}}N - 1$, $s_{tx}(nT_s)$ is the envelope samples of the passband signal, $v(nT_s)$ is the sampled AWGN noise, θ is the random phase noise due to time delay.

Burst Detection and Symbol Timing Estimation. Being the packet composed by a preamble followed by data, the burst detection is performed by estimating the start of the preamble through a correlation method. Specifically, the transmitted preamble, known at the receiver, is cross-correlated with the received data so that the position of the correlation's peak gives an estimated of the preamble start position:

$$\hat{t}_p = \operatorname*{argmax}_{n} \left| \sum_{k=0}^{L-1} y((n + k)T_s)p^*(kT_s) \right| \tag{3}$$

where $\hat{t}_p$ is the estimate of the sample index where the reference preamble p begins, N_{pre} is the preamble's length, $L = f_{s_{rx}}N_{pre}$ since the receiver is working at two samples per symbol (oversampling frequency $f_{s_{rx}} = 2$), and $n = 0, 1, ..., f_{s_{rx}}N - 1$.

Hence, the received signal is shifted in time according to the estimated start of the preamble $\hat{t}_p$ and is equalized with a Wiener filter, that also performs symbol timing improving the delay estimate obtained with (3).

The coefficients $w(i)$ of the filter, with $i = 1, ..., N_f$, are calculated by using the shifted received preamble $y_p(nT_s) = y(nT_s + \hat{t}_p)$ and the known transmitted one $p(nT_s)$ with $n = 0, 1, ..., f_{s_{rx}}N_{pre} - 1$. In more details, the vector $\mathbf{w} = [w_1, w_2, ..., w_{N_f}]$ of the coefficients can be computed by minimizing the mean square error (MSE) between the transmitted and estimated preamble, defined as

$$\epsilon = E\left\{[p(nT_s) - \hat{p}(nT_s)]^2\right\} \tag{4}$$

Setting the following partial derivatives of the error (4) equal to zero

$$\frac{\partial \epsilon}{\partial w_i} = 0, \text{ for } i = 1, 2, ..., N_f \tag{5}$$

we can solve (4), (5) for the coefficients w_i by inverting an autocorrelation matrix of size $N_f \times N_f$, which leads to the following Wiener-Hopf equation

$$\mathbf{w} = \mathbf{R}_{y_p}^{-1}\mathbf{r}_{py_p} \tag{6}$$

where $\mathbf{R}_{y_p} = \{r_{y_p}(k)\}$ is the autocorrelation matrix of the received preamble y_p, whose elements are $r_{y_p}(k) = E\{y_p(i - k)y_p(i)\}$, and $\mathbf{r}_{py_p} = \{r_{py_p}(k)\}$ is the cross-correlation vector between the transmitter preamble p and the received one y_p, whose elements are defined as $r_{py_p}(k) = E\{p(i - k)y_{p_k}(i)\}$, and $i, k = 1, 2, ..., f_{s_{rx}}N_f$.

After calculating the Wiener coefficients using only the preamble, the filter is applied to all the sequence, so that its output is the estimated transmitted sequence $\hat{x}(nT_s)$, expressed as

$$\hat{x}(nT_s) = \sum_{l=0}^{N_f-1} w(lT_s)y((n - l)T_s + \hat{t}_p) \tag{7}$$

After a downsampling operation at one sample per symbol, the BPSK symbol sequence is demapped to a bit sequence and the preamble is removed, thus completing the receiver operations. The obtained bit sequence may be hence compared to the transmitted one for BER calculation.

3.4   Implementation of the GC System

Before evaluating the performance of the overall system with a real tissue-based GC channel, we first test only the transmitter and the receiver, for which the configuration in Fig. 6 is considered. Then, an experimental setup is evaluated with real tissue for GC transmissions as in Fig. 3.

Figure 6 derives from Fig. 3 by substituting the steak with a simple wire connecting the *LINE OUT* sound card's jack of the PC running the Matlab transmitter program with the *LINE IN* jack of the other PC running the receiver program.

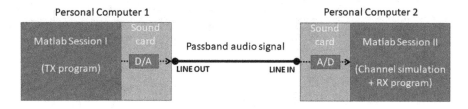

Fig. 6. Audio-band testbed using two PCs and a wire

For the final setting, shown in Figs. 2 and 3, the wire connecting *LINE IN* and *LINE OUT* jacks of the two PCs is cut and each of its two parts are attached to the electrodes of the GC transmitter and receiver, respectively. Since the wire is composed by three electric cables, two of them are connected to the electrodes on each side, while the third one remains floating. Under this configuration, the two transmitter and receiver Matlab session runs in parallel to perform the experimental evaluation detailed in the following section.

4 Experimental Setup and Performance Evaluation

After testing the architecture in the configuration shown in Fig. 6, which have confirmed the feasibility of the proposed transmitter and receiver architecture, we have conducted experiments in the final real scenario shown in Figs. 2 and 3. The parameters setting is detailed in Table 1, and the average BER is calculated over 100 iterations.

Note that we use really small size electrodes (in the order of 0.5 mm) while the SoA is employing 1 cm electrodes [14]. Although such choice would reduce the achievable distance between GC transmitter and receiver, in this way we test a real configuration scenario for future miniaturized implantable devices. The inter-distance between the electrodes at both the transmitter and receiver is set equal to 1 cm, while the distance between the transmitter and receiver is varied during the experiments, together with the transmit power.

Figures 7 and 8 show the transmitted and received signal in the frequency domain, respectively, for 3 cm distance between GC transmitter and receiver. Figure 7 refers to the transmitted signal before being modulated on the carrier frequency, as well as Fig. 8 illustrates the received signal after demodulation and filtering. The comparison between the two figures confirms that the received signal exhibits the same shape of the transmitted one, since the side lobe of the receiver signal is maintained low by the filter being its amplitude around 90 dB less than the main one.

Figure 9 shows BER performance by varying the transmit power for different distance values between transmitter and receiver. As expected, BER performance decreases when increasing the distance, although the performance for 2, 4, 6 cm result to be quite similar. We are able to achieve a BER in the order of 10^{-4} with 9.5 dBm transmit power for 1 cm distance, reaching $7 \cdot 10^{-3}$ for 10 cm, a valuable result considering the small electrode size of 0.5 mm and the simple receiver that

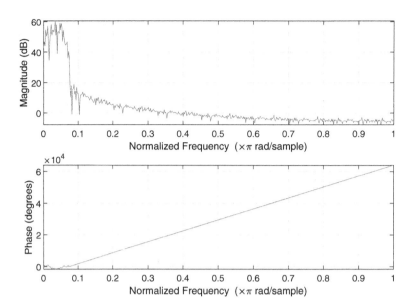

Fig. 7. Transmitted signal in frequency domain

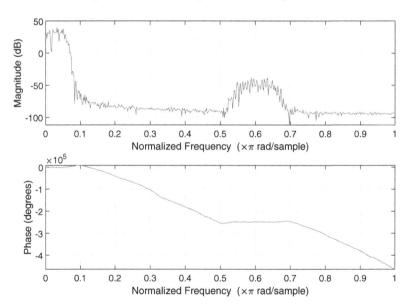

Fig. 8. Received signal after RX filter in frequency domain

is not employing any correction code. More robust receiver may be envisioned based on ultra wideband (UWB) to improve the performance while maintaining simple and energy efficient receiver [22], as required by biomedical implantable devices.

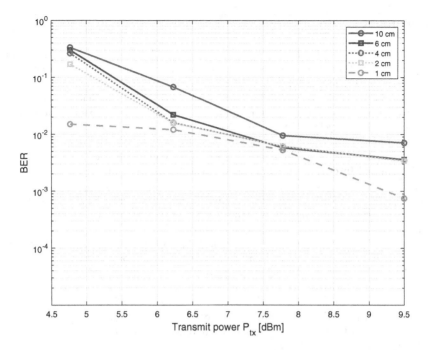

Fig. 9. BER vs transmit power for different distances between GC transmitter and receiver

5   Conclusions

We have proposed a sound card based GC testbed as a quick repeatable platform to carry out experiments. The detailed description of the implemented test system may support the interested researchers in replicating the testbed and thus stimulate further research in the GC field. Experimental tests on real chicken tissue as GC communication channel have been conducted to prove the feasibility of the proposed architecture. We achieve a BER in the order of 10^{-3} with 9.5 dBm transmit power for distances in the range $2-10$ cm, employing an simple receiver and electrodes with really small size (0.5 mm), while the SoA is usually employing 1 cm electrodes. Ongoing works include extensive simulation to evaluate the effect of the carrier frequency, bandwidth, audio sampling frequency, electrodes size, as well as inter-electrodes distance at both the transmitter and receiver. Moreover, we are implementing an extension of the proposed testbed with Arduino platform in order to modulate the signals on a frequency range larger than the audio signals. Future research directions will exploit compressed sensing (CS) and UWB techniques to save time and energy [12,22], a strict requirements in intra-body networks for medical applications.

References

1. Seyedi, M., Kibret, B., Lai, D.T.H., Faulkner, M.: A survey on intrabody communications for body area network applications. IEEE Trans. Biomed. Eng. **60**(8), 2067–2079 (2013)

2. Galluccio, L., Melodia, T., Palazzo, S., Santagati, G.E.: Challenges and implications of using ultrasonic communications in intra-body area networks. In: Proceedings of IEEE Wireless On-demand Network Systems and Services, Courmayeur, Italy, January 2012

3. Park, J., Mercier, P.P.: Magnetic human body communication. In: EMBS, 2015 37th Annual International Conference of the IEEE, pp. 1841–1844, 25–29 August 2015

4. Callejn, M.A., Reina-Tosina, J., Naranjo-Hernndez, D., Roa, L.M.: Galvanic coupling transmission in intrabody communication: a finite element approach. IEEE Trans. Biomed. Eng. **61**(3), 775–783 (2014)

5. Swaminathan, M., Cabrera, F.S., Pujol, J.S., Muncuk, U., Schirner, G., Chowdhury, K.R.: Multi-path model and sensitivity analysis for galvanic coupled intrabody communication through layered tissue. IEEE Trans. Biomed. Circ. Syst. **10**(2), 339–351 (2016)

6. Swaminathan, M., Vizziello, A., Duong, D., Savazzi, P., Chowdhury, K.R.: Beamforming in the body: energy-efficient and collision-free communication for implants. In: IEEE INFOCOM 2017 - IEEE Conference on Computer Communications, Atlanta, GA, pp. 1–9 (2017)

7. Wegmueller, M.S., et al.: Galvanic coupling enabling wireless implant communications. IEEE Trans. Instrum. Meas. **58**(8), 2618–2625 (2009)

8. Wegmueller, M.S., Oberle, M., Felber, N., Kuster, N., Fichtner, W.: Signal transmission by galvanic coupling through the human body. IEEE Trans. Instrum. Meas. **59**(4), 963–969 (2010)

9. Seyedi, M.H., Lai, D.T.H.: A Novel Intrabody Communication Transceiver for Biomedical Applications. Springer, Singapore (2017). https://doi.org/10.1007/978-981-10-2824-3

10. Tomlinson, W.J., Chowdhury, K.R., Yu, C.: Galvanic coupling intra-body communication link for real-time channel assessment. In: 2016 IEEE Conference on Computer Communications Workshops (INFOCOM WKSHPS), San Francisco, CA, 2016, pp. 968–969 (2016)

11. Hwang, J.: Innovative communication design lab based on PC sound card and Matlab: a software-defined-radio OFDM modem example. In: Proceedings of the 2003 IEEE International Conference on Acoustics, Speech, and Signal Processing, 2003, (ICASSP 2003), Hong Kong, pp. III–761 (2003)

12. Banou, S., et al.: Beamforming galvanic coupling signals for IoMT implant-to-relay communication. IEEE Sens. J. **19**(19), 8487–8501 (2019). https://doi.org/10.1109/JSEN.2018.2886561

13. Tomlinson, W.J., Banou, S., Yu, C., Stojanovic, M., Chowdhury, K.R.: Comprehensive survey of galvanic coupling and alternative intra-body communication technologies. IEEE Commun. Surv. Tutor. **21**(2), 1145–1164 (2019). Secondquarter

14. Li, M., et al.: The modeling and simulation of the galvanic coupling intra-body communication via handshake channel. Sensors **17**(4), 863 (2017)

15. Wegmueller, M.S., et al.: An attempt to model the human body as a communication channel. IEEE Trans. Biomed. Eng. **54**(10), 1851–1857 (2007)

16. Song, Y., Zhang, K., Hao, Q., Hu, L., Wang, J., Shang, F.: A finite-element simulation of galvanic coupling intra-body communication based on the whole human body. Sensors **12**, 13567–13582 (2012)
17. Chen, X.M., et al.: Signal transmission through human muscle for implantable medical devices using galvanic intra-body communication technique. In: Proceedings IEEE International Conference Engineering in Medicine and Biology Society, pp. 1651–1654 (2012)
18. Pun, S.H., et al.: Quasi-static modeling of human limb for intra-body communications with experiments. IEEE Trans. Inf. Tech. Biomed. **15**(6), 870–876 (2011)
19. Oberle, M.: Low power systems-on-chip for biomedical applications. Ph.D. dissertation, ETH Zurich, Switzerland (2002)
20. Cho, N., Bae, J., Yoo, H.-J.: A 10.8 mW body channel communication/MICS dual-band transceiver for a unified body sensor network controller. IEEE J. Solid-State Circ. **44**(12), 3459–3468 (2009)
21. Callejn, M.A., Reina-Tosina, J., Naranjo-Hernndez, D., Roa, L.M.: Measurement issues in galvanic intrabody communication: influence of experimental setup. IEEE Trans. Biomed. Eng. **62**(11), 2724–2732 (2015)
22. Alesii, R., Marco, P.D., Santucci, F., Savazzi, P., Valentini, R., Vizziello, A.: Multi-reader multi-tag architecture for UWB/UHF radio frequency identification systems. In: 2015 International EURASIP Workshop on RFID Technology (EURFID), Rosenheim, pp. 28–35 (2015)

Sensitivity of Galvanic Intra-Body Communication Channel to System Parameters

Ahmed E. Khorshid[(✉)], Ibrahim N. Alquaydheb, Ahmed M. Eltawil,
and Fadi Kurdahi

University of California Irvine (UCI), Irvine, USA
Khorshia@uci.edu

Abstract. In this paper, we investigate the sensitivity of the galvanic coupling Intra-Body Communication (IBC) channel to the variation of the basic parameters - being them electrical, geometrical or biological - of the main blocks of the IBC system; the transmitter and receiver nodes, the electrodes used, and the communication channel itself being the human body in this case. The study is performed over the frequency range 100 kHz–100 MHz, providing the system designer with a unique guide for the relationship between the system parameters, thus facilitating the design of an efficient and better matched system components.

Keywords: Body Area Networks · Intra-Body Communication · Galvanic coupling · Channel modeling · Circuit model

1 Introduction

Wearable devices are rapidly being adopted as means of augmenting and improving health care services. In order to provide a cable-free biomedical monitoring system, new wireless technologies associated with sensor applications have been promoted as the next biomedical revolution, yet the size and power requirements of wireless sensors which are typically dominated by the Radio Frequency (RF) section of the associated transceivers, have limited their adoption. To overcome such concerns, system architects proposed designing the system in a way that would allow more than one sensor to share the same wireless gateway, providing a distributed solution, with less power consumption. That approach paved the way for adopting IBC systems where data transmission is carried out through the body (mostly skin layers), rather than through air [1, 2]. This emerging technology would ultimately lead to Body Area Networks (BANs) that operate at extremely low power, with minimal foot print by replacing expensive, power consuming RF front ends, for each individual node with simpler interfaces. IBC can be categorized into two main types; capacitive coupling (near field coupling method) and galvanic coupling. In capacitive coupling, only the signal electrodes of the transmitter and the receiver are attached to the body while the ground (GND) electrodes are left floating in the air. The conductive body forms the forward path while the signal loop is closed through the capacitive return path between the transmitter and the receiver

L. Mucchi et al. (Eds.): BODYNETS 2019, LNICST 297, pp. 150–160, 2019.
https://doi.org/10.1007/978-3-030-34833-5_13

GND electrodes. The second approach, which depends on the galvanic coupling principle, uses a pair of electrodes for both the transmitter and the receiver to propagate the electromagnetic wave. The signal is applied over two coupler electrodes and received by two detector electrodes. In both approaches, it has been shown that the attenuation of the body channel can be much lower than that of the air channel in frequencies up to 100 MHz [3]. An attractive feature of the galvanic coupling approach is that the signal is totally confined to the body, unlike capacitive coupling where the signal return path is established through the air, thus galvanic coupled signals experience minimal interference from other electronic devices, enabling robust and secure data exchanges. In this paper, we study the sensitivity of the galvanic IBC channel to the electrical, geometrical and biological parameters of the system, through observing the channel gain/attenuation profile over the frequency range of interest for IBC; 100 kHz to 100 MHz. In Sect. 1, we explain how we model the different parameters and features of the system using an accurate circuit model. In Sect. 3 we study the sensitivity of the system to the biological/electrical aspects of the communication channel; the body. Sections 4 and 5 then consider the impact of the system design parameters; properties of the electrodes as well as the transmitter (TX) and receiver (RX) nodes.

2 System Model

In [4], we present a simple circuit model for IBC using galvanic coupling, as shown in Fig. 1. In the proposed model, biological parameters are assumed to be variable, taking into consideration the impact of important factors; such as age and weight, on these parameters and thus on the overall attenuation profile. The impedances constituting the model are calculated according to the electrical properties - permittivity and conductivity - of the main five body tissues (fat, muscle, skin, cortical bone and bone marrow), the geometrical aspects of the body organs and finally the electrodes' material and dimensions.

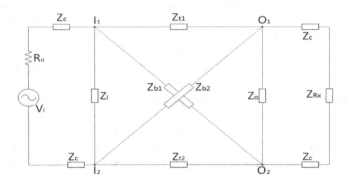

Fig. 1. Circuit model for galvanic coupling, is the signal source at the transmitter, Z_c: the coupling impedance between the electrode and the skin, Z_i: input impedance of the human body. Z_{t1} and Z_{t2} are the transverse impedances of the transmission path, while Z_{b1} and Z_{b2} are the cross impedances, the body output impedance is Z_0, output resistance of the transmitter is R_0 and Z_{RX} is the input impedance of the receiver [4, 5].

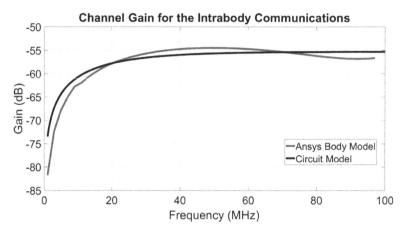

Fig. 2. Comparison between the gain profile for the galvanic IBC channel calculated once through the circuit model then using the FEM model, showing how accurate the circuit model is.

To validate our model, we compared the results we got with experimental measurements reported in the literature [4]. We also validated our model results, by comparing the gain profile calculated using our model with that generated using a full body FEM model developed by NEVA Electromagnetic group, using ANSYS HFSS environment [6]. Results are shown in Fig. 2, showing the accuracy of our proposed circuit model, for galvanic IBC.

3   Tissue's Electrical Properties

In [7], it was shown that electromagnetic waves possess better properties, that can support BAN requirements, versus ultrasonic waves as EM waves experience much less attenuation and delay when traveling through the body which is crucial for system designers. The basic human tissues' properties of concern are those of the complex dielectric properties; namely the permittivity and the conductivity. Thus the first sensitivity analysis test performed was on how the variation in these electrical properties would affect the IBC channel characteristics (gain). We studied the effect of varying the properties of each tissue solely in a range between −20% to 20% of the average nominal values [8], and results are plotted in for skin and muscles in Figs. 3 and 4. The error was also calculated (the deviation of the IBC channel gain from the nominal value, reported in Fig. 2) and summarized in Tables 1 and 2, where the maximum error percentage is reported for each case. As shown from the results, the IBC channel characteristics are much more sensitive to the conductivity of the tissues over the permittivity, since the conductivity mainly accounts for the signal transmission capability through a certain medium. This finding is crucial for applications like phantoms design, for manufacturing more accurate tissue mimicking materials [9]. From a tissue perspective, muscle, skin and fat layers tend to affect the characteristics of the IBC channel more than cortical bone and bone marrow, this is due to: (a) the better conductive properties of the first three tissues, (b) the fact that only a tiny portion of the signal will travel through the bones (since most of the signal is transmitted through the skin, then muscles, as shown in [10]).

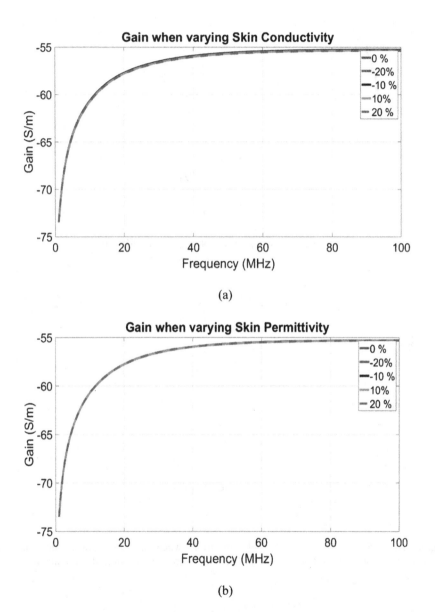

Fig. 3. The variation in the IBC channel gain profile, when varying the; (a) conductivity and (b) permittivity of the skin tissue, within the range −20% to 20% from the nominal measured values [8].

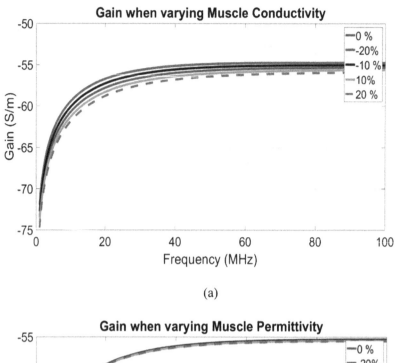

(a)

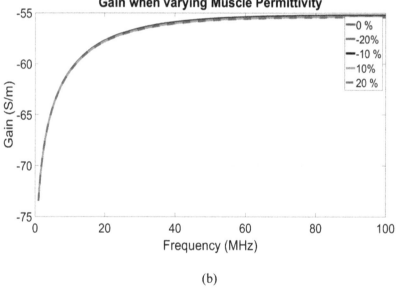

(b)

Fig. 4. The variation in the IBC channel gain profile, when varying the; (a) conductivity and (b) permittivity of the Muscle tissue, within the range −20% to 20% from the nominal measured values [8].

Table 1. Maximum error percentages for the deviation in the IBC channel gain when varying the electrical conductivity of the tissues.

Tissue	Conductivity			
	−20%	−10%	10%	20%
Skin	0.1013%	0.05008%	0.04923%	0.09785%
Fat	0.5278%	0.259%	0.2497%	0.4906%
Muscle	2.194%	1.053%	0.9776%	1.891%
Cortical bone	0.00461%	0.002302%	0.002302%	0.004617%
Bone marrow	0.0014%	0.000697%	0.000697%	0.0014%

Table 2. Maximum error percentages for the deviation in the IBC channel gain when varying the electrical permittivity of the tissues.

Tissue	Permittivity			
	−20%	−20%	−20%	−20%
Skin	0.04311%	0.04311%	0.04311%	0.04311%
Fat	0.03%	0.03%	0.03%	0.03%
Muscle	0.1624%	0.1624%	0.1624%	0.1624%
Cortical bone	0.00127%	0.001275%	0.001275%	0.001275%
Bone marrow	0.00052%	0.000524%	0.000524%	0.000524%

4 Electrodes

Electrodes are responsible for connecting the electronic systems to the human body through transducing ionic currents from the human body into electric currents and vice versa, thus modeling the electrode and electrode-body compact impedance has a significant impact on the overall channel model. Parameters as the electrode size, material, shape, width, thickness …etc. should all be taken into account. Other factors that further determine the value of the electrode-contact impedance include the operating frequency, spacing between each of the electrode pairs (ex: separation between the two electrodes of the transmitter) and the location of the electrodes on the human body. In [11], the authors investigated various techniques to reach an accurate electrical circuit representation of the electrode-body contact. A double order model, shown in Fig. 5, was adopted, since it accurately models the interaction at the interface between the metal electrode and the electrolyte gel solution, as well as that between the electrolyte and the skin. In the model, C_d represents the double layer capacitance between the electrode and the electrolyte solution in the body tissue, R_a is the activation polarization resistance, R_w and C_w represent the diffusion polarization impedance (Warburg impedance), Z is the reaction impedance and Z_t is the impedance of the tissue under the electrode (skin). We first study the effect of using different electrode materials; copper, brass and stainless steel.

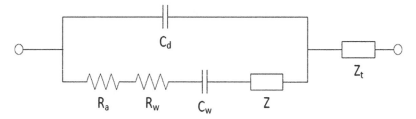

Fig. 5. Contact impedance circuit model proposed in [12], taking into consideration the activation polarization, diffusion polarization, reaction impedance and the body tissue impedance.

Material dependent parameters reported in [12] are used, and results are shown in Fig. 6, showing how sensitive the channel is to the material used (thus the electrode impedance). In Fig. 7, we study the impact of the separation between electrodes of each node, where the separation is varied; 1 cm, 6 cm and 10 cm, while the electrode area and distance between the TX and RX are kept fixed at 20 cm^2 and 10 cm respectively. In Fig. 8, the electrode area is varied; 1 cm^2, 10 cm^2 and 100 cm^2 while the distance between the TX and RX nodes and separation between pair of each node are kept constant at 10 cm and 6 cm respectively. As the electrode area increases, its impedance drops till the body input impedance becomes dominant over it, thus the body input impedance will have the higher impact on the channel profile [11], and matching improves between the body input impedance and the electrode impedance specially at lower frequencies.

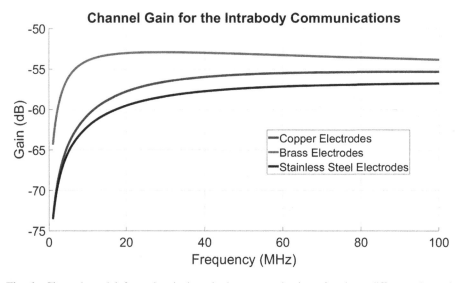

Fig. 6. Channel model for galvanic intra-body communications for three different electrode materials; copper, brass and stainless steel.

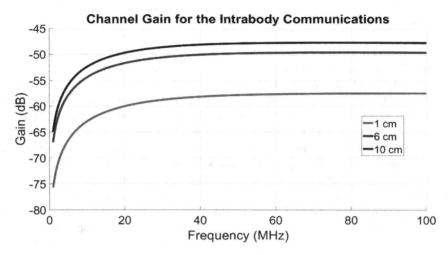

Fig. 7. Varying the separation between electrodes of each node; 1 cm, 6 cm and 10 cm, while both the electrode area and distance between TX and RX are kept constant.

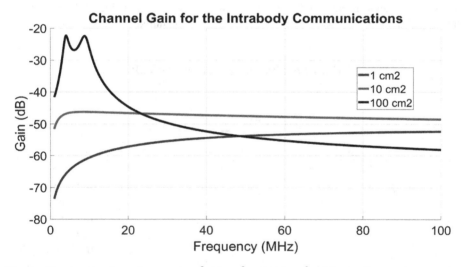

Fig. 8. Varying the electrode area; 1 cm^2, 10 cm^2 and 100 cm^2, while the distance between the TX and RX nodes and separation between pair of each node are kept constant.

Moreover, changing the separation between the electrode pairs at each node, changes the input impedance seen between these two electrodes according to the model proposed in [4], thus the final channel gain will be determined according to the relation between the various impedances (input impedance, electrode impedance, transmission path impedance ...etc.).

5   Transmitter and Receiver Nodes

The final blocks in the IBC system are the transmitter and the receiver nodes. Since the channel characteristics are mostly affected by the relation between the impedances of the basic blocks of the system; an impedance matching issue for maximum power transfer between the electronics system and the body and vice versa, we will investigate the impact of the TX output impedance and the RX input impedance on the IBC channel. In Fig. 9, we vary the magnitude of the RX input impedance between 100, 1K, 10K, 100K and 1M Ω, and observe the channel gain. As expected, the gain of the channel improves as the RX input impedance value increases, as more signal power is delivered to the receiver node. However, after reaching a certain value ($\sim 10K$ in this case) the gain saturates, since the RX input resistance becomes much larger than the system impedance, thus most of the power is transferred from the system (body and electrodes) to the RX anyway. On the TX side, the TX output impedance is our concern, since it partially determines the portion of the power that will be delivered from the source to the system. While 50 Ω would be the nominal value that most devices/circuits try to design according to, for matching purposes, we included other values; 10, 100, 500, 1K, 2K, 5K and 10K Ω to study its impact on the gain of the channel, as shown in Fig. 10. Clearly the gain improves as the value of the resistance drops, as less power is lost in the TX node; more transmitted to the system.

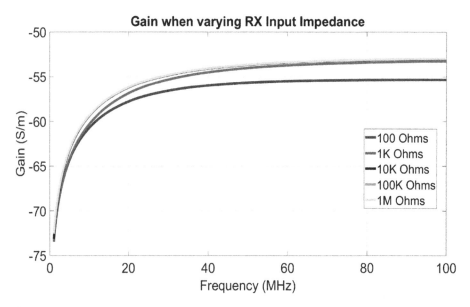

Fig. 9. Gain when varying the value of the RX input impedance; 100, 1K, 10K, 100K and 1M Ω.

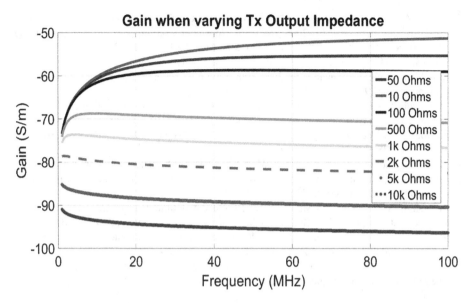

Fig. 10. Gain when varying the value of the TX output resistance; 10, 100, 500, 1K, 2K, 5K and 10K Ω.

6 Conclusion

In this paper, we investigated the relationship between the system's electrical, geometrical, biological parameters and the IBC galvanic coupling channel profile. It was shown how the channel is more sensitive to the tissue's conductivity over their permittivity. Also as expected, the properties of the electrodes impact the channel gain profile significantly. Contribution of the RX input impedance and the TX output resistance was also discussed. The paper provides a basic guideline for the relationships between the basic IBC system blocks, showing how sensitive the channel is to the parameters of each of these blocks, which is crucial for the system architect, to improve the system's efficiency and performance.

Acknowledgments. The authors gratefully acknowledge that this work was supported in part by the National Institute of Justice (NIJ) grant number 2016-R2-CX-0014.

References

1. Zimmerman, T.G.: Personal area networks: near-field intrabody communication. IBM Syst. J. **35**(3.4), 609–617 (1996)
2. Handa, T., Shoji, S., Ike, S., Takeda, S., Sekiguchi, T.: A very low-power consumption wireless ECG monitoring system using body as a signal transmission medium. In: Proceedings of International Solid State Sensors and Actuators Conference (Transducers' 97), vol. 2, pp. 1003–1006. IEEE, June 1997

3. Ruiz, J.A., Xu, J., Shimamoto, S.: Propagation characteristics of intra-body communications for body area networks. In: 2006 3rd IEEE Consumer Communications and Networking Conference 2006, CCNC 2006, vol. 1, pp. 509–513. IEEE, January 2006

4. Khorshid, A.E., Eltawil, A.M., Kurdahi, F.: Intra-body communication model based on variable biological parameters. In: 2015 49th Asilomar Conference on Signals, Systems and Computers, pp. 948–951. IEEE, November 2015

5. Alquaydheb, I.N., Khorshid, A.E., Eltawil, A.M.: Analysis and estimation of intra-body communications path loss for galvanic coupling. In: Fortino, G., Wang, Z. (eds.) Advances in Body Area Networks I. IT, pp. 267–277. Springer, Cham (2019). https://doi.org/10.1007/978-3-030-02819-0_20

6. Song, Y., Hao, Q., Zhang, K., Wang, M., Chu, Y., Kang, B.: The simulation method of the galvanic coupling intrabody communication with different signal transmission paths. IEEE Trans. Instrum. Meas. **60**(4), 1257–1266 (2011)

7. Khorshid, A.E., Eltawil, A.M., Kurdahi, F.: On the optimum data carrier for intra-body communication applications. In: Proceedings of the 11th EAI International Conference on Body Area Networks, pp. 137–140. ICST (Institute for Computer Sciences, Social-Informatics and Telecommunications Engineering), December 2016

8. Gabriel, S., Lau, R.W., Gabriel, C.: The dielectric properties of biological tissues: II. Measurements in the frequency range 10 Hz to 20 GHz. Phys. Med. Biol. **41**(11), 2251 (1996)

9. Khorshid, A.E., Alquaydheb, I.N., Eltawil, A.M., Kurdahi, F.J.: Physical multi-layer phantoms for intra-body communications. IEEE Access **6**, 42812–42821 (2018)

10. Mao, J., Yang, H., Lian, Y., Zhao, B.: A five-tissue-layer human body communication circuit model tunable to individual characteristics. IEEE Trans. Biomed. Circ. Syst. **12**(2), 303–312 (2018)

11. Khorshid, A.E., Alquaydheb, I.N., Eltawil, A.M.: Electrode impedance modeling for channel characterization for intra-body communication. In: Fortino, G., Wang, Z. (eds.) Advances in Body Area Networks I. IT, pp. 253–266. Springer, Cham (2019). https://doi.org/10.1007/978-3-030-02819-0_19

12. Kanai, H., Chatterjee, I., Gandhi, O.P.: Human body impedance for electromagnetic hazard analysis in the VLF to MF band. IEEE Trans. Microw. Theory Tech. **32**(8), 763–772 (1984)

Magnetic Steering of Superparamagnetic Nanoparticles in Duct Flow for Molecular Communication: A Feasibility Study

Niklas Schlechtweg[1], Sebastian Meyer[1], Harald Unterweger[2],
Max Bartunik[1], Doaa Ahmed[1], Wayan Wicke[3], Vahid Jamali[3],
Christoph Alexiou[2], Georg Fischer[1], Robert Weigel[1], Robert Schober[3],
and Jens Kirchner[1(✉)]

[1] Institute for Electronics Engineering,
Friedrich-Alexander-University Erlangen-Nürnberg, 91 058 Erlangen, Germany
`jens.kirchner@fau.de`
[2] Section for Experimental Oncology and Nanomedicine,
University Hospital Erlangen, 91 052 Erlangen, Germany
[3] Institute for Digital Communications,
Friedrich-Alexander-University Erlangen-Nürnberg, 91 058 Erlangen, Germany
`https://lte.techfak.uni-erlangen.de/`
`http://www.hno-klinik.uk-erlangen.de/seon-nanomedizin/`
`https://www.idc.tf.fau.de/`

Abstract. Molecular communication (MC) denotes information transmission by use of molecules and nanosized particles. For the realization of testbeds, superparamagnetic iron oxide nanoparticles (SPIONs) in duct flow have recently been proposed. Here, an experimental setup is provided to direct these particles at a branching of a tube into a specific direction by use of magnetic fields.

For that purpose, gold-coated SPIONs suspended in water at constant flow rate are considered at a Y-shaped connector of tubes. The particles are attracted by use of a custom-made electromagnet, while change of particle concentration in either of the branches is measured by a commercial susceptometer. The approach is evaluated for different flow rates and with the electromagnet both at a fixed position and moving along the tube. Exemplary measurements show that an information transmission is feasible in both approaches and with all tested flow rates.

The feasibility study hence shows that particle steering by use of magnetic fields is a viable approach, which is even robust against flow rate variations. It can thus be used in MC to address different transmission channels as well as to realize differential signal transmission. Furthermore, it might help to improve magnetic drug targeting in future applications.

Supported in part by the Friedrich-Alexander University Erlangen-Nürnberg (FAU) under the Emerging Fields Initiative (EFI), and the STAEDTLER Foundation.

L. Mucchi et al. (Eds.): BODYNETS 2019, LNICST 297, pp. 161–174, 2019.
https://doi.org/10.1007/978-3-030-34833-5_14

Keywords: Superparamagnetic nanoparticles · Particle steering · Magnetic field · Duct flow · Molecular communication

1   Introduction

Molecular communication (MC) encodes and transmits information in the concentration, type or structure of molecules or nanosized particles [9,20]. It thus provides an alternative to conventional electromagnetic- (EM-) based communication on small scale and in applications where EM energy is highly absorbed, e.g. in water and water solutions [6].

To this day, extensive theoretical and simulation-based investigations have been performed that improve the channel modeling in MC systems [1,2,13,14, 27]. In addition to the theoretical work, several experimental setups have been recently proposed [7,8,11,17,18]. These testbeds allow to put theoretical channel models to the test, identify and study the relevant physical processes involved and predict opportunities and limits of future realizations. The first such MC testbed was proposed by Farsad et al. [8], where alcohol is ejected by a nozzle through open air and detected by a sensor at variable distances between 2 and 4 m from the transmitter. The testbed was later extended to MIMO communication by use of two nozzles and two sensors as senders and receivers, respectively [17]. As an alternative approach, Farsad et al. [7] proposed to code information in the pH-level of a fluid by using two complementary pumps, which inject either an acid or a base into the main flow of tube, in order to transmit a bit 0 and 1, respectively, over a length of several decimeters.

Besides the pioneering work of N. Farsad et al., other air-based MC system concepts have been proposed since then [15]. Giannoukus et al. [10] designed an odor emitter, which uses a controlled evaporation of liquid chemicals and carrier gas such as nitrogen; Kennedy et al. [16,22] proposed the transmission and detection of concentration of isopropyl (IPA) alcohol vapor.

While alcohol- and pH-based demonstrators cannot be used for MC in humans, superparamagnetic iron oxide nanoparticles (SPIONs), which were originally developed for cancer therapy and are therefore biocompatible, could fill this gap. A corresponding testbed was presented by the authors [23]. Here, a peristaltic pump allows to inject a suspension of SPIONs into a constant background flow. After a few centimeters, these particles are detected by a susceptometer, which measures the change of inductance of a coil wound around the propagation channel. As a realization of on-off keying, a bit 1 is represented by a particle injection, a bit 0 by no injection.

However, all of the above mentioned approaches, irrespective of the signaling molecules under investigation, make use of mechanical pumps. Due to this very mode of operation, the pumps are limited in speed and granularity of the injected volumes. Furthermore, miniaturization of the testbeds will make these approaches inapplicable and will therefore call for alternatives.

For modulation of pH level, a replacement for the macroscopic pumps has already been proposed by Grebenstein et al. [11], based on Escherichia coli bacteria that, when stimulated by light pulses, emit protons and thus reduce the local pH-level. Another modulator, appropriate for receiver design, was proposed in [18], where a specific signal molecule induces a fluorescence reaction in E. coli bacteria and thus allows interfacing chemical with optical and, by use of a photodetector, electrical domain. For modulation of SPIONs concentration, in contrast, no such alternative has been proposed so far.

In this paper we propose to make use of the superparamagnetic property of the nanoparticles in a tube system. We demonstrate that it is possible to direct the SPIONs into a particular channel at a Y-shaped branching of the tube system, overcoming the counteracting background flow in the tube system. Therefore we display a customized electromagnet that is utilized as steering unit.

For that purpose, the following sections will outline the fundamentals of the particle steering and describe the experimental setup. The results section will provide the first measurements, which demonstrate the feasibility of the approach. A summary of potential applications and future steps of research will conclude the article.

2   Fundamentals

2.1   Generation of Magnetic Fields

In order to steer the SPIONs by use of magnetic fields, an electromagnet is used. The underlying physical principles are formed in the Maxwell's equations, more accurate in Ampère's law. This partial differential equation describes the creation of a magnetic field of intensity H by a surface current density J. Adding the displacement current density D as Maxwell's fixture to the equation, Ampère's law can be written as follows [12]:

$$\nabla \times H = J + \frac{\partial D}{\partial t} \tag{1}$$

In magnetostatics currents are steady and the surrounding electric field is constant[1]. These conditions form a special case of Ampère's law [12]:

$$\frac{\partial D}{\partial t} = 0$$

$$\nabla \times H = J \tag{2}$$

Using Stoke's theorem, Eq. (2) can be transformed from differential to integral form:

$$\oint_{\partial A} H \, dl = \int_A J \, dA = I \tag{3}$$

Equation (3) states that the total current I through a given surface A agrees with the circulation of H around A, i.e., the integral of H along the boundary of A. It can be rewritten in the form of the Biot-Savart law [12]

$$dH(r) = \frac{I}{4\pi} \frac{dl \times (r - l)}{\|r - l\|^2}, \tag{4}$$

---

[1] $D = \varepsilon E$ is known as constitutive relation with the electric field E and the relative permittivity ε.

which specifies the contribution dH to the magnetic field intensity H at point r caused by an infinitesimal piece of wire dl at position l that carries a current I.

Integration of (4) along a path dl allows to determine the magnetic field caused by any current-carrying conductor in general and by an electric coil in particular. Analytical solutions can be derived for simple setups (see, e.g. [3,4,19]), whereas for the study of more complex electromagnets, particularly including core materials, simulation-based approaches are required.

In order to guide the magnetic flux and to increase the magnetic field outside the coil, cores of ferro- or ferrimagnetic materials such as iron are often used. In such magnetic media, an external field H induces a magnetization

$$M = \chi H, \tag{5}$$

which is proportional to the external field H, with the material-dependent magnetic susceptibility χ as proportionality factor. The magnetic induction

$$B = \mu_0(H + M) = \mu_0(1 + \chi)H \tag{6}$$

is then composed of the external field and the magnetization of the material, where $\mu_0 = 4\pi \times 10^{-7} \mathrm{N/A}^2$ is the vacuum permeability.

Depending on the atomic structure of the material, the magnetization aligns against or with the external field, i.e., $\chi < 0$ and $\chi > 0$, respectively. The corresponding materials are denoted as diamagnetic ($\chi < 0$), paramagnetic ($\chi > 0$) and ferromagnetic ($\chi \gg 0$).[2] It is important to note that paramagnetic media do not exhibit remanent magnetization when the external field is turned off, whereas ferromagnetic media do so.

2.2   Superparamagnetic Iron Oxide Nanoparticles

While control of particles within the body by use of magnetic fields is highly desirable, e.g., for drug targeting, neither dia- nor paramagnetic materials could serve this purpose, due to a too low χ-value and therefore negligible reaction to the external magnetic field. Ferromagnetic materials are also not suitable due to the residual magnetization, which boosts agglomeration of the particles in the blood vessels and thus involves a high risk of vascular occlusion.

Superparamagnetic nanoparticles, in contrast, unite the benefits of para- and ferromagnetism. They are made of ferromagnetic material, usually from the iron oxides magnetite or maghemite (then called superparamagnetic iron oxide nanoparticles or short SPIONs), at sizes in the nanometer-range, typically between 10 nm and 100 nm. Due to these small dimensions, the particles do not exhibit remanence, while still offering high susceptibility values. Furthermore, SPIONs are biocompatible and thus applicable for human use. These nanoparticles have therefore been proposed and are investigated for use as diagnostic agents in magnetic resonance imaging and as non-viral gene vectors as well as for cancer therapy by drug targeting and magnetic hyperthermia [5,25].

---

[2] For the sake of simplicity, ferri- and antiferromagnetic materials are neglected here.

2.3   Particle Steering

In order to direct SPIONs into a specific direction from outside the body, an external magnetic field B is applied. Then a particle of volume V_P and susceptibility χ_P within a solution of susceptibility χ_S will be subject to the force [21,24]

$$F = \frac{\chi_P - \chi_S}{\mu_0} V_P (B \cdot \nabla) B, \tag{7}$$

where ∇B denotes the covariant derivative of B, i.e., a tensor of degree 2.

From (7), it follows that F is proportional to the susceptibility of the particle relative to that of the solution, to the volume of the particle, to the strength of the magnetic field and to its gradient. While the former two factors are determined by the application scenario and the manufacturing of the SPIONs, the latter two factors depend on the design of the electromagnet and its position to the particle.

3   Methods

Based on the fundamentals introduced in the previous section, a demonstrator with a customized steering unit for the SPIONs has been developed. In Sect. 3.1 the proposed demonstrator is described in detail. In Sect. 3.2 different settings for the measurements will be introduced.

3.1   Measurement Setup

The setup in Fig. 1a shows a closed-loop flow of a suspension of nanoparticles in distilled water. From a reservoir, the particle suspension flows to the central part of the loop, a Y-shaped connector, which splits the tube into two branches (see also Fig. 1b). Through these branches, the particles flow back to the reservoir, where they can start the next flow cycle. The constant flow is driven by the peristaltic pump REGLO Digital (Ismatec, Wertheim, Germany), which is positioned at the end of the two branches before these enter the reservoir, which assures a symmetric flow in both branches. All tubes used have diameter of 1.5 mm. In order to steadily monitor the particle concentration in one branch of the tube, this branch leads through the detector coil of the susceptometer MS2G (Bartington Instruments, Witney, United Kingdom).

The setup can be regarded as transmission line between a transmitter located at the Y-connector and the susceptometer as receiver. A binary "1" is sent, when an increased particle concentration is induced by the transmitter via magnetic particle steering and measured at the receiver, a binary "0", when a decreased particle concentration is induced. The setup hence forms a single-ended communication line; if the susceptometer is replace by a detector that contemporaneously measures both branches of the Y-connector and by that determines the concentration difference between the two branches, differential signal transmission is obtained.

peristaltic pump

susceptometer

Y-piece with
positioning scale
for the magnet

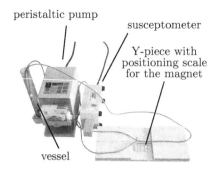

vessel

(a) Measurement setup to steer the SPI-ONs at the Y-shaped branching, to allow measuring the concentration in the desired tube.

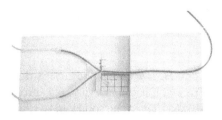

(b) Y-piece (close-up) with identical flow in both tubes.

PVC winding body

iron nail

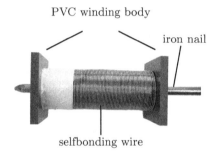

selfbonding wire

(c) Electromagnet used as a steering unit.

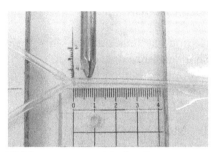

(d) Measurement with the electromagnet in a fixed position. The scaling parallel to the tube defines the x-coordinate, the scaling parallel to the nail defines the y-coordinate of the pointed end of the iron nail.

Fig. 1. Measurement setup.

The electromagnet displayed in Fig. 1c was specially designed as a steering unit for the demonstrator. The winding body was made of a polyvinyl chloride (PVC) tube with a length of 10 cm, an inner diameter of 7 mm and an outer diameter of 12 mm. Two additional PVC plates were mounted to the ends of the tube, to create axial limits for the windings. A selfbonding wire made out of copper with a diameter of 0.9 mm was coiled around the winding in 10 layers of 85 windings each, leading to a total winding number of 851. An iron nail with a length of 21 cm and a diameter of 7 mm was inserted into the winding body acting as core material, as well as focus for the magnetic flux density at the pointed end.

The magnet was operated at a voltage of 4.6 V and a current of 2.5 A max. ($P = 11.5$ W). The control measurement with an FM 302 magnetometer (Projekt Elektronik GmbH, Berlin, Germany) resulted in a magnetic flux density of 200 mT at the pointed end of the nail.

3.2 Measurement

For all the following test settings a new type of SPIONs, provided by the Section for Experimental Oncology and Nanomedicine (SEON) of the University Hospital Erlangen was used. These particles are coated with a golden layer. In Table 1 the parameters of the particles are listed.

Table 1. Parameters of the golden-layered particles (SPIONs).

Parameter	Value
Particle radius	424 nm
Iron concentration	1.12 mg/L
Gold concentration	0.27 mg/L

In Fig. 1d the pointed end of the nail is shown in a fixed position. Behind the tube a cartesian coordinate system is marking the position of the pointed end. Three series of measurements were performed, each with four measurement at different flow rates Q, where Q increased from 4 mL/min to 7 mL/min in steps of 1 mL/min. In each measurement the bit sequence [1, 1, 1, 1, 1, 1] of six consecutive "1" was sent, with a symbol duration of 20 s and a duty cycle of 5 s.

In the first two measurement series, during these 5 s the tip of the electromagnet was moved from point $A(x = 0; y = 0)$ to $B(x = 4; y = 0)$ following the scaling described in Fig. 1d alongside the tube, whereas during the remaining 15 s no magnetic force was exerted on the particle. In the first measurement series, the susceptibility was measured in the branch opposed to the magnet, i.e., in the branch where a decreased susceptibility is expected. In the second measurement series, the susceptometer was positioned around the branch on the same side as the magnet, i.e., the tube where an increase of susceptibility is expected. In the last measurement series, the electromagnet was fixed on position $A(x = 0; y = 0)$ and the tube with the decreasing susceptibility was measured.

3.3 Flow Profile

The efficiency of the particle steering with the setup described beforehand is highly dependent on the balance between the flow profile in the tube, the flow rate of the particles and the applied magnetic field. With the tube diameter of 1.5 mm and the flow rates stated above, it can be shown that the flow follows a laminar flow profile [23, 26], which is characterized by the parabolic velocity profile

$$v(r) = v_0 \left[1 - \left(\frac{r}{R} \right)^2 \right],$$
(8)

where r is the radial coordinate, R the radius of the tube and v_0 the velocity of the particles at the center of the tube. This profile is illustrated in Fig. 2, which shows that the maximum velocity is present in the center of the tube cross section and decreases in radial direction towards the tube wall to zero.

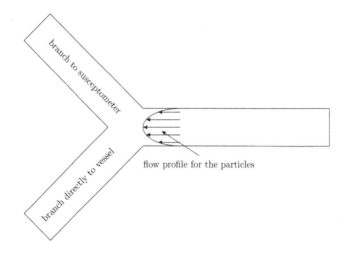

Fig. 2. Schematical illustration of the flow profile for the particles.

Relating the laminar flow profile to the particle concentration, it becomes clear that particles with a radial coordinate $r \approx R$ will stop moving. This means the particle steering unit not only directs the particles into the desired branch of the tube system, it can also force the particles from the tube borders to the center, thus from areas with low to higher velocity, and vice versa. Therefore the strength and position of the electromagnet affect the particle concentration that is lead into the desired branch.

4   Results

Figures 3, 4 and 5 display the results of the test settings described in the previous section. In each figure, the four subfigures show the susceptibility over time for the different flow rates given above. In addition to the raw measured signal, given in dark gray, the smoothed signal, computed by use of a moving average filter of width 5 s, is displayed in red color. The spacing of the abscissa is chosen such that it agrees with the symbol duration of 20 s.

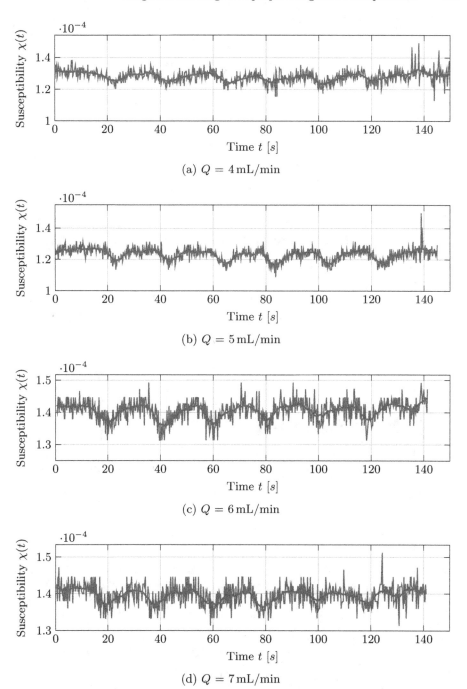

Fig. 3. Received signal due to a transmitted bit sequence for different flow rates Q with moving magnet and measuring the decreasing susceptibility; symbol duration $T = 20\,\text{s}$; transmitted bit sequence: [1, 1, 1, 1, 1, 1]. Raw signal given in gray, smoothed signal in red color (moving average of with 5 s). (Color figure online)

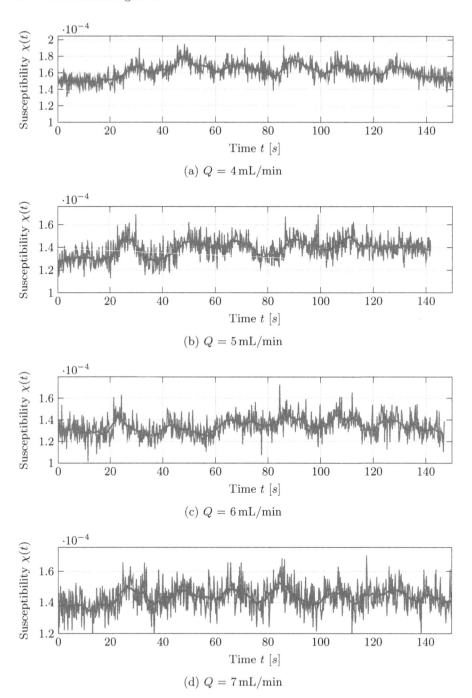

(a) $Q = 4\,\mathrm{mL/min}$

(b) $Q = 5\,\mathrm{mL/min}$

(c) $Q = 6\,\mathrm{mL/min}$

(d) $Q = 7\,\mathrm{mL/min}$

Fig. 4. Received signal due to a transmitted bit sequence for different flow rates Q with moving magnet and measuring the increasing susceptibility; symbol duration $T = 20\,\mathrm{s}$; transmitted bit sequence: [1, 1, 1, 1, 1, 1]. Raw signal given in gray, smoothed signal in red color (moving average of with 5 s). (Color figure online)

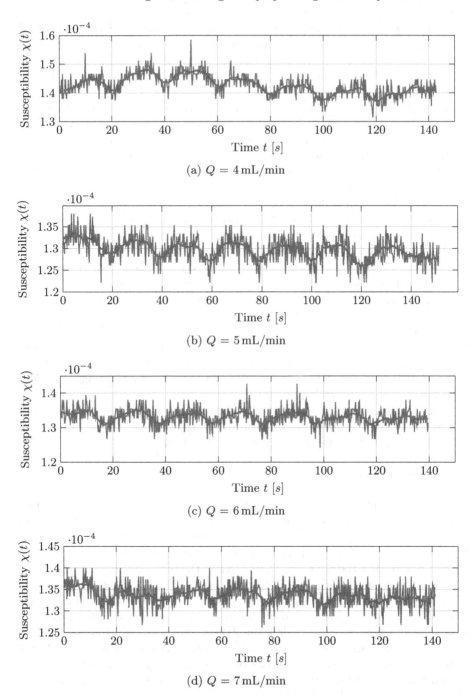

Fig. 5. Received signal due to a transmitted bit sequence for different flow rates Q with fixed magnet and measuring the decreasing susceptibility; symbol duration $T = 20\,\mathrm{s}$; transmitted bit sequence: [1, 1, 1, 1, 1, 1]. Raw signal given in gray, smoothed signal in red color (moving average of with 5 s). (Color figure online)

In each plot a periodic pattern of decrease or increase of the susceptibility, more precise the peaks that correspond to the transmitted bit sequence, are clearly visible. After the duty cycle, the susceptibility always returns to its baseline value. Note that the arrival time of the first peak depends on the flow rate.

Furthermore, the expectations concerning increase and decrease of the particle concentration are met. The branch opposite to the magnet leads exhibits indeed a reduction of the susceptibility, i.e., the magnet detracts the particle from this path (Fig. 3). In contrast, the branch on the same side as the magnet shows an increase in susceptibility, i.e., an accumulation of particles in this branch is observed (Fig. 4).

Due to the laminar flow in the tube, with the zero flow at its boundary, particles tend to get stuck at the surface of the tube wall, when no external magnetic field is operated. This leads to a lower overall particle concentration in both branches together and in the susceptometer in particular, in consequence decreasing peak amplitudes of the bit sequence. This behavior will pose a major challenge on magnetic particle steering and was addressed here in two approaches: by moving the magnet alongside the tube to direct the particles into the desired branch in the first two measurements, and by keeping the electromagnet at a fixed position in the third measurement. The results show that both approaches allow satisfactory transmission behavior. While the fixed-position approach would be easier to realize, an implementation comparable to the approach with the moving magnet, using a series of electromagnets along the tube instead, is possible, too.

The variation of the flow rates in the different setups proves a second thing: that information transmission in the proposed approach is feasible for different flow rates, i.e., it is robust against flow rate variations.

5   Conclusion

The measurements have shown that it is possible to steer superparamagnetic nanoparticles at a branching of a flow channel by use of magnetic fields in such a way that an accumulation of particles is observed in one channel and a diminution in the other. This steering is successful under different flow conditions. However, note that the approach is sensitive to the testbed parameters, viz. flow as well as position and strength of the electromagnet: If not properly balanced, the particles either are not sufficiently deflected or accumulate in front of the branching in the low-flow region of the tube close to the walls. Therefore, the next steps of research will include a simulation-based optimization of the setup, before the next realization of the testbed is tackled. Besides investigation of the said parameters, improvements of the steering unit might be obtained. Here, a second magnet could be added to create a channel switch function, as well as using more magnets alongside the tube, as was suggested in Sect. 4.

With an optimal setup for steering of SPIONs at channel branchings, several applications become possible: First of all, it can replace the original transmitter of the MC testbed described in [23] without the restrictions imposed by mechanical devices. Then one of the branches would be used for signal transmission, while the other, unused branch would direct the particles into a waste bin. Second, in contrast to this single-ended approach, an MC testbed can be realized with differential signaling, i.e., where information is coded in the difference between two parallel tubes rather than in the absolute value of a single tube. In both of these scenarios, the particle steering module would be responsible for the modulation of the SPIONs concentration and thus be the central part of the receiver. It can play yet another role and, third, direct the particles into different channels before modulation takes place, such that different receivers can be addressed. Finally, it should be mentioned that the steering of SPIONs can provide a benefit beyond molecular communication, viz. in cancer therapy, where an optimized targeting of the tumor by drug-loaded nanoparticles could reduce medication dosage and thus side effects of chemotherapy.

References

1. Andrews, S.S.: Accurate particle-based simulation of adsorption, desorption and partial transmission. Phys. Biol. **6**(4), 046015 (2009). https://doi.org/10.1088/1478-3975/6/4/046015
2. Bicen, A.O., Akyildiz, I.F.: Molecular transport in microfluidic channels for flow-induced molecular communication. In: 2013 IEEE International Conference on Communications Workshops (ICC), pp. 766–770, June 2013. https://doi.org/10.1109/ICCW.2013.6649336
3. Dasgupta, B.B.: Magnetic field due to a solenoid. Am. J. Phys. **52**, 258 (1984)
4. Derby, N., Olbert, S.: Cylindrical magnets and ideal solenoids. Am. J. Phys. **78**, 228–235 (2010)
5. Dulińska-Litewka, J., Łazarczyk, A., Hałubiec, P., Szafrański, O., Karnas, K., Karewicz, A.: Superparamagnetic iron oxide nanoparticles–current and prospective medical applications. Materials **12**(4) (2019). https://doi.org/10.3390/ma12040617
6. Eremenko, Z.E., Kuznetsova, E.S., Shubnyi, A.I., Martunov, A.V.: High loss liquid in layered waveguide at microwaves and applications. In: 2018 IEEE 17th International Conference on Mathematical Methods in Electromagnetic Theory (MMET), pp. 246–249, July 2018. https://doi.org/10.1109/MMET.2018.8460267
7. Farsad, N., Pan, D., Goldsmith, A.: A novel experimental platform for in-vessel multi-chemical molecular communications. In: GLOBECOM 2017–2017 IEEE Global Communications Conference, pp. 1–6, December 2017. https://doi.org/10.1109/GLOCOM.2017.8255058
8. Farsad, N., Guo, W., Eckford, A.: Tabletop molecular communication: text messages through chemical signals. Public Libr. Sci. ONE **8**, e82935 (2013)
9. Farsad, N., Yilmaz, B., Eckford, A., Chae, C.B., Guo, W.: A comprehensive survey of recent advancements in molecular communications. IEEE Commun. Surv. Tutor. **18**, 1887–1919 (2016)
10. Giannoukos, S., Marshall, A., Taylor, S., Smith, J.: Molecular communication over gas stream channels using portable mass spectrometry. J. Am. Soc. Mass Spectrom. **28**(11), 2371–2383 (2017). https://doi.org/10.1007/s13361-017-1752-6
11. Grebenstein, L., et al.: Biological optical-to-chemical signal conversion interface: a small-scale modulator for molecular communications. IEEE Trans. Nanobiosci. **18**(1), 31–42 (2019). https://doi.org/10.1109/TNB.2018.2870910

12. Griffiths, D.J.: Introduction to Electrodynamics. Always Learning, 4th edn. Pearson, Boston (2013). International Edition
13. Gul, E., Atakan, B., Akan, O.B.: NanoNS: a nanoscale network simulator framework for molecular communications. Nano Commun. Netw. **1**(2), 138–156 (2010). https://doi.org/10.1016/j.nancom.2010.08.003. http://www.sciencedirect.com/science/article/pii/S1878778910000256
14. Iwasaki, S., Yang, J., Nakano, T.: A mathematical model of non-diffusion-based mobile molecular communication networks. IEEE Commun. Lett. **21**(9), 1969–1972 (2017). https://doi.org/10.1109/LCOMM.2017.2681061
15. Jamali, V., Ahmadzadeh, A., Wicke, W., Noel, A., Schober, R.: Channel modeling for diffusive molecular communication - a tutorial review. CoRR abs/1812.05492 (2018). http://arxiv.org/abs/1812.05492
16. Kennedy, E., Shakya, P., Ozmen, M., Rose, C., Rosenstein, J.K.: Spatiotemporal information preservation in turbulent vapor plumes. Appl. Phys. Lett. **112**(26), 264103 (2018). https://doi.org/10.1063/1.5037710
17. Koo, B., Lee, C., Yilmaz, H.B., Farsad, N., Eckford, A., Chae, C.: Molecular MIMO: from theory to prototype. IEEE J. Sel. Areas Commun. **34**(3), 600–614 (2016)
18. Krishnaswamy, B., et al.: Time-elapse communication: bacterial communication on a microfluidic chip. IEEE Trans. Commun. **61**(12), 5139–5151 (2013). https://doi.org/10.1109/TCOMM.2013.111013.130314
19. Labinac, V., Erceg, N., Kotnik-Karuza, D.: Magnetic field of a cylindrical coil. Am. J. Phys. **74**, 621–627 (2006)
20. Nakano, T., Eckford, A., Haraguchi, T.: Molecular Communication. Cambridge University Press, Cambridge (2013)
21. Rikken, R.S.M., Nolte, R.J.M., Maan, J.C., van Hest, J.C.M., Wilson, D.A., Christianen, P.C.M.: Manipulation of micro- and nanostructure motion with magnetic fields. Soft Matter **10**, 1295–1308 (2014)
22. Shakya, P., Kennedy, E., Rose, C., Rosenstein, J.K.: Correlated transmission and detection of concentration-modulated chemical vapor plumes. IEEE Sens. J. **18**(16), 6504–6509 (2018). https://doi.org/10.1109/JSEN.2018.2850150
23. Unterweger, H., et al.: Experimental molecular communication testbed based on magnetic nanoparticles in duct flow. In: 2018 IEEE 19th International Workshop on Signal Processing Advances in Wireless Communications (SPAWC), pp. 1–5, June 2018. https://doi.org/10.1109/SPAWC.2018.8446011
24. Urbach, A.R., Love, J.C., Prentiss, M.G., Whitesides, G.M.: Sub-100 nm confinement of magnetic nanoparticles using localized magnetic field gradients. J. Am. Chem. Soc. **125**(42), 12704–12705 (2003). https://doi.org/10.1021/ja0378308
25. Wahajuddin, S.A.: Superparamagnetic iron oxide nanoparticles: magnetic nanoplatforms as drug carriers. Int. J. Nanomed. **7**, 3445–3471 (2012). https://doi.org/10.2147/IJN.S30320
26. White, F.: Fluid Mechanics, 7th edn. McGraw-Hill, New York (2011)
27. Yilmaz, H.B., Suk, G., Chae, C.: Chemical propagation pattern for molecular communications. IEEE Wirel. Commun. Lett. **6**(2), 226–229 (2017). https://doi.org/10.1109/LWC.2017.2662689

Fat in the Abdomen Area as a Propagation Medium in WBAN Applications

Mariella Särestöniemi[1(✉)], Carlos Pomalaza Raez[2], Chaïmaâ Kissi[3], Timo Kumpuniemi[1], Marko Sonkki[1], Matti Hämäläinen[1], and Jari Iinatti[1]

[1] Centre for Wireless Communications, University of Oulu, Oulu, Finland
`mariella.sarestoniemi@oulu.fi`
[2] Department of Electrical and Computer Engineering, Purdue University, West Lafayette, USA
[3] Electronics and Telecommunication Systems Research Group, National School of Applied Sciences (ENSA), Ibn Tofail University, Kénitra, Morocco

Abstract. This paper presents a study on the fat in the abdomen area as a propagation medium in wearable and implant communications systems. Propagation via subcutaneous and visceral fat is considered separately. Simulations and measurements are done for both female and male bodies with the on-body antennas designed for in-body communications. Propagation paths are calculated and compared with the simulated and measured impulse responses. Furthermore, we analyze simulated 2D power flow figures, which illustrate the propagation inside the different tissues. It is shown that the signal propagates through the fat layer with minor losses compared to the other tissues of the studied cases. The signal propagates through the fat tissue from the abdomen area to the backside of person with 60 dB power loss. Additionally, the calculated fat layer propagation paths match well with the peaks of the simulated and measured impulse responses. The information about the fat as propagation medium is useful when designing the wireless and wired medical and health monitoring devices.

Keywords: Anatomical voxel model · Capsule endoscopy · Directive antenna · Finite integration technique · Gastrointestinal monitoring · Implant communications · Power distribution · Radio channel · Wireless body area networks

1 Introduction

Recently, wearable and implant communications have been intensively studied topics in the wireless body area networks (WBAN) [1–4]. Smooth design of the communications systems requires comprehensive knowledge of the radio channel characteristics. Hence, in–body channel modeling and propagation within the tissues have been under the scope in e.g. in [5–17].

© ICST Institute for Computer Sciences, Social Informatics and Telecommunications Engineering 2019
Published by Springer Nature Switzerland AG 2019. All Rights Reserved
L. Mucchi et al. (Eds.): BODYNETS 2019, LNICST 297, pp. 175–187, 2019.
https://doi.org/10.1007/978-3-030-34833-5_15

It has been recognized that the signal propagates differently in different tissues due to the variations in dielectric properties [18]. Fat tissue appears to be the easiest tissue for the propagation in terms of propagation velocity and losses [5, 6, 10, 19–21]. Fat as a propagation channel has been a topic for few recent papers [19–21], which have verified by simulation and measurement based studies that the fat tissue is promising propagation medium is the ultra wideband (UWB) based medical applications.

Reference [10] presents a study on the in-body power distribution for abdominal monitoring and implant communication systems. The study is conducted by examining power flow distribution on the anatomical voxel model at different cross section layers in the abdomen area. The presented power results verify that the signal travels through the fat layer for wider areas with minor power loss than in the other tissues.

This paper is a continuation for the power distribution studies presented in [10], focusing now on the propagation in the fat layer. The aim of this paper is to present a study on the fat as a propagation medium in the abdomen area using finite integration technique (FIT) based simulations using an anatomical voxel models. Furthermore, measurement data and propagation path calculations are used in the analysis to validate the results. Both subcutaneous fat and visceral fat are considered separately.

This paper is organized as follows: Sect. 2 presents the study cases describing the simulations, measurements, antennas, and antenna locations. Furthermore, propagation path calculations are described as well. Section 3 presents the propagation through the fat layer with 2D power flow diagrams. Section 4 presents propagation through subcutaneous fat layer with measurement based studies and propagation path calculations. Conclusions are given in Sect. 5.

2 Study Case

2.1 Simulations

Simulations are conducted with electromagnetic simulation software CST MicroWave Studio [22] by using finite integration technique (FIT). CST provides several voxel models, among which we selected anatomical voxel models Laura and Gustav, presented in Fig. 1a–b. Laura correspond to lean female body with resolution of 1.875 mm × 1.875 mm × 1.25 mm. Gustav is a normal-weighted male with the resolution of 2.08 mm × 2.08 mm × 2 mm. Cross section of the voxel models abdomen area on the navel line is shown in Fig. 1c. Subcutaneous and visceral fat, muscles, small intestine (SI), and colon are marked in the Fig. 1c.

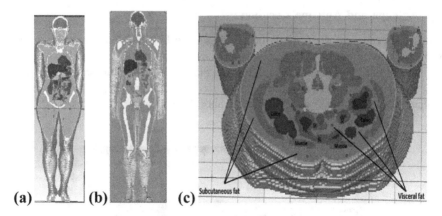

Fig. 1. (a) Anatomical voxel model Laura, (b) Gustav, (c) cross cut of the abdomen area presenting the subcutaneous and visceral fat.

2.2 Measurements

The measurements were conducted in an anechoic chamber in University of Oulu by using Agilent 8720ES vector network analyzer (VNA). The measured frequency band was the full UWB band 3.1–10.6 GHz, according to IEEE802.15.6 standard [23]. We also used a large bandwidth to achieve good time resolution for the measurements. Transmitted power was selected to be +5 dBm, which does not cause harm for human tissues.

The antenna prototypes were connected to the VNA by using 8 m long phase stable Huber + Suhner SUCOFLEX 104PEA measurement cables. A proper calibration was performed before the measurements to neglect cable effect. The VNA was set to sweep 100 times for each scenario, collecting 1601 frequency points per sweep for each measurement setup. The measurements were conducted in the frequency domain to obtain radio channel frequency responses (S21 parameters), which were later transformed into the time domain in Matlab using inverse fast Fourier transform (IFFT). After IFFT, radio channel impulse response (IR) is obtained.

In this paper, we use the measurement data of two human volunteers, one male (M3) and one female (F1), with different body sizes and body balances. The details of the volunteers are presented in [7], but here we repeat the information in Table 1, which is relevant for the propagation studies through the fat layer.

Table 1. Information about the volunteers.

Volunteer	Waist [cm]	Visceral fat [%]	Overall fat [%]	Muscle [%]
Female F1	76	5	29	34
Male M3	103	14	32	31

2.3   Antenna and Antenna Location

In this study case, we use a cavity-backed low-band UWB on-body antenna designed for in-body communications. The antenna's simulation model and the prototype are presented in Fig. 2a–b, respectively [24]. On the studied simulation and measurement scenarios, transmitter (Tx) antenna is on the navel, and the receiver (Rx) antenna is on the flank. This scenario is conceivable for abdominal monitoring scenarios.

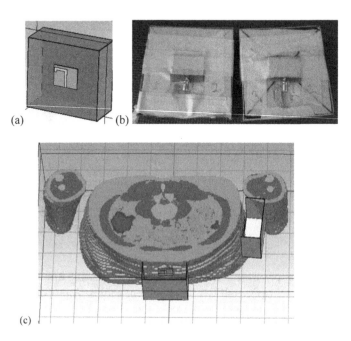

Fig. 2. (a) Cavity-backed low-band UWB antenna designed for in–body communications, (b) prototypes used in the measurements, (c) location of the antennas

2.4   Propagation Path Calculations

In [5], we presented the idea for calculating the propagation paths when signal is passing through different tissues. In this paper, we just focus on the propagation paths through the fat layer, either subcutaneous or visceral fat – or as combination. As discussed in [5], the propagation time t_d is calculated taking into account the frequency f, the distance d that the signal travels through tissue, and the wavelength in the tissue λ as

$$t_d = \frac{d}{v} = \frac{d}{f\lambda} \tag{1}$$

Wavelengths on the different tissues are presented in Table 2. As one can note, wavelength, and hence the propagation speed v in the tissue may vary significantly between different tissues. For instance, wavelength in the fat tissue is remarkable

Table 2. Thickness of the layers on the navel area and wavelengths in the tissues.

Tissue	Thickness [cm]	Wavelength [λ]
Skin	0.15	0.012
Subcutaneous fat	2.5	0.0033
Muscle	1.2	0.010
Visceral fat	2.0	0.0033
SI wall	0.1	0.010
SI content	2.0	0.010

different from other tissues. Hence, the propagation speed is much higher in fat than for instance in muscle layer. The Table 2 includes also the estimated thicknesses of the tissue layers on the navel area of the voxel model.

3   Propagation Through Fat Layers with 2D Power Flows

In this section, we evaluate the propagation through the fat layer by studying the 2D power flow diagrams and Poynting vector values in different areas of the abdomen area. This study is continuation for power distribution studies presented in [10], however, now we focus especially on the propagation through the fat layer.

First, we study the 2D power flow representations for the horizontal and vertical cross sections as presented in Fig. 3a–b. The power flow is normalized for −60 dB– 0 dB range for the clarity. Similar power flow figures are presented in the in-body power distribution results in [10] but they are repeated here for the fat propagation channel analysis. The power flow arrow representation describes well how the signal propagates in the vicinity and inside the human body. Signal propagates along the body surface, as creeping waves [25], but on the way, the part of the signal also passes the skin surface and propagates inside the tissues. One can easily notice the propagation through the fat layer both in the horizontal and vertical cross sections. In the horizontal cross section, the back area can easily be reached within the maximum attenuation −60 dB as the signal propagates through the subcutaneous fat layer. Instead, attenuation is strong in the intestine area and thus no power arrays are visible behind the intestine area. From the vertical cross section in Fig. 3b, one can easily note how the propagation travels vertically through the fat layer over a wide area. Within the plotted dB range from −60 dB to 0 dB, the area from the upper parts of the leg until the stomach can be covered.

Next, we will investigate the power values in different parts of the subcutaneous fat as well as in the intestine area. Table 3 summarizes the relative power values at $f = 4$ GHz. The values are normalized so that the power is 0 dB just before the skin layer below the Tx-antenna. This way we can easily observe the propagation loss within the tissues. Points A–H correspond the power values in the fat layer on the path from the navel to the back. In the point A, the power is −4 dB and at H is −74 dB. As the power flow arrows describe, the signal in the fat layer consist of the signal passing through the skin (from creeping waves) as well as the signal propagated through fat layer from the antenna. The power decreases gradually as the distance from the Tx antenna increases. Surprisingly, the power is at the points F and G −48.5 dB and −48.0 dB, respectively.

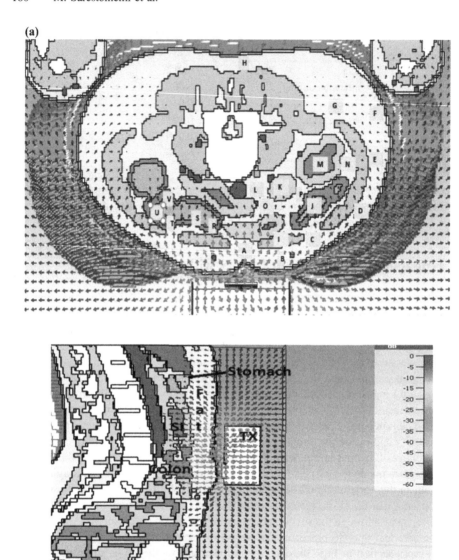

Fig. 3. (a) Power flow diagram of the on the cross-cut A with the antenna location option 1, (b) power flow diagram with the vertical cross section

The power is slightly higher at G, since there is more power summed from the larger area of propagation through the fat layer compared to the point F, whose power consists mostly the power arriving through the skin.

Table 3. Power at different points in the abdominal area.

Subcutaneous fat points	A	B	C	D	E	F	G	H
Power [dB]	−4	−5	−18	−33	−43	−48.5	−48.1	−74
GI/Visceral fat points	I	J	K	L	M	N	O	P
Power [dB]	−10	−40	−51	−49	−68	−54	−39	−46
Colon points	R	S	T	U	V			
Power [dB]	−16	−32	−22	−36	−41			

Next, we compare the power values inside different parts of the intestine and visceral fat area. It is interesting to note how the power is remarkable higher in the points on the visceral fat area compared to the points on the intestine area although the distance from the transmitter antenna is the same. For instance, in the furthest point of the small intestine M the power is −68 dB, whereas in the visceral fat point N, which is next to M, the power is −54 dB. It is also interesting to note that the power in G is approximately 20 dB higher than in M, although M is clearly closer to the Tx antenna than point G. Similarly, as we compare visceral fat point value P and small intestine point K, we can note that the power is 5 dB higher at P than in K. At the visceral fat point L and SI point K, the difference is only 2 dB.

The impact of the fat to the propagation path in the signal strength can easily be noticed when evaluating power values in the left colon points: R, S, T, and U. At the point R, where part of the signal has a direct path from the on-body antenna through the fat layer, the power is −16 dB. Whereas at point S, the power level is −32 dB. The loss in the colon tissue is high and, thus, the power difference between the points R and S are remarkable. At the point T, the power is again higher, −22 dB, since the signal can reach the colon from the left side of the abdominal muscle directly through the fat layer. At the points U and V, the power is again significantly lower: −36 dB and −41 dB, respectively.

These power studies verify that the signal propagates with minor losses in the fat tissue. Additionally, the averaged power is higher in the small intestine points, which are in the vicinity of the subcutaneous or visceral fat.

4 Propagation Through Subcutaneous Fat with the Channel Simulations and Measurement Data

In this section, we evaluate the propagation through the fat layer by comparing the propagation path calculations to the simulated and measured data. The part of the data has been published in [7], in which we present the channel characteristics on the abdomen area. Some of the impulse responses are repeated here to ease the analysis for the fat as a propagation medium but also to ease the comparison between the channel responses and propagation path calculations.

4.1   Simulation Results

First, we evaluate the channel characteristics using Gustav-voxel model and verify it with the corresponding propagation path calculations. Propagation paths are calculated using the dimensions obtained from the Gustav's cross section, presented in Fig. 4. The thicknesses of the subcutaneous fat layers below the Tx antenna (on the navel) is $df = 2.5$ cm, and below the Rx antenna (on the flank) is $ds = 2$ cm. Based on the power flow figures presented in the previous section, the signal is assumed to travel through the subcutaneous fat layer, both outer part of the subcutaneous fat (Path1) as well as inner part of the subcutaneous fat (Path2). Propagation distance of Path1 is estimated to be $d1 = 25.5$ cm. Propagation distance of Path2 ($d2$) is estimated to be $d2 = d1 + ds + df$. Obviously, there is a propagation between these limits, in the middle part of the fat layer. Besides there is a path, in which the signal travels cross the subcutaneous fat layer towards intestine area until reaching the visceral fat layer, and then travels via visceral fat until reaching the area where the abdominal muscle layer is thinner, and returns back to the subcutaneous fat layer continuing towards the Rx antenna on the flank. Path 3 is the propagation path, which travel around the abdominal muscle on the right side and then merges to the Path 2 in the point A. The length of this round trip in the visceral fat layer $dsur$ is estimated to be 8 cm and hence, the total length of the Path3 is $d3 = d2' + dsur$, where $d2'$ is the distance from the point A until the Rx antenna via Path 2. Additionally, the signal can travel similarly around the left abdominal muscle resulting in the $d4 = d2 + dsul$, which is denoted as Path 4.

Next, the propagation times are calculated for the explained propagation paths. The propagation times are summarized in Table 4. For the value presented in the Table 2, we have added the propagation time which $tskin = 2*0.06$ ns, which takes when the signal passes the skin layer until the fat layer. Now, when we compare the obtained propagation times with the IRs presented in Fig. 5, we can see a clear correspondence between the location of the strongest peaks of the IR and the calculated propagation times. In this antenna location option, there is no clear line-of-sight (LOS) component since the antennas are towards the different directions. Thus, the IR consists of the peaks arriving through the creeping waves [25] as well as via the propagation within the tissues. In this study, we focus on the propagation through fat layer. The strongest peak of the IR arrives at time instant of 2 ns, which corresponds to the propagation path through the outer subcutaneous fat Path1. The width of the first peak is 1.1 ns, starting from 1.5 ns until 2.6 ns. Propagation time for the Path2 is calculated to be 2.4 ns, which is inside the first peak's range. The second strongest peak arrives at 2.4 ns, which corresponds to the Path3. Propagation time for Path 4 is calculated to be 3.8 ns, which also can be found from the IR. The rest of the IR peaks belong to the propagation paths travelling through other tissues as well as propagation via body surface, but those are out of scope in this paper.

The obtained propagation paths match well with the peaks appearing in the simulated IR. Some of the peaks are wider than the others. This is because there are several indistinguishable paths in the fat layer as well. Signal may bounce back and forth from the muscle and SI layers making the propagation distance slightly longer. Next, we will verify the simulated results with the measurement data.

Table 4. Propagation times with Gustav-voxel

Paths through the fat	Path1	Path2	Path3	Path4
Propagation distance in fat [cm]	25.5	31	34	50
Propagation time [ns]	2	2.4	2.6	3.8

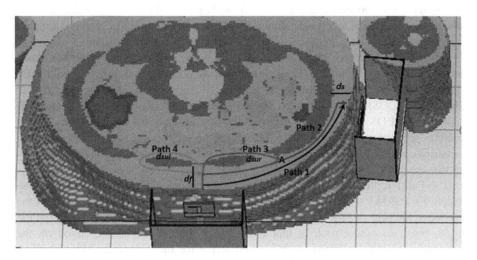

Fig. 4. Dimensions on Gustav-voxel's cross section and propagation path 1-4.

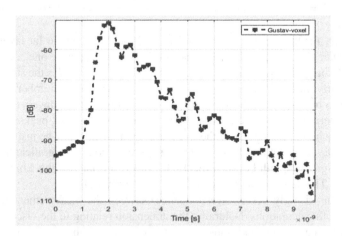

Fig. 5. Impulse response obtained with the Gustav-voxel.

4.2   Measurement Results

In the measurements, the antenna separation distance for the female volunteer F1 was 24.5 cm and for the male volunteer M3 is 27.5 cm. The differences in the distances are due the different sizes of the waists of the volunteers. The distances ds and df are estimated in this case since there was no tools to measure exact thicknesses of the subcutaneous fat layers of the volunteers. The corresponding dimensions of the voxel models were used to estimate the dimensions. For the volunteer F1, ds and df were estimated to be 2.5 cm and for the volunteer M3, 6 cm. Additionally, $d$sur and $d$sul are estimated to same as for the Gustav model, 7 cm and 8 cm, respectively.

Propagation times are summarized in Table 5. Next, we compare the calculated propagation times presented in Table 3 with the IRs obtained with different volunteers which are presented in Fig. 3. As in the case of the simulation results, there is no clear line-of-sight (LOS) component between the antennas. By free-space propagation calculations, the LOS signal should arrive at the time instants 0.8 ns and 0.9 ns for the antenna separation distances 24.5 cm and 27.5 cm, respectively. The impulse responses consist of the peaks due to creeping waves [25] as well as propagation within the tissues.

The Path1 (outer part of the subcutaneous fat) is calculated to arrive for the volunteers F1 and M3 at the time instants 1.8 ns and 2.2 ns, as we take account also the time when the signals pass the skin layer as well (at 0.06 ns). As one can note from the Fig. 6, there is a clear peak at that time instant for the volunteers. Based on the propagation path calculations, Path2 would arrive for the volunteers M3 and F1 at 3.0 ns and 2.4 ns, respectively. These peaks can also be clearly found from the both IRs as well. Path3 and Path4 arrive for the volunteer F1 at 2.6 ns and 3.5 ns and for the M3 the both paths 3 and 4 at 3.6 ns. Also, in this case the match with the measured IRs is good. Additionally, in the measured IRs, one can note several peaks around these time instants.

The reason for this is that the signal travels through the whole fat layer, not just inner and outer fat layers, which can be seen as several peaks one after another. Volunteer M3 has more peaks at the time range 3–4.5 ns and besides the strength of the peaks are clearly higher than those of the volunteer F1. The larger number of the peaks are assumed to be due to the thicker subcutaneous and visceral fat layers the volunteer M3 has. Furthermore, there is clear difference of the level of the IR peaks: M3's peaks are remarkably higher than those of the F1. The reason for this may be just the tilting of the antennas: Even the small tilts towards different direction can significantly decrease the received signal strength between the Tx-Rx link, especially in this kind of antenna configuration. This appear due to the antenna directivity [24].

There is surprisingly good correspondence between the measurement results and propagation path calculations. Naturally, the dimension relating to the visceral fat layer are just estimated values and thus there is some uncertainties in the data. The knowledge about the fat as a propagation channel is useful when designing the monitoring antennas and especially the antenna locations for on-in body communication links. The signal may travel from the intestine area through the visceral and subcutaneous fat with reasonable losses if the antennas are located in the area where there is less muscle layer between the visceral and subcutaneous fat layers.

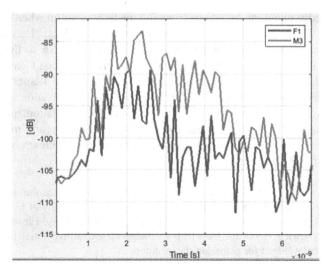

Fig. 6. Impulse response obtained with the volunteer F1 and M3.

Table 5. Propagation times in the fat layer for the volunteers F1 and M3

Paths through the fat	Path1	Path2	Path3	Path4
Propagation distance in fat [cm]	F1: 25.5	F1: 31.5	F1: 34.5	F1: 45.5
	M3:27.5	M3:44.5	M3: 47.5	M3: 47.5
Propagation time [ns]	F1: 1.8	F1: 2.4	F1: 2.6	F1: 3.5
	M3: 2.2	M3: 3	M3: 3.6	M3: 3.6

5 Conclusions

This paper presents a study of the fat in the abdomen area as a propagation medium in WBAN applications. Propagation via subcutaneous and visceral fat is considered separately. The study was conducted via simulations with anatomical voxel models evaluating the channel characteristics between two on-body antennas designed for in-body communications as well as via corresponding on-body measurements. Simulations and measurements were done for both female and male bodies with the on-body antennas designed for in-body communications. Propagation paths were calculated and compared with the simulated and measured impulse responses. Furthermore, we analyzed simulated 2D power flow figures, which illustrate the propagation inside the different tissues.

It was shown that the signal propagates through fat layer with minor loss compared to the other tissues. The signal propagates through the fat tissue from the abdomen area to the backside of person with 60 dB power loss. Additionally, the timing of the calculated propagation paths through the fat layer match well with the peaks of the simulated and measured impulse responses.

The knowledge about the fat as a propagation medium is useful when designing the wireless and wired medical and health monitoring devices. Location of the antennas/sensor nodes for the monitoring devices can be establish so that the propagation through the fat layer can be maximized. Appropriate antenna locations can also facilitate that the signal may reach deeper inside the abdominal tissues via subcutaneous and visceral fat, which is useful for the implant communication systems. As a future work, we plan to continue the study by using the simulation models having different thickness of the subcutaneous and visceral fat. Furthermore, more measurements will be conducted with different antenna locations and with several volunteers having different body balance.

Acknowledgements. This research has been financially supported by the project WBAN Communications in the Congested Environments and in part by Academy of Finland 6Genesis Flagship (grant 318927). Ilkka Virtanen, Timo Mäkinen, and Jari Sillanpää from University of Oulu deserve acknowledgement for their help to enable the exhaustive simulations. Dr. Sami Myllymäki is acknowledged for preparing the prototypes.

References

1. Teshome, A., Kibret, B., Lai, D.T.H.: A review of implant communication technology in WBAN, progresses and challenges. IEEE Rev. Biomed. Eng. **12**, 88–99 (2018)
2. Schires, E., Georgiou, P., Lande, T.S.: Vital sign monitoring through back using an UWB impulse radar with body coupled antennas. IEEE Trans. Biomed. Circ. Syst. **12**(2), 292–302 (2018)
3. Wei, Y., Zahid, A., Heidari, H., Imran, M., Abbasi, Q.H.: A compact non- invasive wearable vital signal monitoring system. In: IEEE Asia Pasific Conference on Postgraduate Research in Microelectronics and Electronics (2018)
4. Leelatien, P., Ito, K., Saito, K., Sharma, M., Alomainy, A.: Channel characteristics and wireless telemetry performance of transplanted organ monitoring system using ultrawide-band communication. IEEE J. Electromag. RF Microw. Med. Biol. **2**(2), 94–101 (2018)
5. Särestöniemi, M., Pomalaza-Raez, C., Kumpuniemi, T., Hämäläinen, M., Iinatti, J.: Measurement data based study on the intra-body propagation in the presence of the sternotomy wires and aortic valve implant. Trans. Antennas Propag. **67**(8), 4989–5001 (2019)
6. Särestöniemi, M., et al.: Comprehensive study on the impact of the sternotomy wires on the UWB WBAN channel characteristics. IEEE Access (2019)
7. Särestöniemi, M.: Measurement and simulation based study on the UWB channel characteristics on the abdomen area. In: ISMICT (2019)
8. Särestöniemi, M., Kissi, C., Pomalaza-Raez, C., Hämäläinen, M., Iinatti, J.: Impact of the antenna-body distance on the UWB on-body channel characteristics. In: ISMICT (2019)
9. Särestöniemi, M., Kissi, C., Pomalaza Raez, C., Hämäläinen, M., Iinatti, J.: Propagation and UWB channel characteristics on human abdomen area. In: EUCAP (2019)
10. Särestöniemi, M., Pomalaza-Raez, C., Berg, M., Kissi, C., Hämäläinen, M., Iinatti, J.: In-body power distribution for abdominal monitoring and implant communications systems. In: ISWCS, September 2019
11. Demir, A.F., et al.: Anatomical region-specific in vivo wireless communication channel characterization. IEEE J. Biomed. Health Inf. **21**(5), 1254–1262 (2017)

12. Chávez-Santiago, R., et al.: Experimental path loss models for in-body communications within 2.36–2.5 GHz. IEEE J. Biomed. Health Inf. **19**(3), 920–937 (2015)
13. Li, J., Nie, Z., Liu, Y., Wang, L., Hao, Y.: Characterization of in-body radio channels for wireless implants. IEEE Sens. J. **17**(5), 152–1537 (2017)
14. Khaleghi, A., Balansingham, I., Chavez-Santiago, R.: Computational study of ultra wideband wave propagation into the human chest. Antennas Propag., IET Microwaves (2009)
15. Turalchuk, P., Munina, I., Pleskachev, V., Kirillov, V., Vendik, O., Vendik, I.: In-body and on-body wave propagation: modeling and measurements. In: International Workshop on Antenna Technology: Small Antennas, Innovative Structures, and Applications (iWAT) (2017)
16. El-Saboni, Y., Conway, G.A., Cotton, S.L., Scanlon, W.G.: Radiowave propagation characteristics in the intra_body channel at 2.38 GHz. IEEE International Conference on Wearable and Implantable Body Sensor Networks (BSN) (2017)
17. Alomainy, A., Hao, Y., Yuan, Y., Liu, Y.: Modelling and characterization of radio propagation from wireless implants at different frequencies. In: European Conference on Wireless Technology (2009)
18. https://www.itis.ethz.ch/virtual-population/tissue-properties/database
19. Asan, N.B., et al.: Intra-body microwave communication through adipose tissue. Healthc. Technol. Lett. **4**(4), 115–121 (2017)
20. Asan, N.B., et al.: Characterization of fat channel for intra-body communication at R-band frequencies. MDPI Sens. **18**(9), 2752 (2018)
21. Asan, N.B., et al.: Reliability of the fat tissue channel for intra-body microwave communication. In: 2017 IEEE Conference on Antenna Measurements & Applications (2017)
22. CST Microwave Studio. http://www.cst.com
23. Astrin, A.: IEEE standard for local and metropolitan area networks _part 15.6: wireless body area networks. In: IEEE Std 802.15.6 2012, pp. 1–271 (2012)
24. Kissi, C., Särestöniemi, M., Pomalaza-Raez, C., Sonkki, M., Srifi, M.N.: Low-UWB directive antenna for wireless capsule endoscopy localization. In: BodyNets2018 Conference (2018)
25. Kumpuniemi, T., Hämäläinen, M., Mäkelä, J.P., Iinatti, J.: Path loss modeling for UWB creeping waves around human body. In: ISMICT, Portugal (2017)

On-Body Communications

Optical Wireless Data Transfer Through Biotissues: Practical Evidence and Initial Results

Iqrar Ahmed[1](✉), Alexander Bykov[2], Alexey Popov[2],
Igor Meglinski[2], and Marcos Katz[1]

[1] Centre for Wireless Communications, University of Oulu, Oulu, Finland
iqrar.ahmed@oulu.fi
[2] Opto-Electronics and Measurement Techniques,
University of Oulu, Oulu, Finland

Abstract. Light has been used in many medical applications to monitor health status and diagnose diseases. Examples include optical sensing through near-infrared (NIR) spectroscopy, optical coherence tomography, and pulse oximetry. In this article, we propose and demonstrate digital communications through biological tissues using near-infrared light. There are many possible uses to an optical system transmitting information across tissues. In current practices, implants predominantly use radio frequency (RF) radiation for communication. However, molecular biology restricts use of the RF in terms of power, frequency etc., while interference and security issues represent technological challenges in RF communication. In this paper, we demonstrate a novel way of employing NIR light for wireless transmission of data through biological tissues. A phantom mimicking a biological tissue is illuminated with a NIR 810 nm wavelength light-emitting diode (LED), and a light detector with line-of-sight alignment is placed on receiving end. An experimental testbed for Optical Communications through Biotissue (OCBT) was designed and implemented using mostly off-the-shelf components. Measurements for different levels of optical output power and thicknesses were carried out. Transmission rates as high as several tens of kilobits-per-second across several millimeters of tissues were achieved. Hardware limitations in modulating the baseband signal prevented achieving higher data rates. In addition, a high-resolution picture was successfully transmitted through biotissue. The communication system as well as details of the testbed implementations are presented in this paper. Moreover, initial performance measures as well as suggestions for potential use of this optical communication system are also presented and discussed.

Keywords: Near-infrared communications · Biological tissue · Optical wireless communications · Implantable medical devices · Medical wireless communications · Medical technology · WBAN

© ICST Institute for Computer Sciences, Social Informatics and Telecommunications Engineering 2019
Published by Springer Nature Switzerland AG 2019. All Rights Reserved
L. Mucchi et al. (Eds.): BODYNETS 2019, LNICST 297, pp. 191–205, 2019.
https://doi.org/10.1007/978-3-030-34833-5_16

1 Introduction

In the past decades, there has been an increasing interest in applying wireless communications to the field of medical ICT. Examples include the development of wireless personal and body area networks (WPAN and WBAN, respectively). On-body and in-body wireless sensors can be deployed on and in the patient's body to monitor physiological variables and further relay this information to a processing node. Radio technology is predominantly used for transmitting data within hospitals and for personalized healthcare monitoring. Medical implant communication systems (MICS), WBANs and WPANs typically exploit radio to communicate with implants and sensors for patient diagnostics, and treatment [1–4].

In recent years, the types and roles of controllable body implants have significantly increased. IMD, implantable medical device, is the generic name to refer to these electronic implants. Typical applications of IMD include monitoring and treatment of cardiac, neurologic and sensory problems as well as automatic deliver of medication. In general, IMDs can be controlled wirelessly to change settings or operating modes, to activate functionalities, etc. As radio communications is the typical way to communicate with electronic implants, these devices are vulnerable to cyber-attacks (i.e., unauthorized use), as it has been demonstrated recently in a number of planned attacks to demonstrate the real risk of commercial devices are prone to encounter [5–7]. The term "brainjacking" has been recently coined to describe a security breach allowing a remote user to control a brain implant [8].

In this paper, we demonstrate the potential of utilizing light instead of radio to carry out wireless communications to and from IMDs. In particular, we use near infrared (NIR) as at these wavelengths, propagation through biotissues is significantly more favorable compared to the case of visible light. Optical communications have numerous advantages over the RF, such as security and privacy, i.e., it cannot be hacked remotely; safety i.e., there is no radiation exposure to human body; non-interference nature i.e., it does not interfere with RF devices, etc. Light-emitting diodes (LEDs) are inexpensive and can emit a broad range of wavelength spectrum. Moreover, power consumption of optical transceivers could be very low. We show that a NIR LED of 810 nm can transmit data through a dense layer of biotissues. A line-of- sight (LOS) communication link is established between a LED source and photodiode receiver, where a biotissue works as the optical channel. We successfully transmitted a high-resolution image file through the phantom. For the experiments, optical phantoms as well as real bio tissues (e.g., skull) were used. There are numerous challenges in transmitting data through biotissues. Indeed, biotissues are characterized by very high attenuation due to light absorption, reflection within the dense tissue layers and anisotropic properties of biotissues. The photothermal effect due to illumination of organ is worth mentioning, when biotissues are illuminated for a long time. The photothermal effect can increase tissue temperature [9], thus prevention practices are recommended by ICNIRP [10].

In this paper, we describe an experimental testbed that was implemented as a proof of concept. Practical performance measurements were carried out and results are also reported and discussed here. In general, results suggest that transmitting optical information over biotissues is possible. Basic performance measures such as data throughput and range can be enhanced by increasing transmitted optical power, though particular care should be taken with the maximum allowed power density.

This paper is organized as follows. Section 2 presents the system model considered in this paper. In Sect. 3 the developed testbed is introduced, including its key parts, namely the front end for wireless data transmission as well as the biotissue- mimicking phantom. Section 4 presents some performance results of the system, while Sect. 5 discusses use cases and applications. Discussions are presented in Sect. 6. Finally, in Sect. 7 the conclusions of this work are presented.

2 System Model

Figure 1 depicts the basic concept considered in this paper. Two cases are described. First, an IMD connected to an external node through optical links. Transmission can be in both directions, namely to-body (e.g., control signal transmitted to the IMD) and from body (information or sensor reading transmitted from the IMD for further analysis). The second case considers intra-body communications, where two in-body devices (IMDs, sensors or nodes of a network) exchange information, for instance. While the first case has more immediate applications as the use of IMD is growing rapidly, it is expected that the second case will become also very relevant, as advancement in in-body communications and the concept of internet of human body further develop. The range of the optical links is expected to be from millimeters to centimeters.

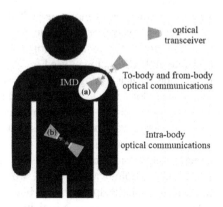

Fig. 1. Wireless optical communications: (a) to and from an IMD and (b) intra-body communications.

A. Optical Communications Link

The simplified block diagram of the optical transceiver needed to create the communications links is shown in Fig. 2. Note that this picture describes a generic two-directional communication system. Means to control optical power as well as duty cycle are also incorporated, as they have a direct impact on the quality and range of the established optical links. Details of the implementation of an experimental testbed are presented in next section. For the purpose of this feasibility study, only a single communication branch was implemented in our testbed.

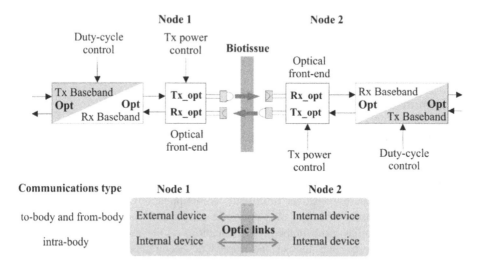

Fig. 2. Block diagram of the optical transceiver considered in this paper.

B. Biotissue as an Optical Media

Light propagation in a turbid media such as biotissue is challenging. Such medium is characterized by very strong absorption and scattering. Understanding light behavior in biotissues is important due to the multiple applications of light in healthcare. Light, both visible and NIR, is today used for biomedical diagnosis and treatment. Applications include optical tomography, laser surgery, photodynamic therapy. NIR spectroscopy is predominant in transcranial [11] and hemodynamics [12] applications. Numerous non-invasive spectroscopy techniques [13–20] have been studied over the past decades to exploit the harmless nature of light to examine optical properties of biotissue, perform diagnosis as well as to treat malignant tissues. In some cases, therapeutic applications using visible and infrared light have been demonstrated to alleviate pathological disorders, wound healing, pain, and inflammation [21, 22]. These therapeutic applications either utilize low-level light, termed as low-level light therapy (LLLT) or non-ionizing light sources termed as photobiomodulation (PBM). The aim of using low level light is to stimulate photochemical and photophysical effects in biotissues for remedy and to alleviate the photothermic response from biotissues [21, 23, 24].

Light interaction with biotissues has been extensively studied to reveal tissue properties such as absorption, scattering, anisotropy [25–27] and further used in modelling. The useful optical or therapeutic window lies between 700 nm to 1100 nm, where the NIR light faces minimal absorption and scattering, hence maximum penetration in biotissues. Scattering, the dominant phenomenon in biotissues, causes light dispersion, reducing rapidly energy density as light propagates. The initial step in utilizing NIR light is to understand the relationship of wavelength and its interaction with biotissues. Next, to study this relationship we utilize a phantom mimicking the biotissue in our experimentations. The characteristics of the phantom must match the optical characteristics of the tissue it is mimicking. Nowadays, these phantoms are fabricated utilizing different biopolymers mixed with numerous dyes and particles [28, 29]. As light interact with biotissues, particular care is needed to avoid any possible damage to the tissue. Light energy- and power-density need to be below certain limits to avoid harmful effects [30].

In this paper, we propose and demonstrate the use of biotissues as optical channels for transmitting information. Communication across biotissues has numerous applications as use cases, as discussed later in this paper.

3   Testbed Implementation

In this section, we briefly introduce our testbed, the front-end components we utilized for transmitting and receiving data. Next, we discuss the modulation scheme we implemented for modulating the baseband carrier. Finally, we describe the phantom we utilized in our testing.

3.1   System Overview

We developed our testbed utilizing mostly off-the-shelf electronics. We utilized USRP modules (Universal Software Radio Peripheral) to implement the receiver and transmitter. GNU radio software was used and we implemented the GNU radio tunnel example [31]. The software is available freely and does not need any licensing to implement. The GNU radio tunnel example creates a tunnel between source and receiving nodes, the software comprises several blocks connected to each other. Among several modulation options available in GNU radio, we chose and implemented Gaussian minimum-shift keying (GMSK) modulation. GMSK is a constant envelope scheme that performs better than other modulation schemes e.g., quadrature phase-shift keying (QPSK) etc., in the optical communications. The slowness of LED to follow the abrupt phase changes in the externally modulated optical signal deteriorates the performance of QPSK [31].

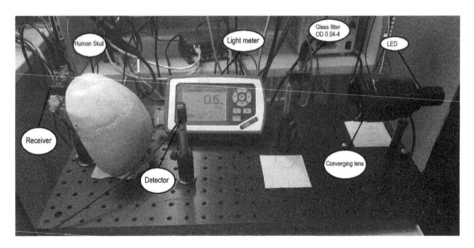

Fig. 3. Overview of the testbed, including optical transmitter (right), optical receiver (left) and tissue (skull).

Figure 3 shows the testbed components; the transmitting end on the right transmits data-modulated light (NIR) and the receiving end on the left side receives and further process the optical signal. An optical phantom or real tissue is placed between transmitter and receiver.

3.2   Transmitter Characteristics

We have used Thorlabs 810 nm mounted IR LED [32], the LED has a maximum output power of 325 mW and has a radiation spot of 1 mm^2. The maximum supplied current to the LED is 500 mA. To modulate the LED input current, we have used the Thorlabs DC2200 LED driver [33]. The LED driver comprises a single channel and can supply the LED with as high as 10 A current providing the input voltage to the driver of 50 V. The LED driver also supports external modulation, termed as Small Signal Bandwidth by Thorlabs. The driver can handle sine wave and has a limitation of handling baseband modulated signal within the range from DC-250 kHz. The external modulated signal from USRP is fed to DC bias-Tee that can operate between 100 kHz to 4200 MHz at 0 to 5 V. The bias-Tee adds the DC voltage to RF signal from USRP. Output of bias-Tee is then fed to DC2200 LED driver, the driver feeds the equivalent current to LED. The input current to LED is converted by driver based on modulation coefficient formulae by Thorlabs. The specification sheet of DC 2200 tells that per 1 V, the driver feeds 400 mA current to LED. The LED can handle between 0 to 3.6 V forward voltage, so we maintained the DC bias to 3.6 V when illuminating the LED with full scale. The input to LED can be controlled by changing the applied voltage to bias-Tee. The LED brightness is directly proportional to the percentage of current fed by LED driver.

The beam collimation is performed by Thorlabs SM2F32B anti-reflective (AR) lens [34]. The lens with adjustable collimation can operate within the range of 650–1050 nm and the reflective coating is used to alleviate reflection.

3.3   Receiver Characteristics

The receiver of our testbed comprises silicon avalanche photodetector APD120A from Thorlabs [35]. The operating range for this detector is from 400-1000 nm. The sensitivity of the detector peaks at 800 nm, the active area of detector is 1 mm^2 while it can be increased by attaching a lens to the detector. The output of the receiver is connected to USRP. The signal from the receiver is then demodulated on receiver's end for further processing.

3.4   Biotissue-Mimicking Phantom

Rigorous experimentation needs to be carried out when measuring optical properties of biotissues. The properties of biotissues degrade over time, thus use of stable biotissue-mimicking phantoms with present properties are of high importance. The phantoms are fabricated in our laboratories using polyvinyl chloride-plastisol (PVCP) and zinc oxide (ZnO) nanoparticles, the properties of the phantom remain the same at least over four months [28, 29]. The optical properties i.e., absorption coefficient μa, scattering coefficient μs, scattering anisotropy g, thickness L and refractive index n of the phantom are tuned to match the properties of the biotissue it mimics.

Transmittance, reflectance, and collimated transmittance of the fabricated phantom are measured and the mentioned optical properties are reconstructed by inverse adding-doubling (IAD) method. The phantoms we used in our experiments mimic skin. We added multiple layers of phantoms to mimic the complex structure of skin.

4   System Evaluation

As discussed in Sect. 3.2, a Thorlabs NIR LED was employed, where the LED's input current was modulated through an LED driver DC2200. The output/brightness of the LED is proportional to the input current supplied. When an externally modulated voltage signal is applied to the LED driver, it converts the voltage to an input current for the LED based on modulation coefficient. 1 V is converted into 400 mA current. The maximum output of the LED is 325 mW generated at 500 mA when an externally modulated voltage of 3.6 V is applied to LED driver. The output of the LED can be reduced by varying the modulating signal, to avoid damaging the biotissue when exposed for longer durations, due to the photothermal effect. ANSI.Z136.1-2007 [36] standard on laser safety states that for 830 nm wavelength an exposure for 1 s that can generate 2 W/cm2 power is safe. We measured the optical power applied to the phantom at varying input levels. Table 1 gives an overview of the measured optical power at the phantom at varying input current, the values are well within the safe limit.

Table 1. The amount of optical power delivered to the phantom.

LED Input Current (mA)	Optical Power to Phantom (mW/mm^2)
10	5.3
50	22.15
100	49.5
200	102.8
300	147
400	195.4
500	239.1

We utilized Thorlabs NDC-100C-4 Unmounted Round Variable Density Filter (Uncoated). This linear attenuation filter has 100 mm in diameter and the optical density (OD) of the filter ranges between 0.04–4. The filter is utilized to investigate the optical communication at varying OD, as OD corresponds to tissue thickness. Figure 4 shows the amount of power transmitted through filter at different OD, measured at the receiver. These power values are well below the safe limit set by ANSI. Transmitted signal cannot go through for values of OD larger than 3. The top horizontal axis in red represents the equivalent depth of bloodless dermis.

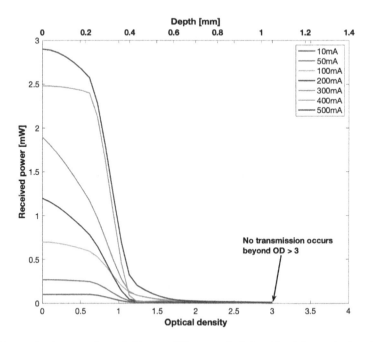

Fig. 4. Transmitted power through filter at different optical densities. The equivalent depth for bloodless dermis presented in top (red) horizontal axis (Color figure online).

Figure 5 shows the relationship between thickness and OD for white matter, grey matter, bloodless dermis, muscles and breast. OD is expressed in term of exponential decrease in optical intensity when transmitted through biotissues, for OD equal to 1, the incident optical intensity will be decreased 2.71. For grey matter, 0.2 mm thickness will decrease incident intensity to 2.71 times, similarly 0.6 mm slab will provide the OD equivalent to 2. We estimated the light attenuation for 5 different types of media from which light can pass through. Figure 6 shows that increasing LED output will result in light passing through an increased thickness, this is advantageous when transmitting data with high energy pulses of short duty cycle, in this way data can be transmitted through thicker slabs of phantoms while keeping operating safety below the obligatory limits.

In the experiments, a data throughput of several tens of Kbps was attained. The current testbed set some practical limitations on the maximum achievable data throughput. In our future work, we plan to experiment with more advanced hardware systems. We expect a considerable increase in data rate support.

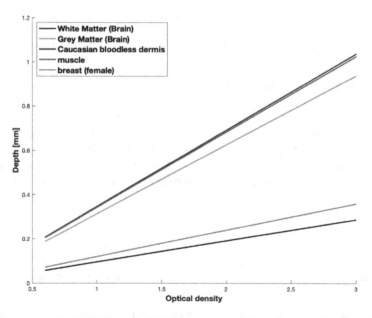

Fig. 5. Penetration depth (thickness) of different types of biotissue as a function of optical density.

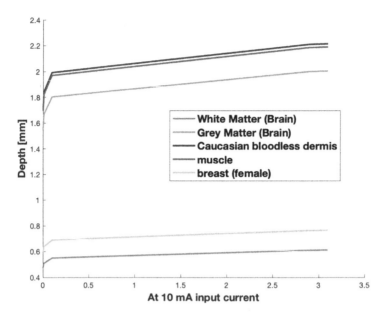

Fig. 6. Relationship between the achievable tissue depth and LED input current.

5 Use Cases and Applications

Optical Communications through Biotissue (OCBT) has numerous use cases and applications. As discussed, the most immediate application is providing wireless connectivity to IMD. Representative IMDs include cardiac devices (pacemakers and implantable cardioverter defibrillators), neurostimulators (e.g., deep brain stimulators, gastric electrical stimulators, spinal cord stimulators, brain implants, etc.) and medical delivery pumps (e.g., delivering medicines, fluids, nutrients, etc.) Over the years, the types and applications of IMD have increased rapidly.

OCBT offers a number of benefits over RF communications, as summarized next

Security and privacy are some of the most relevant advantages of OCBT; eavesdropping, jamming the communication link or accessing illegally the IMD is extremely difficult as accessing an IMD needs to be done locally, in some cases requiring proximity of the order of centimeters.

Safety: Radio exposure is not an issue when using OCTB. However, biotissues and organs could also be damaged by light if high-power light sources are used. Low power light and pulse-modulated carriers are in general preferred for OCBT.

Interference: Radio-based links are prone to be interfered by other radio systems. This is particularly true in uncontrolled environments, e.g., home, where other radio systems could be located in the vicinity. In controlled environments, e.g., hospitals, radio links could eventually create interference to highly sensitive equipment. OCBT does not suffer from these limitations.

Energy: Power requirements of optical transceivers can be very low, and this is an important advantage particularly for energy-limited IMD. Furthermore, in some applications where range is very short, e.g., subcutaneous IMD, the same light used to transmit information can be used to power up the complete IMD or some of its functionalities. The possibility of energy harvesting is a unique advantage of OCBT.

Integration to Other Light-based Applications: In principle, this approach can be combined with already well-established light-based healthcare applications. For instance, light from node A to node B could be used to make a diagnosis of the tissue between these nodes. Node B, after making the diagnosis, transmits these results digitally to node A.

Hybrid Networks: In order to enhance performance and have a much more flexible connectivity solution (e.g., increase reliability, data rate) OCBT can be combined radio-based transmissions [31, 37].

In-body Connectivity: In addition to providing connectivity to IMDs, OCBT can be used to create in-body networks, from simple point-to-point wireless connections to more sophisticated networks involving sensing nodes, gateways, repeaters, and other processing units. In principle in-body nodes as well as IMDs can be nodes of a WBAN.

6 Discussions

In this section, we further discuss the results and prospects for the concepts proposed in this paper. We highlight the fact that the above results are exploratory, and additional measurements will be carried out to better characterize the suitability of biotissues as optical media for data transmission. However, results so far are encouraging, and we can already say that even with low optical power, low data rate information can be transmitted through biotissues across some reasonable distances (e.g., centimeters). Using higher optical power and pulsed communications is expected to increase data throughput and range.

There are some limitations associated with the current testbed, which are mostly due to hardware. The use of commercial off-the-shelf components (Thorlabs and National Instruments) limits the achievable data transmission rate in our initial experiments. However, this low data rate is enough for transmitting packets of data as those required by some IMDs. Some IMD applications might require substantially higher data rates. For that, in addition to increasing transmitted power, one can use more advanced modulation schemes. In our experiments, we successfully transmitted a 14 MB of high-resolution image through the biotissue-mimicking phantom.

Since OCBT is a novel technique to transmit data through biotissues, several technological challenges need to be tackled. Moreover, extensive experimentation on phantoms needs to be carried out to further understand this medium. Performance of the optical link can be enhanced by exploiting different techniques. Next, some of these techniques are discussed to improve energy efficiency, reliability and range.

Energy Efficiency. The OCBT sensors up-fronts i.e., receiver and transmitter, can be configured to work in an interactive mode keeping the up-front in sleep mode for conserving energy. In the battery-operated OCBT sensors, the power consumption needs to be kept as low as possible. The size of the up-front circuitry should be kept small and interactive communication would help to reduce power drainage. The overall size of the sensor and electronic circuitry is important; the package should be kept small to preserve energy for prolonged battery life.

High Reliability/Integrity. The reliability of data is of utmost importance; possible errors due to partial data reception need be checked and corrected. Reliability can be addressed in many ways, and this needs to be further investigated in this scenario. Increasing transmission power is not a straightforward solution as there are limits on the maximum energy that be radiated into biotissue. The use of diversity is a promising approach, and diversity can be exploited in multiple domains. The sensitivity of the detector can be increased to handle lower power.

Range: In some cases, such as in-body communications or when IMD are deeply implanted, the communications range might become an issue. Increasing transmission power to increase range is not a straightforward solution, as the transmission must comply with regulations limiting the transmitted optical power.

7 Conclusions

In this paper, we proposed and demonstrated the use of light to transmit digital information across biotissues. A near infrared LED was used as a light source, as propagation of NIR light in biotissues is more favorable than at other wavelengths. An experimental testbed was implemented, consisting of an optical transmitter, a phantom/biotissue and an optical receiver. The demonstrated *Optical Communication through Biotissue (OCBT)* technique offers potential benefits over radio, because, among others, the optical communication is secure and safe compared to radio. We discussed the architecture of OCBT used in this study. The data signal modulating the IR LED is controlled through a LED driver. We utilized GMSK modulation in our measurements. In our testbed, proven and inexpensive technology was used. Bidirectional communicational is also possible and it depends on sensor package.

Measurements show that it is feasible to use light to securely transmit information across biotissues. Initial results show that tens of Kbps can be easily achieved in a range of several millimeters. This is enough for many applications with IMD, as they are located well within the demonstrated range. The range and data throughput can be increased by using more advanced modulation schemes. This will be further investigated in the future. In addition, we plan to study the use of pulsed transmission to increase the range of the transmission. Extensive experimentation with different phantoms/tissues will also be carried out to characterize the transmission medium in more detail.

Several challenges need to be overcome in OCBT to create a truly practical system. Building and embedding the proposed communication system into a small package using system-on-chip (SoC) or other integrated circuit technology is required in order to have a practically usable system. Miniaturization of the optical transceiver is quite feasible, as the communication system is quite simple, for low-rate systems operating over several millimeters. The potential benefits of security and user safety in OCBT make the demonstrated system promising for future medical applications.

Acknowledgement. This research has been funded by Academy of Finland HERONET project and partially funded by Academy of Finland (6Genesis Flagship - grant 318927 and grants 290596, 314369).

References

1. Bradley, P.D.: An ultra low power, high performance medical implant communication system (MICS) transceiver for implantable devices. In: 2006 IEEE Biomedical Circuits and Systems Conference, pp. 158–161. IEEE (2006)
2. Chow, E.Y., Morris, M.M., Irazoqui, P.P.: Implantable RF medical devices: the benefits of high-speed communication and much greater communication distances in biomedical applications. IEEE Microwave Mag. **14**(4), 64–73 (2013)
3. Chen, Z.N., Liu, G.C., See, T.S.: Transmission of RF signals between MICS loop antennas in free space and implanted in the human head. IEEE Trans. Antennas Propag. **57**(6), 1850–1854 (2009)
4. Karvonen, H., Mikhaylov, K., Hämäläinen, M., Iinatti, J., Pomalaza-Ráez, C.: Interference of wireless technologies on BLE based WBANs in hospital scenarios. In: Proceedings of the 2017 IEEE 28th Annual International Symposium on Personal, Indoor, and Mobile Radio Communications (PIMRC), pp. 1–6, IEEE, Montreal (2017)
5. Camara, C., Peris-Lopez, P., Tapiadora, J.E.: Security and privacy issues in implantable medical devices: A comprehensive survey. J. Biomed. Inform. **55**, 272–289 (2015)
6. Beavers, J.L., Faulks, M., Marchang, J.: Hacking NHS pacemakers: a feasibility study. In: 2019 IEEE 12th International Conference on Global Security, Safety and Sustainability (ICGS3), London, UK, 16–18 January 2019 (2019)
7. Tabasum, A., Safi, Z., AlKhater, W., Shikfa, A.: Cybersecurity issues in implanted medical devices In: 2018 International Conference on Computer and Applications (ICCA) (2018)
8. Pycroft, L., et al.: Brainjacking: implant security issues in invasive neuromodulation. World Neurosurg. **92**, 454–462 (2016)
9. Bozkurt, A., Onaral, B.: Safety assessment of near infrared light emitting diodes for diffuse optical measurements. Biomed. Eng. **3**(1), 9 (2004)
10. International Commission on Non-Ionizing Radiation Protection: ICNIRP guidelines on limits of exposure to incoherent visible and infrared radiation. Health Phys. **105**(1), 74–96 (2013)
11. Jagdeo, J.R., Adams, L.E., Brody, N.I., Siegel, D.M.: Transcranial red and near infrared light transmission in a cadaveric model. PLoS ONE **7**(10), e47460 (2012)
12. Zhang, H., Salo, D.C., Kim, D.M., Komarov, S., Tai, Y.C., Berezin, M.Y.: Penetration depth of photons in biological tissues from hyperspectral imaging in shortwave infrared in transmission and reflection geometries. J. Biomed. Opt. **21**(12), 126006 (2016)
13. Mil'Shtein, S.: Infrared scanning for biomedical applications. Scanning **28**(5), 274–277 (2006)

14. Myllylä, T., Harju, M., Korhonen, V., Bykov, A., Kiviniemi, V., Meglinski, I.: Assessment of the dynamics of human glymphatic system by near-infrared spectroscopy. J. Biophotonics 11(8), e201700123 (2018)

15. Korhonen, V.O., et al.: Light propagation in NIR spectroscopy of the human brain. IEEE J. Sel. Top. Quant. Electron. 20(2), 289–298 (2014)

16. Alarousu, E., et al.: Noninvasive glucose sensing in scattering media using OCT, PAS, and TOF techniques. In: Saratov Fall Meeting 2003: Optical Technologies in Biophysics and Medicine, vol. 5474, pp. 33–42) (2003). International Society for Optics and Photonics

17. Bykov, A., et al.: Imaging of subchondral bone by optical coherence tomography upon optical clearing of articular cartilage. J. Biophotonics 9(3), 270–275 (2016)

18. Popov, A.P., et al.: High-resolution deep-tissue optical imaging using anti-Stokes phosphors. In: European Conference on Biomedical Optics, p. 88010C (2013). Optical Society of America

19. Meglinsky, I.V., Matcher, S.J.: Modelling the sampling volume for skin blood oxygenation measurements. Med. Biol. Eng. Comput. 39(1), 44–50 (2001)

20. Bonesi, M., Proskurin, S.G., Meglinski, I.V.: Imaging of subcutaneous blood vessels and flow velocity profiles by optical coherence tomography. Laser Phys. 20(4), 891–899 (2010)

21. Tsai, S.R., Hamblin, M.R.: Biological effects and medical applications of infrared radiation. J. Photochem. Photobiol. B Biol. 170, 197–207 (2017)

22. Henderson, T.A., Morries, L.D.: Near-infrared photonic energy penetration: can infrared phototherapy effectively reach the human brain? Neuropsychiatric Dis. Treat. 11, 2191 (2015)

23. de Freitas, L.F., Hamblin, M.R.: Proposed mechanisms of photobiomodulation or low-level light therapy. IEEE J. Sel. Top. Quant. Electron. 22(3), 348–364 (2016)

24. Anders, J.J., Lanzafame, R.J. Arany, P.R.: Low-level light/laser therapy versus photo-biomodulation therapy (2015)

25. Kim, N.J., Lim, H.S.: Measurements of absorption coefficients within biological tissue in vitro. In: Proceedings of the 20th Annual International Conference of the IEEE Engineering in Medicine and Biology Society. Vol. 20 Biomedical Engineering Towards the Year 2000 and Beyond (Cat. No. 98CH36286), vol. 6, pp. 2960–2962. IEEE (1998)

26. Ntziachristos, V., Ripoll, J., Weissleder, R.: Would near-infrared fluorescence signals propagate through large human organs for clinical studies? Opt. Lett. 27(5), 333–335 (2002)

27. Jacques, S.L.: Optical properties of biological tissues: a review. Phys. Med. Biol. 58(11), R37 (2013)

28. Wróbel, M.S., Popov, A.P., Bykov, A.V., Kinnunen, M., Jędrzejewska-Szczerska, M., Tuchin, V.V.: Multi-layered tissue head phantoms for noninvasive optical diagnostics. J. Innov. Opt. Health Sci. 8(03), 1541005 (2015)

29. Wróbel, M.S., Popov, A.P., Bykov, A.V., Kinnunen, M., Jędrzejewska-Szczerska, M., Tuchin, V.V.: Measurements of fundamental properties of homogeneous tissue phantoms. J. Biomed. Opt. 20(4), 045004 (2015)

30. International Commission on Non-Ionizing Radiation Protection. ICNIRP statement on light-emitting diodes (LEDs) and laser diodes: implications for hazard assessment. Health Phys. 78(6), 744–752 (2000)

31. Saud, M.S., Ahmed, I., Kumpuniemi, T., Katz, M.: Reconfigurable optical-radio wireless networks: Meeting the most stringent requirements of future communication systems. Trans. Emerg. Telecommun. Technol. 30(2), e3562 (2019)

32. https://www.thorlabs.com/drawings/b1ef4257936da4d4-4B402694-0F84-14D6-72D3E2437 F4E3C75/M810L3-SpecSheet.pdf
33. https://www.thorlabs.com/drawings/b1ef4257936da4d4-4B402694-0F84-14D6-72D3E2437 F4E3C75/DC2200-Manual.pdf
34. https://www.thorlabs.com/thorproduct.cfm?partnumber=SM2F32-B
35. https://www.thorlabs.com/drawings/b1ef4257936da4d4-4B402694-0F84-14D6-72D3E2437 F4E3C75/APD120A_M-Manual.pdf
36. https://assets.lia.org/s3fs-public/pdf/ansi-standards/samples/ANSI%20Z136.1_sample.pdf
37. Ahmed, I., Kumpuniemi, T., Katz, M.: A hybrid optical-radio wireless network concept for the hospital of the future (2018)

Estimation of Skin Conductance Response Through Adaptive Filtering

Pietro Savazzi[1(✉)] [ID], Floriana Vasile[1], Natascia Brondino[2] [ID], Marco Vercesi[2], and Pierluigi Politi[2] [ID]

[1] Department of Electrical, Computer and Biomedical Engineering,
University of Pavia, Pavia, Italy
`pietro.savazzi@unipv.it, vasilefloriana@gmail.com`
[2] Department of Brain and Behavioral Sciences, University of Pavia, Pavia, Italy
`{natascia.brondino,pierluigi.politi}@unipv.it,`
`marco.vercesi01@universitadipavia.it`

Abstract. The importance of medical wearable sensors is increasing in aiding both diagnostic and therapeutic protocols, in a wide area of health applications. Among them, the acquisition and analysis of electrodermal activity (EDA) may help in detecting seizures and different human emotional states. Nonnegative deconvolution represents an important step needed for decomposing the measured galvanic skin response (GSR) in its tonic and phasic components. In particular, the phasic component, also known as skin conductance response (SCR), is related to the sympathetic nervous system (SNS) activity, since it can be modeled as the linear convolution between the SCR driver events, modeled by sparse impulse signals, with an impulse response representing the sudomotor SNS innervation. In this paper, we propose a novel method for implementing this deconvolution by an adaptive filter, determined by solving a linear prediction problem, which results independent on the impulse response parameters, usually represented by sampling the biexponential Bateman function. The performance of the proposed approach is evaluated by using both synthetic and experimental data.

Keywords: Galvanic skin response · Electrodermal activity · Skin conductance response · Adaptive filter · Wearable sensor

1 Introduction

Galvanic skin response (GSR) may be recorded by measuring the conductance variations over a person's skin in response to sweat secretions. This electrodermal activity (EDA) is due to sweat secretion which alters the electrical property of the skin [4], in response to emotional states like arousal [13], since the GSR signal carries significant information related to neuron firing [10].

By means of modern wearable devices, like the Emaptica E4 [9] bracelet or the Affectiva Q sensor [8], it is possible measuring GSR signals during everyday

L. Mucchi et al. (Eds.): BODYNETS 2019, LNICST 297, pp. 206–217, 2019.
https://doi.org/10.1007/978-3-030-34833-5_17

human activities, allowing interesting medical application especially, but not only, in the field of psychiatry for aiding mental health diagnosis and therapies [12].

A GSR signal may be represented by the sum of two different components [2,6,7]:

- a tonic component, also known as skin conductance level (SCL), a slowly varying signal which is not caused by instantaneous external stimuli but it could be related to the level of attention;
- a phasic or skin conductance response (SCR) component which is caused by sympathetic nervous system (SNS) sporadic stimuli and it usually lasts for a few seconds.

Summarizing, while the SCL represents a measure of the complete absorption of sweat in the human' skin, SCR signals measure discrete and sporadic sweat production events driven by external stimuli caused by user's excitement or any other emotional state variation. Following this reasoning, the primary objective of EDA signal analysis is to extract the SCR components in order to firstly identifying and, in a second step, classifying the different emotional states.

The extraction of SCR events may bu pursued by empirical peak detection techniques that they not take into accounts the effects of closely superimposing SCR responses. For this reason, many literature works focus on deconvolution techniques, usually taking into account nonnegative constraints and signal pre-analysis in order to jointly estimate both SCL and SCR components, see [2] and references therein.

Recently, the sparse nature of SCR signals suggests to use compressed sensing (CS) techniques to determine the driven event impulses by mean of convex optimization [6,7], often exploiting CS reconstruction algorithm constraints for the joint estimation of the tonic and phasic signals.

Since CS reconstruction algorithms are mainly based in convex optimization analysis performed offline after the signal acquisition, in this work we are mainly interested in looking for alternative solutions that could be easily implemented in wearable devices able to provide real-time outputs. These outcomes may be useful on order to rapidly use this information for therapeutic purposes like behavioral interventions in several mental health disorders.

On this purpose, we started from more traditional deconvolution techniques by deriving an adaptive filter which is independent on the specific SCR impulse model parameters, by anyway using an optimization criterion based on the signal sparsity.

The rest of this paper is organized as follows: Sect. 2 is devoted to describe the GSR signal model used in this work, while in Sect. 3 we describe the proposed algorithm derivation. Finally, after exposing the obtained simulated and experimental data results, respectively in Sects. 4 and 5, some final concluding comments and perspective of future works end the paper.

2   EDA Signal Generation Model

2.1   Continuous-Time Model

Following the GSR signal decomposition in its tonic and phasic components, the acquired sensor signal in the continuous-time domain may be represented as:

$$y(t) = h_{ct}(t) * x(t) + b(t) + n(t) \tag{1}$$

where the phasic component is modeled ad the linear convolution between the unknown sparse driver $x(t)$, corresponding to the sudomotor SNS innervation, and the impulse response $h_{ct}(t)$; $b(t)$ denotes the tonic slowly varying component, while $n(t)$ represents the electrical thermal noise contribution, modeled as additive white Gaussian noise (AWGN).

The impulse reponse $h_{ct}(t)$ is commonly modeled by the so called Bateman function [3, 15]:

$$h_{ct}(t) = g \left(e^{-\frac{t}{\tau_1}} - e^{-\frac{t}{\tau_2}} \right) \tag{2}$$

where g is a gain factor, while the authors of [15] used the following parameter values for all the analyzed data in their paper: $\tau_1 = 0.75$ s, and $\tau_2 = 2$ s.

2.2   Discrete-Time Model

In the following, we consider the discrete-time equivalent of Eq. (1)

$$\mathbf{y} = \mathbf{h} * \mathbf{x} + \mathbf{b} + \mathbf{n} \tag{3}$$

by taking sequences of length NT_s seconds, where N is length of $\mathbf{y}$ in number of samples, and T_s the sampling time.

The continuous impulse response of Eq. (2) becomes

$$h(n) \equiv h_{ct}(nT_s) = g \left(e^{-\frac{nT_s}{\tau_1}} - e^{-\frac{nT_s}{\tau_2}} \right) \tag{4}$$

with $\mathbf{h} = [h(0), h(1), ..., h(N-1)]$. Usually the EDA sensor output is sampled at a frequency $\frac{1}{T_s} \geq 4$ Hz.

3   Adaptive Filtering

3.1   Deconvolution Filter

The SCR impulse response in Eq. (4) may be represented as an infinite impulse response (IIR) linear system whose z-transform is

$$H(z) = \frac{gz^{-1}\left(e^{-\alpha_1} + e^{-\alpha_2}\right)}{1 - \left(e^{-\alpha_1} + e^{-\alpha_2}\right)z^{-1} + e^{-\alpha_1-\alpha_2}z^{-2}} \tag{5}$$

where $\alpha_1 = \frac{T_s}{\tau_1}$, $\alpha_2 = \frac{T_s}{\tau_2}$.

According to Eq. (5) and initially neglecting, as usually done in the cited literature, both the tonic and noise components, the deconvolution of the EDA signal $y(n)$ can be performed by filtering each measured sequence $\mathbf{y}$ by the following finite impulse response (FIR) filter

$$\mathbf{b} = [1, - \left(e^{-\alpha_1} + e^{-\alpha_2}\right) z^{-1}, e^{-\alpha_1 - \alpha_2} z^{-2}] \tag{6}$$

3.2   Adaptive Filter Derivation

The discrete-time difference equation corresponding to (5) can be written as

$$\beta x(n-1) = y(n) + w(1)y(n-1) + w(2)y(n-2) \tag{7}$$

where

$$\beta = g\left(e^{-\alpha_1} + e^{-\alpha_2}\right)$$
$$w(1) = -\left(e^{-\alpha_1} + e^{-\alpha_2}\right)$$
$$w(2) = e^{-\alpha_1 - \alpha_2}$$

Since the actual shape of the impulse $h(n)$ in unknown, and the real SCR response could be generated by overlapped pulses with different time lengths, see for instance how in [6] the same problem is faced by a multiscale analysis, we may assume a filter length equal to $p+1$ that could be greater than 3. Following this reasoning, we may define a new difference equation

$$\beta x(n-1) = y(n) + \sum_{i=1}^{p} w(p)y(n-p) \tag{8}$$

In order to look for a sparse solution for $x(n)$ we may find the filter coefficients $w(k)$ which minimize

$$E\left\{x^2(n)\right\}, \tag{9}$$

by computing

$$E\left\{\frac{\partial x^2(n-1)}{\partial w(k)}\right\} = 0 \tag{10}$$

where E denotes the expectation operator, and $\frac{\partial}{\partial w(k)}$ the partial derivative with respect to the filter coefficient $w(k)$.

The solution of (10), using (8), is given by the following Wiener-Hopf equations [5]

$$\mathbf{w} = \mathbf{R}_y^{-1}\mathbf{r}_y \tag{11}$$

where

$$\mathbf{w} = [w(1), w(2), ...w(p)], \tag{12}$$

$$\mathbf{r}_y = [r_y(1), r_y(2), ..., r_y(p)], \tag{13}$$

and

$$\mathbf{R}_y = \begin{bmatrix} r_y(0) & \cdots & r_y(p-1) \\ \vdots & \ddots & \vdots \\ r_y(p-1) & \cdots & r_y(0) \end{bmatrix} \tag{14}$$

where $r_y(k) = E\{y(n)y(n-k)\}$ is the autocorrelation of the EDA signal $y(t)$.

It is interesting to note that the constraint in (8), derived from (5), (7), and corresponding to $w(0) = 1$, actually makes the Wiener-Hopf solution equivalent to one of a linear predictor of order p.

The filter coefficients may be computed by solving Eq. (11) over a suitable time window, or, with a lower computational complexity, by the correspondent stochastic gradient solution

$$\mathbf{w}_{n+1} = \mathbf{w}_n + \mu x(n-1)\mathbf{y}_n \tag{15}$$

where $\mathbf{w}_n$ denotes the filter coefficient vector at the discrete time instant n, $\mathbf{y}_n = [y(n), y(n-1), \cdots, y(n-p)]$, and μ is a suitable step size.

Finally, the sparse impulse signal $x(n)$ may be computed by (8), while the nonnegative constraint has been taken into account by setting $x(n) = 0$ when $x(n) = m < 0$, by considering the tonic signal $b(n) = -m$.

4   Simulation Results

For synthetic data experiments, we have taken into account the generation model, described in [7], which considers a baseline component, i.e., the tonic one, inspired by the fact that wearable sensor movements may cause changes in the measured EDA signal.

Considering the discrete-time SCR signal $\mathbf{x}$ of (3) with a length of N samples, we may assume a number of ideal pulses different from zero equal to s, which denotes the SCR driven signal sparsity. According to this premise, the SCR ideal pulses lie in the set

$$X(s, \delta) = \{\mathbf{x} | \mathbf{x} \in \mathbb{R}^N, \|\mathbf{x} - \mathbf{x}_s\|_1 \le \delta\} \tag{16}$$

where δ is a suitable constant threshold, and $\mathbf{x}_s$ has exactly s non zeros elements corresponding to the s largest components of $\mathbf{x}$. $\| \cdot \|_1$ represents the L^1 norm.

In a similar manner, it is possible to define the baseline signal $\mathbf{b}$ to lie in the set

$$B(c, \lambda) = \{\mathbf{b} | \mathbf{b} \in \mathbb{R}^N, \|\mathbf{D}\mathbf{b} - \mathbf{D}\mathbf{b}_c\|_1 \le \lambda\} \tag{17}$$

where c and λ have a similar meaning to respectively s and δ, and $\mathbf{D}$ is the pairwise difference matrix defined in [7], so that $\mathbf{D}\mathbf{b}$ corresponds to the first discrete derivative of $\mathbf{b}$. Moreover, the parameter c denotes the number of baseline jumps due to sensor movements.

4.1 Simulation Parameters

We have considered multiple repetitions of the EDA signal $\mathbf{y}$ with a length equal to 400 samples and the sampling frequency equal to 4 Hz, corresponding to a time duration of 100 s. The parameters λ, δ of (16), (17), have been all set to 0.01, and the added Gaussian noise corresponds to a signal-to-noise ratio of 15 dB. We have found that the value of the adaptive filter order p which gets the best simulated and experimental results is in the interval $(2, 10)$. The following results have been obtained by setting $p = 10$.

4.2 Mean-Square Error Performance

Since we know the event signal $x(n)$, in order to assess the algorithm performance for the simulated data we may use the average mean-square error (MSE), defined as

$$\xi = \frac{E\left\{(\mathbf{x} - \hat{\mathbf{x}})^2\right\}}{E\left\{\mathbf{x}^2\right\}} \tag{18}$$

with $\hat{\mathbf{x}}$ the estimated event signal.

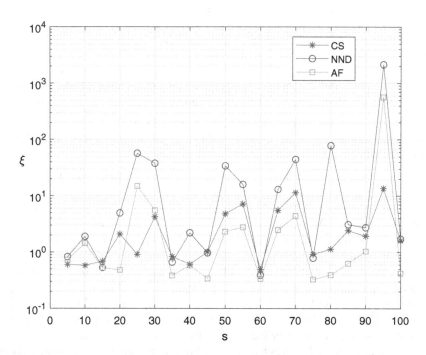

Fig. 1. ξ versus the number of event pulses s, $c = 1$, CS: compressed sensing, NND: nonnegative deconvolution, AF: adaptive filter

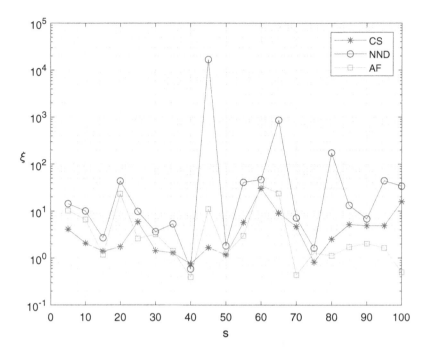

Fig. 2. ξ versus the number of event pulses s, $c = 5$, CS: compressed sensing, NND: nonnegative deconvolution, AF: adaptive filter

In Figs. 1, 2, 3 and 4, the average MSE versus the number of sparsity degree s of the SCR event signal $\mathbf{x}$ is shown for the three compared algorithms:

- CS: the compressed sensing algorithm presented in [7];
- NND: the nonnegative deconvolution filtering technique described in [3];
- AF: the adaptive filter method proposed in this work.

The EDA synthetic signal has been generated by considering positive random values for the parameters τ_1, τ_2 with their means equal to respectively 10 and 1, while for the two algorithms that assume to know the information about the impulse response $h(n)$, i.e., CS and NND, $\tau_1 = 10$, and $\tau_2 = 1$. In this way, we have considered a sort of pulse shape variations that could better represent the real data behavior.

The performance of the proposed algorithm looks better, especially for lower values of c and higher ones for the sparsity degree s. It is important to note that since the synthetic model represents the main assumptions used by the CS algorithm, we think that this can justify why the CS algorithm performs better in some cases, especially for lower values of s. In the next section, we will consider a real data analysis in order to get more insights about the algorithm comparison.

5   Experimental Data Results

In order to test the described algorithm with real-world EDA signals, we have considered a video and reading stimuli experiment. In more details, the experi-

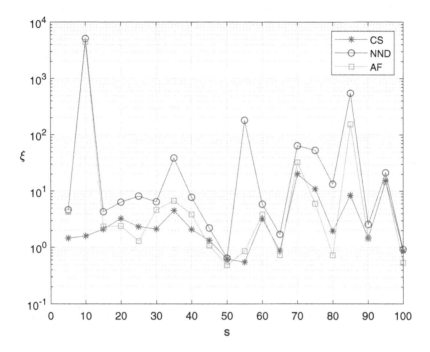

Fig. 3. ξ versus the number of event pulses s, $c = 10$, CS: compressed sensing, NND: nonnegative deconvolution, AF: adaptive filter

ment has been conducted in the three following step: a first neutral EDA measurement without stimuli, a second period of measurement with an erotic content video as stimulus, and, finally, the subjects under test were asked to read a brief erotic story.

5.1   Qualitative Results

As a first look at the experimental results, we consider the measured EDA signal, and the corresponding algorithm outputs, of one of the subjects participating to the experiment.

From Figs. 5, 6 and 7, it seems that the proposed adaptive filter solution produces an estimated event signal which is more sparse with respect to the estimates of the other two algorithms.

5.2   Quantitative Performance Evaluation

In order to verify if each of the two different non-neutral stimuli outputs a different EDA signal, we have counted the estimated number of SCR events by taking the mean of the obtained responses, for each subject under test.

In Fig. 8, it can be seen that all the three techniques are able to well discriminate the video stimulus from the others, for the four tested subjects. The

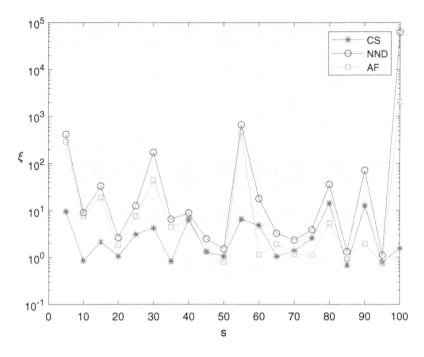

Fig. 4. ξ versus the number of event pulses s, $c = 20$, CS: compressed sensing, NND: nonnegative deconvolution, AF: adaptive filter

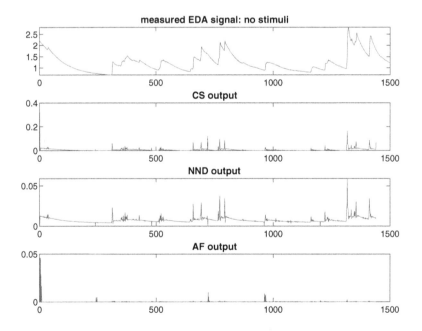

Fig. 5. Example of a subject measured and estimated responses without stimuli

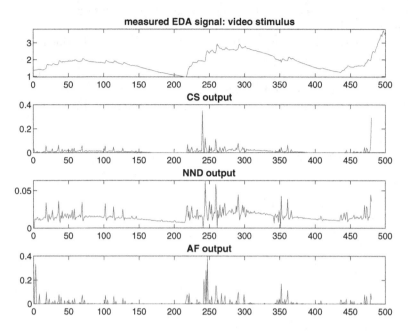

Fig. 6. Example of a subject measured and estimated responses with a video stimulus

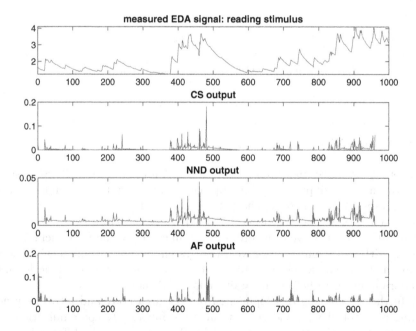

Fig. 7. Example of a subject measured and estimated responses with a reading stimulus

proposed techniques seems to be able to also address a difference between the neutral and reading stimulus.

Ongoing works will be devoted to better characterize this classification ability by considering alternative methods for counting the number of event pulses: as an example, a threshold with a more sophisticated method to count the number of pulses could provide more feasible results. Possible ways to face this problem may be derived from the spike signal processing literature [11].

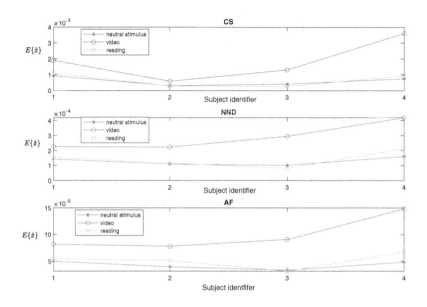

Fig. 8. Estimated SCR response mean per each subject

6   Conclusion

In this work, we have presented a novel method for estimating the SCR signal events through an adaptive filtering approach, which results independent on the impulse response parameters. The performance of the proposed approach has been proven by using both synthetic and experimental data.

Interesting perspective of future research lines may come from including the novel algorithm in a multi sensor wearable system, where the different measured outputs may be combined and processed, for instance, by a machine learning procedure in order to help medical diagnoses and therapies [12].

A further interesting development, from the area-body and intra-body networking point of view, could come from using intra-body communication systems, like [1,14], in order to optimize the collecting process of differently posed sensor measurements.

References

1. Banou, S., et al.: Beamforming galvanic coupling signals for IOMT implant-to-relay communication. IEEE Sen. J. 1 (2019). https://doi.org/10.1109/JSEN.2018.2886561
2. Benedek, M., Kaernbach, C.: A continuous measure of phasic electrodermal activity. J. Neurosci. Methods **190**(1), 80–91 (2010)
3. Benedek, M., Kaernbach, C.: Decomposition of skin conductance data by means of nonnegative deconvolution. Psychophysiology **47**(4), 647–658 (2010)
4. Boucsein, W.: Electrodermal Activity. Springer, New York (2012). https://doi.org/10.1007/978-1-4614-1126-0
5. Haykin, S.: Adaptive Filter Theory, 4th edn. Prentice Hall, Upper Saddle River (2002)
6. Hernando-Gallego, F., Luengo, D., Arts-Rodrguez, A.: Feature extraction of galvanic skin responses by nonnegative sparse deconvolution. IEEE J. Biomed. Health Inform. **22**(5), 1385–1394 (2018). https://doi.org/10.1109/JBHI.2017.2780252
7. Jain, S., Oswal, U., Xu, K.S., Eriksson, B., Haupt, J.: A compressed sensing based decomposition of electrodermal activity signals. IEEE Trans. Biomed. Eng. **64**(9), 2142–2151 (2017). https://doi.org/10.1109/TBME.2016.2632523
8. Kappas, A., Kster, D., Basedow, C., Dente, P.: A validation study of the affective q-sensor in different social laboratory situations (2013)
9. McCarthy, C., Pradhan, N., Redpath, C., Adler, A.: Validation of the empatica E4 wristband. In: 2016 IEEE EMBS International Student Conference (ISC), pp. 1–4, May 2016. https://doi.org/10.1109/EMBSISC.2016.7508621
10. Nishiyama, T., Sugenoya, J., Matsumoto, T., Iwase, S., Mano, T.: Irregular activation of individual sweat glands in human sole observed by a videomicroscopy. Auton. Neurosci. **88**(1–2), 117–126 (2001)
11. Park, I.M., Seth, S., Paiva, A.R.C., Li, L., Principe, J.C.: Kernel methods on spike train space for neuroscience: a tutorial. IEEE Signal Process. Mag. **30**(4), 149–160 (2013). https://doi.org/10.1109/MSP.2013.2251072
12. Sano, A., et al.: Identifying objective physiological markers and modifiable behaviors for self-reported stress and mental health status using wearable sensors and mobile phones: observational study. J. Med. Internet Res. **20**(6), e210 (2018)
13. Sidis, B.: The nature and cause of the galvanic phenomenon. J. Abnorm. Psychol. **5**(2), 6974 (1910). https://doi.org/10.1037/h0075352
14. Swaminathan, M., Vizziello, A., Duong, D., Savazzi, P., Chowdhury, K.R.: Beamforming in the body: energy-efficient and collision-free communication for implants. In: IEEE INFOCOM 2017 - IEEE Conference on Computer Communications, pp. 1–9, May 2017. https://doi.org/10.1109/INFOCOM.2017.8056989
15. Wright, J.J., et al.: Toward an integrated continuum model of cerebral dynamics: the cerebral rhythms, synchronous oscillation and cortical stability. BioSystems **63**(1–3), 71–88 (2001)

Capacitive Body-Coupled Communication in the 400–500 MHz Frequency Band

Robin Benarrouch[1,2,3(✉)], Arno Thielens[3,4], Andreia Cathelin[1],
Antoine Frappé[2], Andreas Kaiser[2], and Jan Rabaey[3]

[1] STMicroelectronics, Technology and Design Platforms, 38920 Crolles, France
`robin.benarrouch@st.com`
[2] Univ. Lille, CNRS, Centrale Lille, ISEN, Univ. Valenciennes,
UMR 8520 - IEMN, 59000 Lille, France
[3] University of California Berkeley, Berkeley, CA 94704, USA
[4] Ghent University, imec, Department of Information Technology,
9052 Ghent, Belgium

Abstract. One approach to enable wireless communication between body-worn nodes is to use capacitive body-coupled communication (C-BCC). This technique, which uses capacitive electrodes as transducing elements, has previously been demonstrated at relatively low frequencies (<200 MHz) and hence also low bandwidths. This work presents a theoretical analysis of wireless C-BCC, between body worn electrodes at higher frequencies (420–510 MHz), offering the potential for higher data rates. The theory is confirmed both by numerical simulations (performed on a human body phantom), and actual wireless communication between two prototypes on the arm of a real human.

Keywords: Body area network · Capacitive Body Coupled Communication · Radio frequency · Propagation

1 Introduction

Body Area Networks (BAN) are an attractive field of research with a wide variety of applications, including medical- and wellness-oriented systems. A standard for wireless radio-frequency (RF) communication in BANs exists [11]. In this standard, communication within BANs are split in four categories: (1) on-body to in-body to enable the communication with an implanted device; (2) implant to implant communication, (3) on-body to off-body to upload data to a base station for instance, and (4) on-body to on-body communication allowing data exchange between two points over the human body [11].

An interesting concept within BANs, the Human Intranet, introduced in [19], describes the minimum requirements to implement a network dedicated to the human body. The dynamic variations of shape and geometry of such a network raise the need for coverage robustness and reliability. As the network

© ICST Institute for Computer Sciences, Social Informatics and Telecommunications Engineering 2019
Published by Springer Nature Switzerland AG 2019. All Rights Reserved
L. Mucchi et al. (Eds.): BODYNETS 2019, LNICST 297, pp. 218–235, 2019.
https://doi.org/10.1007/978-3-030-34833-5_18

will be connecting a diverse assortment of sensors and actuators (movement, temperature sensors, smart prosthetics, insulin pumps...) with different needs in terms of data rate and latency, a target of multiple tens of Mbps is required in terms of aggregated data rate. Ultimately, the communications must be secured due to the sensitive nature of the transmitted information.

Multiple technical solutions, like standardized RF (Bluetooth...) [6,11], ultrasonic [4], optical [8] or Body Coupled Communication (BCC) [3] could be considered to implement such a system. This manuscript will focus on the latter and more specifically on Capacitive Body Coupled Communication (C-BCC), analyzing and exploring its propagation mechanism. One of the main advantages of C-BCC is the convenient form factor of the on-body capacitive electrodes used for this technology in comparison to on-body antennas which operate at the same frequency. Consequently, this work can be situated in the fourth category described in the IEEE BAN standard [11]. Several papers have already studied and described C-BCC at lower frequencies (below 200 MHz) [1,2,5,13,14,17], with relatively large electrode form factor [2,5,13,14]. Only [13] performed electromagnetic simulations to analyze the impact of the reference electrode on the channel loss in a single on-body configuration. However, up to date, most systems are either impractical for real on-body usage or operate at a carrier frequency that is not high enough to provide the necessary bandwidth and data rates required for the Human Intranet. Therefore, this manuscript focuses on exploring C-BCC using relatively compact electrodes at carrier frequencies higher than the state of the art. Pushing RF communication to higher frequencies does come at a cost: propagation distances will become larger relative to the smaller wavelengths, which in general leads to higher propagation losses at a fixed (on-body) distance [18]. Additionally, the tissues that make up the human body show RF losses that increase over frequency [10]. These considerations led us to target a frequency range of 420–510 MHz offering a good compromise between bandwidth availability and on-body propagation loss [11].

The novelties and main contributions of this manuscript are the following: first, a demonstration of C-BCC at a higher frequency range of investigation than what has previously been demonstrated in literature: 420–510 MHz, second this study on C-BCC considers the theory, numerical simulations, prototyping, measurements and correlates the results.

2   Theory and State of the Art

Capacitive coupling can occur between at least two pieces of conductive material which are not connected together, one used as a reference (called the "reference electrode") and the other(s) connected to the signal feed (referred as the "signal electrode(s)"), see Fig. 1. When another electrode pair is in proximity of such a pair of electrodes there will be coupling between both capacitive electrode pairs. This coupling occurs via several paths. In C-BCC the most common configuration is a stacked architecture where the signal electrode is in contact or in close vicinity to the surface of the body while the reference electrode is stacked on top, both electrically insulated by a dielectric material (see Fig. 1).

A very common way of representing C-BCC in this point of view, is to assume a capacitive return path between both reference electrodes (one on each end, the transmitter (Tx) and the receiver (Rx)) which are floating and an external reference plane, usually the earth ground, as pictured in Fig. 1. In [7] the authors investigated and highlighted the conditions in terms of frequency range and distances under which no power is radiated out of the human body in this configuration. In other words, the conditions where the assumption illustrated in Fig. 1 is applicable. The authors of [7] concluded that the frequency of operation must be below 21 MHz (which is not compatible with the envisioned project highlighted in Sect. 1) in order to keep the communication confined within the human body.

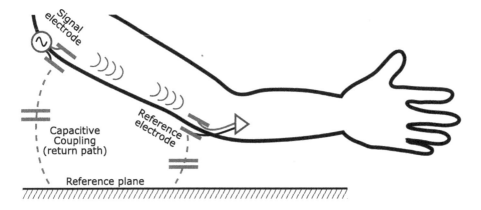

Fig. 1. Common representation of Capacitive Body Coupled Communication mechanism.

Besides this capacitive coupling, there is also electromagnetic wave propagation between both pairs of electrodes. In this aspect, the electrodes can be described as electrically small dipoles at wavelengths that are relatively large in comparison to the electrode dimensions [3]. In free space, there exists a theoretical formulation for the magnitude of the electric field E_z in the plane (XY) (see Fig. 2) at a distance r from such a source (dipole parallel to the Z axis in a Cartesian coordinate system at $z = 0$) [3]:

$$|E_Z| = \left| \frac{I \cdot dz \cdot k^3}{4\pi\omega\epsilon_0} i \left[\frac{1}{r} + i \cdot \frac{1}{r^2} - \frac{1}{k} \cdot \frac{1}{r^3} \right] \cdot e^{-ikr} \right| \tag{1}$$

With I the current fed to the dipole, dz the length of the dipole, k the magnitude of the wave vector, ω the angular frequency and ϵ_0 the permittivity of free space. When r is relatively small, the $1/r^3$ term is dominant. On the contrary, the term $1/r$ is dominant further away from the source.

The electromagnetic fields surrounding such a small dipole on an infinite conductive surface located at z values below the Z-coordinate of the bottom

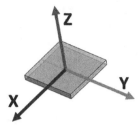

Fig. 2. Parallel plate capacitor in free space centered in a Cartesian coordinate system.

electrode, see Fig. 2, can be expressed theoretically [15,16]. The amplitude of the electric field strength (Ez) at the interface between air and the conducting surface in the direction parallel to the dipole (the dominant polarization [15], when the receiver is also located at the air-conductor interface, the Z direction in Fig. 2) at a distance r from the transmitting dipole can be expressed using [3]:

$$|E_Z| = 2|k \cdot S \cdot \frac{1}{r} + i \cdot \frac{1}{r^2} - \frac{1}{k} \cdot \frac{1}{r^3}| \qquad (2)$$

where S is a term that depends on the frequency and the dielectric properties of the conducting surface. The first term in $1/r$ corresponds to surface wave propagation, while those in $1/r^2$ and $1/r^3$ highlight the induction field and quasi-static coupling respectively. By plotting the weight of those different propagation mechanisms at the frequency range of interest (i.e. 400–500 MHz), it is clear that the surface wave becomes dominant when the distance considered is greater than 13–15 cm. The results are shown in Fig. 3 for S computed for muscle tissue with parameters obtained from the Gabriel database [10].

The theories and investigation on C-BCC described above suggest that we will operate using a communication mechanism dominated by surface wave propagation. This can be advantageous as the communication is less sensitive to changes in the return path. In addition, [7] shows the limits of the representation shown in Fig. 1, and highlights that our electrodes cannot be modeled as an electric circuit only but requires a full-wave electromagnetic simulation to describe the transmission.

3   Materials and Methods

3.1   Numerical Simulations

In order to verify whether the proposed theory [3,15,16] corresponds to transmission between two body-worn electrodes in our studied frequency band (420–510 MHz), we executed two types of numerical simulations: (1) simulations with electrodes in free-space, and (2) simulations with electrodes on a so-called

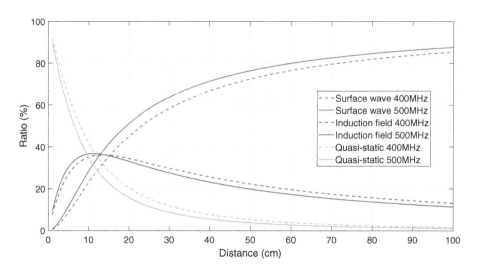

Fig. 3. Contribution of each mechanism as a proportion of the total electric field for 400 MHz (dotted lines) and 500 MHz (solid lines).

phantom. A phantom is a proxy for the human body; in this case, we chose to work with a cuboid that mimics the limbs of the human body.

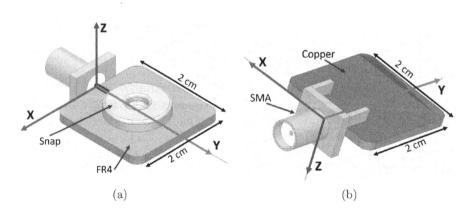

Fig. 4. 3D electrode model. (a) top view, (b) bottom view.

Figure 4 shows the model of the studied electrodes. The dielectric properties assigned to the different layers were taken from software Ansoft HFSS. The model consisted out of a $2 \times 2\,\text{cm}^2$ FR4 (Relative permittivity = 4.4, Relative Permeability = 1 Bulk conductivity = 0 S/m) board substrate, 1.6 mm thick, covered by a 35 μm copper (Relative permittivity = 1, Relative Permeability = 0.99,

Bulk conductivity $= 5.8 \cdot 10^7$ S/m) layer on one side. On the other face, a stainless steel (Relative permittivity $= 1$, Relative Permeability $= 1$, Bulk conductivity $= 1.1 \cdot 10^6$ S/m) snap connector with a diameter of 12 mm and 1 mm in height was glued. The snap was connected to the central conductor of a side-mounted SMA connector modeled in brass (Relative permittivity $= 1$, Relative Permeability $= 1$, Bulk conductivity $= 1.5 \cdot 10^7$ S/m), while the connectors ground pads were connected to the copper layer on top of the FR4 board. The SMA and the snap were connected together with a copper wire of 0.8 mm in diameter. The female snap connector was connected to its male counterpart (also modeled as stainless steel). This male snap connector was in its turn connected to a wet electrode (modeled from a standard pre-gelled disposable medical electrode from Covidien: Kendall Arbo H124SH [21]) which was modeled as a conductive dielectric with properties and water (Relative permittivity $= 81$, Relative Permeability $= 0.99$, Bulk conductivity $= 0.01$ S/m).

The phantom is a cuboid shape, with a 50×50 mm^2 square section and a length of 4 m (see Fig. 5). This latter value was selected, so that no simulation artifacts from the edges are observed. The section dimensions were chosen to represent a human arm. The phantom was assigned frequency-dependent dielectric properties corresponding to muscle in the Gabriel database [10].

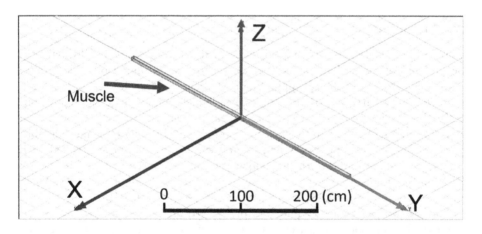

Fig. 5. 3D representation of the cuboid shaped phantom.

In our simulations, the elements of interest (electrodes and arm) are surrounded by a box of air of the following size: $3 \times 3 \times 6$ m^3. These electrodes were excited by a lumped port with impedance 50 Ω and voltage 1 V, placed in between the coaxial conductor and the mantle of the SMA connector. The FEM method implemented in Ansoft HFSS was used to calculate the electromagnetic fields surrounding the electrodes when they were fed a voltage at a frequency of 300–600 MHz.

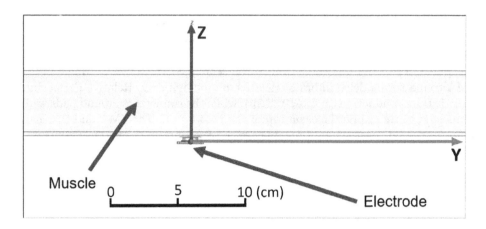

Fig. 6. Electrode positioned on muscle (YZ) plane.

The frequencies of interest were set every 50 MHz from 300 MHz to 600 MHz. In parallel, an interpolating frequency sweep over the same range with 10 MHz steps was enabled. We retained values in the 420–510 MHz frequency band.

3.2   Measurement Set-Up

In order to measure the attenuation under realistic conditions, a fully battery-powered prototype was implemented. Battery-powered operation is key for a standalone wireless on-body application. Moreover, this solution allows for a separation between the two reference planes, which cannot be achieved by connecting those with two cables to the same measurement instrument [1], even with the introduction of baluns in the measurement circuit. In order to achieve flexibility, adaptability and repeatability the signal was generated and controlled with a sub-GHz radio available with the following evaluation kit: STEVAL-FKI433V2 [22] from STMicroelectronics. The signal type was a continuous wave (CW) at a frequency swept from 420 MHz to 510 MHz by steps of 10 MHz.

The electrodes (connector and skin pre-gelled) are shown in Fig. 7.

Lastly, the on-body measurements were performed along the arm of a male subject, standing still, and arms along the body. The transmitter (Tx) was positioned on the left wrist. The receiver (Rx) was placed on the same arm, at a distance d from Tx. The covered range was the following: 5 cm to 55 cm by steps of 5 cm. For every step, the received power at the Rx was computed by collecting 220 samples for frequencies from 420–510 MHz in steps of 10 MHz. These measurements were split for each harmonic frequency and fed into a log-linear least-square fit according to the following channel loss (L) model [3]:

$$L = \begin{cases} L_0 & d = d_0 \\ L_0 + \alpha_0(d - d_0) & d_0 < d < d_1 \\ L_1 + \alpha_1(d - d_1) & d_1 < d \end{cases} \quad (3)$$

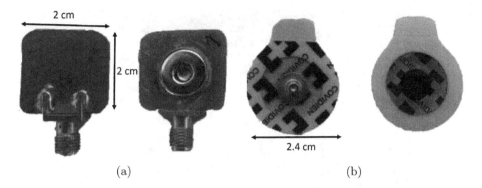

Fig. 7. C-BCC electrode. (a) connector (2×2 cm), (b) skin pre-gelled.

with d the inter-electrode distance, L_0 the baseline channel loss at the shortest measured inter-electrode distance (d_0, 5 cm in this case), d_1 is the boundary distance where the transition between the quasi-static (QS) and surface wave regimes occur. Following the analysis shown in Fig. 3, a boundary distance $d_1 = 15$ cm was determined for the studied frequencies on muscle. Hence, this value was chosen in the fit to determine the channel losses per unit distance α_0 and α_1 in both regimes.

The setup, hardware and measurement conditions were strictly identical to the one described in [20].

4   Results and Discussion

4.1   Free Space Simulation Results

In order to understand the electrode behavior, a single electrode was simulated in the air. The simulation parameters were those described in Sect. 3.1. All plots and figure are in the plane (YZ) (see Fig. 5) since the electrodes are symmetric (except for the SMA) and such representation eases the comparison with the simulation on the phantom.

Figure 8(a) shows the electric field (E-field) radiated by the electrode in air at 450 MHz. The magnitude of the E-field is maximum in the center and fades as the distance increases. Figure 8(b) shows the E-field strength along the positive Y-axis together with two fits: a near field approximation using $1/r^3$ and a far field approximation using $1/r$.

According to theory, the electrode should behave as a small electric dipole in free space with electric field strength according to Eq. (1) with the $1/r^3$ term dominating the near field and the $1/r$ term dominating the far-field behavior. The simulation results highlighted in Fig. 8(b) show a good agreement with the theory presented in Eq. 1 since there is a good correspondence between the fits and the simulation results Fig. 8(a) shows that the magnitude of the E-field is the greatest in the direction parallel to the conductive material (XY plane).

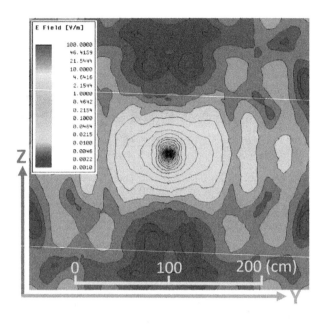

(a)

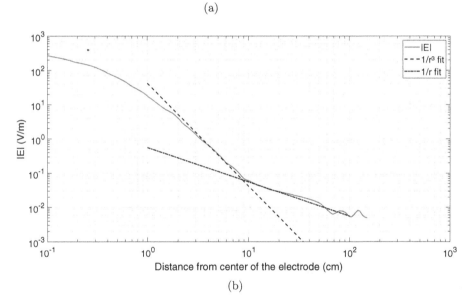

(b)

Fig. 8. E-field radiated by one electrode in air at 450 MHz, (a) in the (YZ) plane, (b) along the positive Y-axis.

Hence, this is the direction of optimal communication. This is in line with the envisioned communication strategy outlined in Fig. 1 and thus shows that these electrodes are good candidates for C-BCC.

4.2 "On-phantom" Simulation Results

The "on-body" simulations were based on the same configuration as the free-space simulation for comparison purposes. A cuboid modeled as muscle was added as described in Sect. 3.1. The electrode was positioned in contact below the muscle, as described Fig. 6.

Figure 9 represents the E-field in the (YZ) plane while a single electrode was positioned on-body at 450 MHz. From this figure, we can observe that in the Y direction the E-field travels further distance than in free-space. For example at 50 cm from the center of the electrode the E-field strength at 450 MHz is 0.26 V/m on the phantom and 0.01 V/m in free space, for the same input power.

As the simulation was conducted in the exact same condition than in free-space, it is clear that the E-field propagates along the phantom model. The electric fields also penetrate the muscle phantom. Figure 9 demonstrates that the fields inside the phantom are out of phase with the ones outside the phantom. The minima of the internal E-fields occur at those propagation distances where the external fields show a local maxima and vice versa.

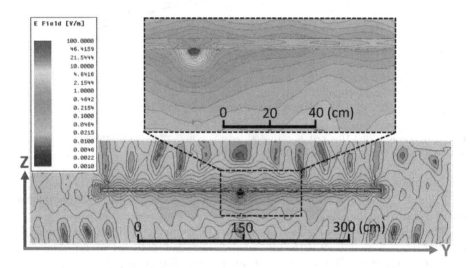

Fig. 9. E-field radiated by a single electrode on muscle at 450 MHz in the (YZ) plane.

For the standard phantom size ($50 \times 50 \times 4000\,\text{mm}^3$), multiple frequencies of excitation from 420 MHz to 510 MHz by steps of 30 MHz were simulated. We performed a comparison between theory (Eq. 2) and simulation of an electrode positioned on a phantom modeled as a cuboid shape with muscle dielectric properties. These results are highlighted Fig. 10 which shows the electric field along the Y-axis for the specified frequency set. Additionally, two fits are shown for the results at 450 MHz, $1/r$ for the surface wave and $1/r^3$ for the quasi-static field.

The far-field electric field at 450 MHz showed a $1/r$ dependency (Fig. 10) and matches the theory. However the simulation in the near field is only accurate in a very limited range (3 to 5 cm). This could be explained by the electrode's edge positioned at 1 cm from the center, whereas the theory assumes the dipole does not have any width. The E-field strength at a fixed distance for the frequencies of interest (420 MHz to 510 MHz) showed very little fluctuation, less than a factor of 1.5.

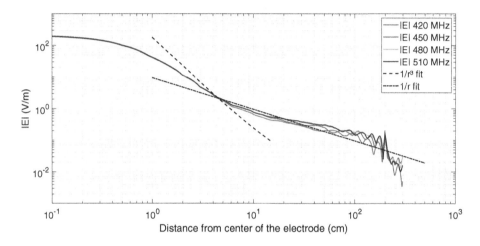

Fig. 10. E-field along the Y-axis radiated by a single electrode on muscle for multiple frequencies on a $50 \times 50\,\mathrm{mm}^2$ phantom cross section.

Figure 11 shows the E-field strength at 5 distances along the Y-axis over the full studied frequency band.

The E-field strength at a fix distance for the frequencies of interest (420 MHz to 510 MHz) showed very little fluctuation, less than a factor of 1.5. This is a desirable property of the communication channel, since this indicates that for a fixed human body limb size a 90 MHz band width with very small fluctuations in channel loss might be available. In order to validate whether this is also the case in reality, these results will be compared with on-body measurements results within the next sub-Section.

In our simulations, the human is represented as a cuboid modeled with the dielectric properties of muscle. Its base-dimensions are $50 \times 50 \times 4000\,\mathrm{mm}^3$ as described Sect. 3.1. However, the arbitrary section size may vary from body to body. In order to better understand the impact of such a variation, the section side-length (as it is a square) was swept from $30 \times 30\,\mathrm{mm}^2$ to $80 \times 80\,\mathrm{mm}^2$ by steps of 10 mm in square edge size. The results are presented Fig. 12.

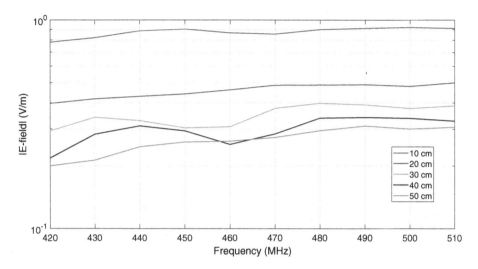

Fig. 11. E-field radiated along the Y-axis by a single electrode on muscle over frequency for multiple distances.

The variations observed in electric field strength are larger when the phantom's section changes at a fixed frequency in comparison to changing the frequency for a fixed section. For example at 50 cm from the electrode, a change in frequency from 420 to 510 MHz, results in a maximal difference of a factor 1.5. On the other hand, at a fixed frequency of 450 MHz we see changes up to a factor of 5 if the phantom's section is changed from $30 \times 30\,\text{mm}^2$ to $80 \times 80\,\text{mm}^2$. These results suggest that the factor S in Eq. 2 does not only depend on the dielectric properties as suggested in [3] but also on the geometry of the phantom.

The polarization of the E-field at the interface air/muscle is plotted in Fig. 13. More than 98% of the total magnitude of the E-field is contained along the Z component of E for propagation distances <200 cm which will be approximately the maximal propagation distance on most human bodies. This shows a strong polarization of the E-field and consequently of the electrode according to the Z direction. It is worth noting that the Z direction in our design is perpendicular to both conductive plates forming the electrode This is again in agreement with the theory presented in Sect. 2.

4.3   On-Body Measurement Results

Figure 14 shows the measured channel losses at 450 MHz as a function of distance along the arm of the subject. The baseline channel loss at 5 cm L_0 is −47 dB, while the loss at the transition point $L_1 = -55$ dB. The fit resulted in two distinctly different slopes defined by the channel losses per distance $\alpha_0 = -0.94\,\text{dB/cm}$ and $\alpha_1 = -0.37\,\text{dB/cm}$. The standard deviation (σ, see

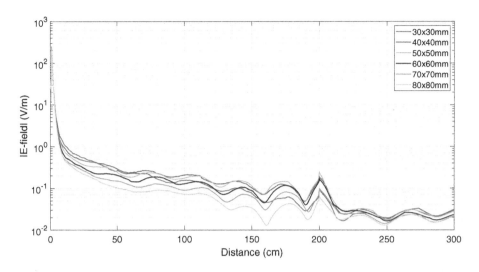

Fig. 12. E-field radiated by a single electrode along the Y-axis on muscle for multiple phantom cross sections at 450 MHz.

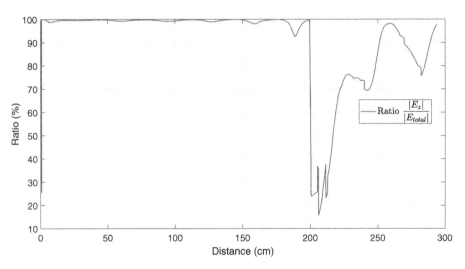

Fig. 13. Ratio of the total electric field along Z direction at 450 MHz with the electrode positioned on muscle.

Eq. 3) on the channel loss model is 6.5 dB. The results of this fit are in line with the model proposed in Eq. 2 with a dominant QS wave near the electrodes that decays stronger over distance than the surface wave which is dominant further away from the electrodes.

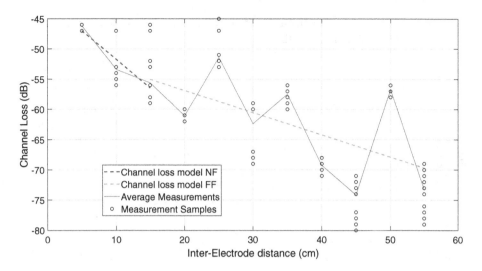

Fig. 14. Channel loss measurements along the arm of a human subject at 450 MHz (black markers). The red and green lines show the two-slope channel loss model described in Eq. 3, fitted to the measurement data. (Color figure online)

Table 1 lists the parameters values of the fit described in Eq. 3 for the following frequencies: 420 MHz, 450 MHz, 480 MHz and 510 MHz.

Table 1. Channel loss parameters.

	420 MHz	450 MHz	480 MHz	510 MHz
L_0 (dB)	−43	−47	−49	−52
α_0 (dB/cm)	−1.2	−0.95	−2.1	−0.79
L_1 (dB)	−54	−55	−62	−59
α_1 (dB/cm)	−0.41	−0.37	−0.19	−0.45
σ (dB)	6.8	6.5	5.8	5.9

Baseline channel loss increased with frequency which is in line with [20]. Near-field losses over distance between 0.8 and 2 dB/cm were measured. These were higher than the far-field losses which were between 0.2 and 0.5 dB/cm. These results are in line with the theoretical model detailed in Sect. 2. It is also interesting to note that the human body is not an homogeneous medium which is the main cause of such an important variance in our measurement results (see Table 1). In fact, the spikes in the channel loss plot in Fig. 14 occur at 25 cm, 35 cm and 50 cm which match the elbow join, the middle of the biceps and the shoulder join of the subject respectively.

Figure 15 shows the Received Signal Strength Indicator (RSSI) while performing on-body measurements for multiple distances over the frequency range of interest. In this case, the RSSI could be seen as a channel loss since the Tx board was set to transmit at 0 dBm.

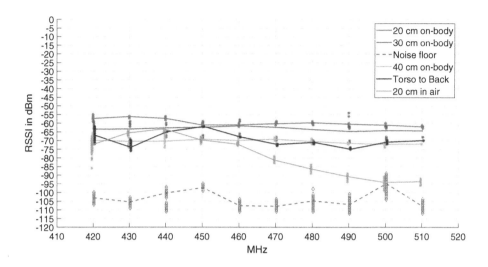

Fig. 15. On-body channel loss for multiple distances.

Figure 15 shows that the variation in on-body channel loss over frequency is relatively small, less than 5 dB over the considered bandwidth over the configurations. This trend over frequency is well aligned with the simulations results from Fig. 11.

Additionally, Fig. 15 shows that the on-body measurements are significantly higher (>30 dB) than the measured noise. This proves that good signal-to-noise can be achieved using C-BCC at these frequencies. To validate the feasibility of C-BCC in conditions where body shielding might occur – such conditions generally lead to the highest on-body channel losses [20] - channel loss was also measured in a back to the torso configuration. The RSSI was found to be higher than the noise and the channel loss did not exceed the one found at 40 cm separation distance. While this result is promising, further research in more non-line of sight conditions has to show whether C-BCC is indeed a good candidate for such communication scenarios. Finally, Fig. 15 also shows the RSSI measured at a separation distance of 20 cm in the air. These were lower than what was measured at 20 cm on the body. This is in line with our numerical simulations and implies that either the electrodes are less efficient in the air or the electrodes are exciting a more efficient communication channel on the body than in the air.

Most previous studies of on-body channel loss at similar frequencies as the ones studied in this manuscript use a channel loss model that is an adaptation of the Friis path loss model with an amended path loss exponent. However, some studies presented on-body propagation measurements at similar frequencies and separation distances as considered in this work, which can be used to extract average losses per distance. [18] presents numerical values of path loss along the body at 400 MHz that amount to average losses of 0.29 dB/cm between 20 and 55 cm separation distance, reducing to 0.11 dB/cm for larger separation distances between 55 and 100 cm. [9] use a theoretical model that predicts losses for propagation around a cylinder. They found losses per unit distance of 1.1 dB/cm between 20 and 35 cm separation distance at 400 MHz. Finally, using the data that form the basis for the IEEE WBAN standard, presented in [12], a loss per distance of 0.39 dB/cm can be obtained when using the measurements between 40 and 60 cm at 400 MHz. In this work we found far-field losses in between 0.19 dB/cm and 0.45 dB/cm. These values are lower than what is found in [9] since we mainly consider propagation in a relatively straight line. The values found in [18] and [12] fall right in between our measurements.

There are previous studies that have investigated C-BCC. Table 2 shows the comparison of those with this work:

Table 2. Comparison with the State of the Art.

	This work	[17]	[2]	[5]	[13]
BCC Type	Capacitive	Capacitive	Capacitive	Capacitive	Capacitive
Op. freq.	400–500 MHz	0.1–100 MHz	DC-25 MHz	0.1–100 MHz	1–40 MHz
Prop. theory	Yes	No	No	No	No
FS sim.	Yes	No	No	No	No
Phant. sim.	Yes	No	No	No	Yes
Circ. model	No	Yes	No	Yes	No
On-body meas.	Yes	Yes	Yes	Yes	Yes
Bat.powered	Yes (Full)	No	No	Hybrid	No
Elec. size	2×2 cm	2×2 cm	3×3 cm	6×4 cm	$\geq 4 \times 4$ cm
Attenuation	65 dB–30 cm 450 MHz	20 dB–30 cm 100 MHz	75 dB–70 cm @ 25 MHz	45 dB–40 cm @ 100 MHz	25 dB–30 cm @ 40 MHz

5   Perspective and Conclusion

Body Coupled Communication has been demonstrated in a frequency band of 420–510 MHz using three complementary methodologies: theory of radio-frequency (RF) propagation along conductive surfaces such as the human body, simulations of RF propagation along a cuboid muscle phantom, and measurements using a battery-powered prototype on the human body.

The theoretical analysis showed that surface wave excitation is dominant in the envisioned frequency band, leading to a mathematical formulation for the electric fields along the human body. In the far-field of the electrodes, a good agreement is found between this theory and our numerical simulation results.

Ultimately, since the propagation mechanism is dominated by surface waves phenomena at 450 MHz (the frequency of interest), a system implementation with the same frequency of operation would enable a communication less sensitive to changes of environment since the return path would have almost no impact at this frequency of operation.

Our numerical simulations demonstrated that propagation along a human body phantom depends on the phantoms cross-section and the frequency of operation. The former being a stronger factor.

Finally, we executed on-body channel loss measurements using electrodes and wireless nodes created using off-the-shelf components. These showed higher channel losses in the near field (0.79–2.1 dB/cm) than in the far-field (0.19–0.45 dB/cm), which is in line with theory and our numerical simulations.

Moreover, our measurements demonstrated that in the studied scenario, the received powers are significantly higher than the noise, indicating that wireless communication using this mechanism is suitable to build the human intranet. In addition, C-BCC does not suffer the Body shadowing effect as it is the case for most RF communication solutions.

From a bandwidth perspective, at the frequency of interest (i.e: 450 MHz) the simulations as well as the measurements results highlighted a minimum bandwidth available of 100 MHz over which the attenuation is very close to be constant. This interesting result could benefit our targeted data rate of tens of Mbps and is compatible with ultra-low power wide band solutions.

Future research will focus on electrode development and optimization in order to reduce the base-line channel loss, development of an ASIC and optimization of an on-body network of C-BCC nodes.

References

1. Anderson, G.S., Sodini, C.G.: Body coupled communication: the channel and implantable sensors. In: 2013 IEEE International Conference on Body Sensor Networks, pp. 1–5. IEEE (2013)
2. Arenas, G.M., Gordillo, A.C.: Design and implementation of a body coupled communication system for streaming music. In: 2016 IEEE ANDESCON, pp. 1–4. IEEE (2016)
3. Bae, J., Cho, H., Song, K., Lee, H., Yoo, H.J.: The signal transmission mechanism on the surface of human body for body channel communication. IEEE Trans. Microw. Theory Tech. **60**(3), 582–593 (2012)
4. Chang, T.C., Weber, M.J., Charthad, J., Baltsavias, S., Arbabian, A.: Scaling of ultrasound-powered receivers for sub-millimeter wireless implants. In: 2017 IEEE Biomedical Circuits and Systems Conference (BioCAS), pp. 1–4. IEEE (2017)
5. Cho, N., Yoo, J., Song, S.J., Lee, J., Jeon, S., Yoo, H.J.: The human body characteristics as a signal transmission medium for intrabody communication. IEEE Trans. Microw. Theory Tech. **55**(5), 1080–1086 (2007)
6. Cotton, S.L., D'Errico, R., Oestges, C.: A review of radio channel models for body centric communications. Radio Sci. **49**(6), 371–388 (2014)
7. Das, D., Maity, S., Chatterjee, B., Sen, S.: Enabling covert body area network using electro-quasistatic human body communication. Sci. Rep. **9**(1), 4160 (2019)
8. Elgala, H., Mesleh, R., Haas, H.: Indoor optical wireless communication: potential and state-of-the-art. IEEE Commun. Mag. **49**(9), 56–62 (2011)

9. Fort, A., Keshmiri, F., Crusats, G.R., Craeye, C., Oestges, C.: A body area prop-
    agation model derived from fundamental principles: analytical analysis and com-
    parison with measurements. IEEE Trans. Antennas Propag. **58**(2), 503–514 (2009)
10. Gabriel, S., Lau, R., Gabriel, C.: The dielectric properties of biological tissues: III.
    pParametric models for the dielectric spectrum of tissues. Phys. Med. Biol. **41**(11),
    2271 (1996)
11. IEEE, P802.15 Working Group for Wireless Personal Area Networks (WPANs):
    Channel Model for Body Area Network (BAN), IEEE P802.15-08-0780-09-0006
    (2009)
12. Katayama, N., Takizawa, K., Aoyagi, T., Takada, J.I., Li, H.B., Kohno, R.: Channel
    model on various frequency bands for wearable body area network. IEICE Trans.
    Commun. **92**(2), 418–424 (2009)
13. Mao, J., Yang, H., Zhao, B.: An investigation on ground electrodes of capacitive
    coupling human body communication. IEEE Trans. Biomed. Circuits Syst. **11**(4),
    910–919 (2017)
14. Mazloum, N.S.: Body-Coupled Communications: Experimental Characterization,
    Channel Modelling and Physical Layer Design. Chalmers University of Technology
    (2008)
15. Norton, K.: The propagation of radio waves over the surface of the earth and in
    the upper atmosphere. Proc. Inst. Radio Eng. **24**(10), 1367–1387 (1936)
16. Norton, K.A.: The propagation of radio waves over the surface of the earth and in
    the upper atmosphere. Proc. Inst. Radio Eng. **25**(9), 1203–1236 (1937)
17. Pereira, M.D., Alvarez-Botero, G.A., de Sousa, F.R.: Characterization and model-
    ing of the capacitive HBC channel. IEEE Trans. Instrum. Meas. **64**(10), 2626–2635
    (2015)
18. Petrillo, L., Mavridis, T., Sarrazin, J., Dricot, J.M., Benlarbi-Delai, A., De Doncker,
    P.: Ban working frequency: a trade-off between antenna efficiency and propagation
    losses. In: The 8th European Conference on Antennas and Propagation (EuCAP
    2014), pp. 3368–3369. IEEE (2014)
19. Rabaey, J.M.: The human intranet-where swarms and humans meet. IEEE Perva-
    sive Comput. **14**(1), 78–83 (2015)
20. Thielens, A., et al.: A comparative study of on-body radio-frequency links in the
    420 MHZ-2.4 GHZ range. Sensors **18**(12), 4165 (2018)
21. Mouser website: Covidien. Kendall ECG electrodes product data sheet. https://
    www.mouser.com/datasheet/2/813/H124SG-1022817.pdf. Accessed 29 May 2019
22. ST Microelectronics website: Sub-GHZ (430–470 MHz) transceiver development
    kit based on S2-LP. https://www.st.com/resource/en/data_brief/steval-fki433v2.
    pdf. Accessed 14 May 2019

Security, Privacy and Performance Evaluation

SmartBAN Performance Evaluation
for Diverse Applications

Rida Khan[(⊠)] and Muhammad Mahtab Alam

Thomas Johann Seebeck Department of Electronics,
Tallinn University of Technology, Tallinn, Estonia
{rikhan,muhammad.alam}@ttu.ee

Abstract. Wireless Body Area Networks (WBANs) envision the realization of several applications which involve the physiological monitoring and/or feedback generations according to the monitored vital signs. These applications range from telehealth or telemedicine to sports and entertainment. SmartBAN provides the physical (PHY) and medium access control (MAC) layer specifications for a simplified and efficient execution of these applications. This paper provides an overview of the existing WBAN use-cases and categorizes them according to their data rate requirements. The SmartBAN performance is thoroughly investigated for the implementation of these diverse applications. For performance evaluation, packet reception rate (PRR), aggregated throughput and latency are taken as the primary quality of service (QoS) criteria. We assume two different channel models, namely static CM3B (S-CM3B) and realistic CM3B (R-CM3B), and different options for the slot durations to further comprehend the results. The simulation results indicate that smaller slot duration performs better in terms of PRR and latency while longer slot durations are more effective to support high data rate application throughput requirements.

Keywords: Wireless body area network (WBAN) · SmartBAN · Data rate · Packet reception rate (PRR) · Throughput · Latency

1 Introduction

Telemedicine and telehealth monitoring systems require the collection of vital information, and in some cases transmission of appropriate feedback, from/to remote patients or subjects through a central hub. Wireless body area network (WBAN) is a set of sensor nodes placed on/inside the subject body for collecting

This research was supported in part by the European Union's Horizon 2020 Research and Innovation Program under Grant 668995, in part by the European Union Regional Development Fund through the framework of the Tallinn University of Technology Development Program 2016–2022, and in part by the Estonian Research Council under Grant PUT-PRG424.

© ICST Institute for Computer Sciences, Social Informatics and Telecommunications Engineering 2019
Published by Springer Nature Switzerland AG 2019. All Rights Reserved
L. Mucchi et al. (Eds.): BODYNETS 2019, LNICST 297, pp. 239–251, 2019.
https://doi.org/10.1007/978-3-030-34833-5_19

physiological information, actuators for receiving the feedback information and a central hub for managing WBAN functioning and communicating with the gateway [1]. Initially, some generic mesh-topology based low power and reduced data rate standards, like IEEE 802.15.4 [2,3], were considered as potential candidates for WBAN applications. But the first attempt to standardize the WBAN physical (PHY) and medium access control (MAC) layer operations was made by IEEE, resulting in the release of IEEE 802.15.6 WBAN standard [4]. European Telecommunication Standard Institute (ETSI) later introduced another WBAN specific standard, called SmartBAN, with rather simplified and energy efficient network structure [5]. Other important features exclusively provided by SmartBAN include faster channel acquisitions, interoperability with other network nodes, hub-to-hub communication or inter-hub relay and coexistence management by coordinator [5].

WBAN can expedite several medical and non-medical applications such as stress monitoring, cardiac monitoring, sports and entertainment [1]. The application requirements vary according to the types of sensor nodes employed, number of nodes, urgency of data delivery, information sampling rate and bit resolution. Some use-cases require only few kilo bits per second (kbps) of data rate while some use-cases demand a throughput as high as hundreds of kbps. A SmartBAN is designed to handle these high variations in data transmission rates while satisfying the other quality of service (QoS) parameters like packet reception rate (PRR) and latency.

In the view of the above discussion, we aim to make the following contributions in this paper:

- We categorize the WBAN use-cases into three categories according to their respective throughput requirements, as low, medium and high data rate applications.
- We evaluate each of these use-cases in terms of PRR, attainable throughput and latency as key performance indicators.
- For a better analysis of associated results, we take static IEEE CM3B (S-CM3B) [6] as well as realistic IEEE CM3B (R-CM3B) [7] channel models. Moreover, different options for slot durations in SmartBAN are also considered for performance evaluation.

The remaining paper is organized in the following way: Sect. 2 describes the SmartBAN PHY and MAC layer specifications and Sect. 3 explains the inherent system model. In Sect. 4, numerical results are investigated and Sect. 5 concludes the paper along with the future work.

2   SmartBAN PHY and MAC Layer Specifications

This section elaborates the ultra low power PHY layer and simplified scheduled access MAC layer structures in SmartBAN.

2.1   Ultra Low Power PHY Layer

SmartBAN operates on 2.4 GHz unlicensed spectrum with 2 MHz bandwidth for each individual channel. The employed modulation scheme is Gaussian Frequency Shift Keying (GSFK) with a bandwidth-bit period product $BT = 0.5$, and modulation index $h = 0.5$. An optional systematic Bose-Chaudhuri Hocquenghem (BCH) code is also provided for the error correction control of MAC-layer protocol data unit (MPDU). SmartBAN proposes the utilization of one, two and four physical-layer protocol data unit (PPDU) repetitions for improving the PRR performance [8].

2.2   Scheduled Access MAC Layer

SmartBAN mainly supports star topology for communication between sensors and central hub. Separate control and data channels are used to enable faster channel acquisitions and simplify the MAC layer operation. Once a sensor node joins SmartBAN, all the communication between the hub and node takes place on data channel. Each inter-beacon interval (IBI) on data channel starts with the D-Beacon, followed by the scheduled access, control and management (C/M) and inactive durations. Scheduled access period involves the data transmission by sensor nodes and the reception of corresponding acknowledgements from hub. C/M period is used for other WBAN operations such as connection establishment, connection modification and connection termination. Inactive period is provided to enable the sleep mode and power saving in SmartBAN [9].

Each scheduled access or C/M slot consists of PPDU transmissions and PPDU acknowledgements separated by inter-frame spacing (IFS). The actual data or control information payload is present in MAC frame body, that is appended with MAC header and frame parity to generate an MPDU. For uncoded transmission, an MPDU becomes physical-layer service data unit (PSDU). PSDU, along with physical-layer convergence protocol (PLCP) header and preamble, constitutes a complete PPDU. In scheduled access mode with two and four repetitions, the transmitted PPDU is repeated twice and four times, respectively, within the assigned time slot duration for each node, resulting in a decrease of the maximum allowed payload size for each slot transmission. Figures 1 and 2 respectively illustrate the IBI formats for no repetition and 2-repetition transmission scenarios [9].

The slot duration T_{slot} for each slot in the IBI on data channel is determined by the parameter L_{slot} as $T_{slot} = L_{slot} \times T_{min}$, where $L_{slot} = \{1, 2, 4, 8, 16, 32\}$ and T_{min} is the minimum slot duration. The slot duration is broadcast in control channel beacon and all the connected sensors transmit their data at this pre-defined slot length in each IBI, after connection establishment with their corresponding central hub. A longer slot length can accommodate more payload, with lesser PHY-MAC layer overheads and acknowledgement transmissions, and facilitates higher throughput whereas a shorter slot duration is sufficient to support low data rate applications. Further details about the SmartBAN PHY and MAC layer specifications are given in [8] and [9].

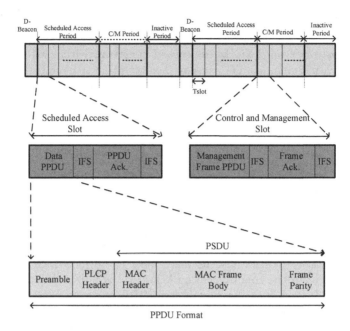

Fig. 1. IBI format with no PPDU repetitions in scheduled access and C/M durations.

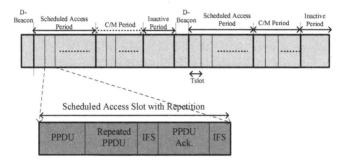

Fig. 2. IBI format with two PPDU repetitions in scheduled access duration.

3   System Model

This section explains the related physical channel and application-specific details of the system model, utilized for carrying out the simulations. Additionally, the simulation setup details are also provided.

3.1   Channel, Mobility and Radio Link Modeling

We take two different channel models for computing the pathloss values which include static IEEE CM3B (S-CM3B) channel with additive white Gaussian noise (AWGN) [6] and realistic IEEE CM3B (R-CM3B) channel with AWGN

[7]. The distances related to each on-body link between the sensor node and hub remain the same in static CM3B model and pathloss is calculated for those constant distances. In the realistic channel model with AWGN, dynamic distances and link types are generated for different on-body links using a biomechanical mobility trace file. Dynamic distances and link types, as defined by a specific mobility scenario like walking, running or sit-stand, are taken as inputs for pathloss calculations. The space-time varying link types identify a particular on-body link as either line of sight (LOS) or non-line of sight (NLOS). An additional NLOS factor of 13% is added to the resultant pathloss value with time-varying distances, for NLOS link status, otherwise the pathloss remains unchanged [7].

After computing the static as well as realistic pathloss values, radio link modeling is performed which includes signal-to-noise ratio (SNR), bit error ratio (BER) and packet error ratio (PER) computations. The theoretical expression for the GFSK BER calculation at SmartBAN PHY layer is given in [10] for a single PPDU transmission scenario. Whereas, for finding BER with two and four PPDU repetitions, SNR calculations are performed according to the diversity technique used for integrating the repetition gain. We assume the maximal ratio combining (MRC) diversity scheme with statistically independent channels for repetition scenarios, therefore, the resulting SNR is the summation of instantaneous link SNRs during each round of the identical PPDU transmission [11]. Subsequently, BER for the repeated PPDU transmissions is computed using the similar BER expression, as mentioned in [7]. Further details about the inherent radio link modeling and the packet reception rate (PRR) analysis are provided in [7].

3.2   WBAN Application-Specific Requirements

A number of medical and consumer electronics use-cases can be identified as potential scenarios for SmartBAN PHY and MAC layer implementation. Each use-case has its own data rate and latency requirements that are peculiar to the number of nodes, sampling rate and quantization, urgency of the data delivery and types of the nodes present in the given use-case. Generally SmartBAN supports a nominal data rate of 100 kbps and a maximum transmission rate of up to 1 Mbps at the PHY layer. The maximum node capacity is 16 nodes per WBAN but typically up to 8 nodes are present in a SmartBAN. For real time high priority traffic, 10 ms latency can be facilitated while for regular traffic 125 ms latency is required [5].

We take three different use-cases classified according to their throughput requirements as low, medium and high data rate applications. A safety and fall monitoring medical use-case is assumed as a low rate application in which patch-type sensors are attached on an elderly adult body. An alert signal is transmitted to the data server when the elder feels physically sick or falls during the regular everyday activities. A rescue and emergency management use-case is considered as medium data rate WBAN application in which sensor data is used to monitor the physical conditions, surrounding environment and location of the rescue workers. A precise athlete monitoring use-case is taken as a high rate application to measure the electrical activity of the muscles and for checking the pitching form in an athlete. All the relevant information about these use-cases is summarized in Table 1.

Table 1. Low, medium and high data rate example use-cases [5, 12, 13].

Safety and fall monitoring (low-data rate)				
Sensor type	Sampling rate/ Quantization	Data rate	Number of sensors	Real time/ Non-real time
Pulse Wave/ ECG	10–16 bit, 64 Hz–1 kHz	640 bps– 16 kbps	1	Real time
Accelerometer/ Gyroscopic sensor	10–16 bit, 64 Hz–1 kHz	640 bps– 16 kbps	3	Real time
Rescue and emergency management (medium-data rate)				
Pulse Wave	10–16 bit, 64 Hz–1 kHz	640 bps– 16 kbps	1	Real time
Accelerometer/ Gyroscopic sensor	10–16 bit, 64 Hz–1 kHz	640 bps– 16 kbps	2	Real time
Voice Command	-	50 kbps– 100 kbps	1	Real time
Ambient sensor	10–16 bit, 64 Hz–1 kHz	640 bps– 16 kbps	1	Real time
GPS node	-	96 bps	1	Real time
Precise athlete monitoring (high-data rate)				
EMG	6–12 bit, 10 kHz–50 kHz	60 kbps– 600 kbps	1	Real time
Accelerometer/ Gyroscopic sensor	10–16 bit, 64 Hz–1 kHz	640 bps– 16 kbps	4	Real time

According to Table 1, all example applications require a maximum 10 ms latency whereas the aggregated throughput requirements range from 2.56 kbps–64 kbps, 52.656 kbps–164.096 kbps and 62.56 kbps–664 kbps for low, medium and high data rate applications respectively. The PRR should be above 90% for all the given use-cases.

3.3   Simulation Setup

Table 2 mentions all the SmartBAN PHY and MAC layer parameters assumed during the simulation. We allocate a single scheduled access slot per sensor node while there are two slots in both the C/M period and inactive durations for all the given use-cases. Therefore, safety and fall monitoring application has four scheduled access slots in its IBI, rescue and emergency management application employs six scheduled access slots and precise athlete monitoring application requires five scheduled access slots. The trace file that provides space-time varying distances and link types for the R-CM3B channel model assessment of the safety and fall monitoring use-case is about 59 s long and contains walking, sitting and hand motions mobility patterns. For the rescue and emergency management and precise athlete monitoring use-cases, the mobility trace file is 63 s long and includes walking, sit-stand and running mobility scenarios. The pathloss values for the S-CM3B channel models are repeated for the similar durations to ensure the performance evaluation at a similar time span. The simulations with the given trace files are repeated 100 times to give performance outcomes with more certainty. All the simulations are carried out in the MATLAB run-time environment.

Table 2. Simulation setup parameters [8,9].

RF parameters	
Transmitted Power (dBm)	$-10, -7.5, -5, -2.5, 0$
Receiver Sensitivity (dBm)	-92.5
Bandwidth per channel (MHz)	2
Information Rate (kbps)	1000
Modulation	GFSK $(BT = 0.5, h = 0.5)$
PHY/MAC parameters	
Minimum slot length (T_{min})	$625\,\mu s$
Slot duration (T_{slot})	0.625 ms, 1.25 ms, 2.5 ms
Interframe spacing (IFS)	$150\,\mu s$
Symbol Rate (R_{Sym})	10^6 symbols/sec
MAC header (N_{MAC})	7 octets
Frame Parity (N_{par})	2 octets
PLCP header(N_{PLCP})	5 octets
PLCP Preamble $(N_{preamble})$	2 octets
PPDU repetition	1, 2 and 4

4   Performance Evaluation

This section analyzes the simulation results to comprehend the QoS obtained using SmartBAN system specifications, for various use-cases.

4.1 Packet Reception Rate (PRR)

The average PRR results for low, medium and high data rate applications are illustrated in Figs. 3, 4 and 5. For low data rate use-case, the smallest slot duration of 0.625 ms, represented by $L_{slot} = 1$ in Fig. 3, can achieve a PRR above 90% under all transmission power levels, single PPDU transmission and both the channel models. PPDU repetitions with smallest slot duration are not possible because the amount of related PHY-MAC overheads to constitute a complete PPDU cannot be transmitted more than once. For 1.25 ms and 2.5 ms slot durations, respectively indicated by $L_{slot} = 2$ and $L_{slot} = 4$ in Fig. 3, the transmission power should be -7.5 dBm or above to obtain the required PRR for single transmission while with PPDU repetitions, all transmission power levels result in the target PRR. In Figs. 4 and 5 for medium and high data rate applications respectively, the PRR values are not significantly affected by the PPDU repetition scheme or transmission power levels for S-CM3B channel. However the transmission power levels above -2.5 dBm are generally required to achieve the target PRR for all slot durations and repetition schemes. Furthermore, larger slot durations, despite carrying more payload with less PHY-MAC overheads, can have decreased PRR because of the increase in overall packet size [10]. The reason for lower PRR values, with realistic CM3B (R-CM3B) channel model in Figs. 3, 4 and 5, is that the R-CM3B model integrates the NLOS or human body shadowing losses as well in radio link modeling, while computing the pathloss, SNR, BER and PER values. The channel losses due to human body shadowing or NLOS conditions are not considered in static CM3B (S-CM3B) channel model and pathloss calculations are performed only for the fixed hub-node link distances. Consequently, the impact of human mobility on PRR performance is not evident with the S-CM3B channel model.

4.2 Throughput

The effective throughput under the given static and realistic CM3B channel conditions can be computed as $Th_{pr} = \frac{N_{Rx}}{T_{trace}}$, where N_{Rx} is the total number of received bits for each node in the given time span and the T_{trace} is complete duration of the pathloss file, as mentioned in Subsect. 3.3. We assume that the maximum allowed payload size, as determined by the slot duration (L_{slot}) is transmitted for each use-case or application. The aggregated throughput results of all the sensor nodes for all the considered use-cases are shown in Figs. 6, 7 and 8. We evaluate the throughput results for -2.5 dBm transmitter power since it ensures the PRR above 90% in almost all of the scenarios, as discussed in Subsect. 4.1. Considering the safety and fall monitoring application, the smallest slot duration 0.625 ms would be enough to satisfy the throughput QoS requirements, as given in Subsect. 3.2. However for medium data rate application, which requires 52.656 kbps–164.096 kbps data rate, 1.25 ms and 2.5 ms slot durations are more suitable with single PPDU transmission and two PPDU repetitions. Finally, for high data rate application throughput requirements, 2.5 ms slot duration with single PPDU transmission and two PPDU repetitions serves as the best

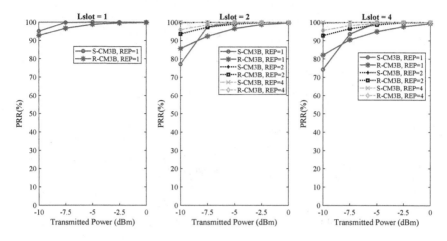

Fig. 3. Packet reception rate (PRR) (%) w.r.t transmission power (dBm) for safety and fall monitoring application (low-data rate), at (a) $L_{slot} = 1$, 2, 4 or $T_{slot} = 0.625$ ms, 1.25 ms, 2.5 ms (b) $REP = 1$, 2, 4 (c) static CM3B (S-CM3B) and realistic CM3B (R-CM3B).

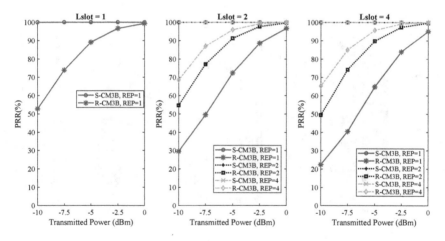

Fig. 4. Packet reception rate (PRR) (%) w.r.t transmission power (dBm) for rescue and emergency management application (medium-data rate), at (a) $L_{slot} = 1$, 2, 4 or $T_{slot} = 0.625$ ms, 1.25 ms, 2.5 ms (b) $REP = 1$, 2, 4 (c) static CM3B (S-CM3B) and realistic CM3B (R-CM3B).

option since it enables the transmission of more payload at once. The increase in throughput with the increase in slot duration (L_{slot}) can be explained by the phenomenon that larger L_{slot} values allow the transmission of more payload with the same PHY-MAC overheads, as compared to the smaller L_{slot} values, in a single transmission.

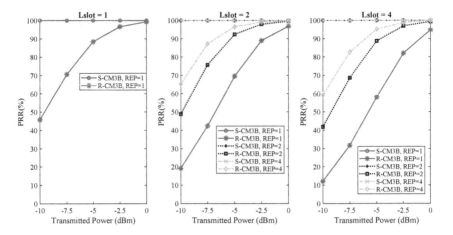

Fig. 5. Packet reception rate (PRR) (%) w.r.t transmission power (dBm) for precise athlete monitoring application (high-data rate), at (a) $L_{slot} = 1, 2, 4$ or $T_{slot} = 0.625\,ms$, $1.25\,ms$, $2.5\,ms$ (b) $REP = 1, 2, 4$ (c) static CM3B (S-CM3B) and realistic CM3B (R-CM3B).

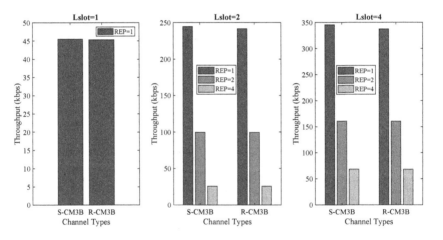

Fig. 6. Throughput (kbps) for safety and fall monitoring application (low-data rate), at (a) $L_{slot} = 1, 2, 4$ or $T_{slot} = 0.625\,ms$, $1.25\,ms$, $2.5\,ms$ (b) $REP = 1, 2, 4$ (c) static CM3B (S-CM3B) and realistic CM3B (R-CM3B) (d) $-2.5\,dBm$ transmission power.

4.3   Latency

The packet latency is calculated as the time difference between the data packet generation and its successful reception. Table 3 enlists the latency values for all the given use-cases with different slot durations. It should be noted that the repetition scheme or the channel types do not affect the obtained latency values since the latency is computed only for the successfully received packets. The latency values increase with the increase in slot durations because larger slot

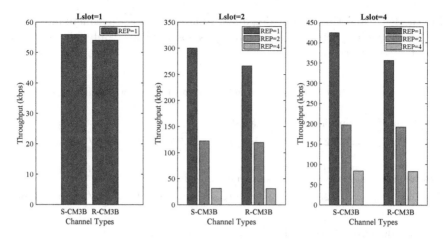

Fig. 7. Throughput (kbps) for rescue and emergency management application (medium-data rate), at (a) $L_{slot} = 1$, 2, 4 or $T_{slot} = 0.625$ ms, 1.25 ms, 2.5 ms (b) REP = 1, 2, 4 (c) static CM3B (S-CM3B) and realistic CM3B (R-CM3B) (d) -2.5 dBm transmission power.

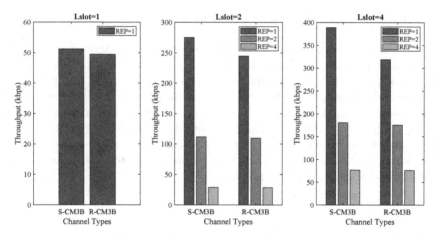

Fig. 8. Throughput (kbps) for precise athlete monitoring application (high-data rate), at (a) $L_{slot} = 1$, 2, 4 or $T_{slot} = 0.625$ ms, 1.25 ms, 2.5 ms (b) $REP = 1$, 2, 4 (c) static CM3B (S-CM3B) and realistic CM3B (R-CM3B) (d) -2.5 dBm transmission power.

durations have longer IBIs. Also the latency values are the highest for the rescue and emergency management application since it has the largest number of sensor nodes and the assigned scheduled access slots. For safety and fall monitoring application, the PRR and throughput requirements are met with the 0.625 ms slot duration, so using this slot duration can guarantee the minimum possible latency for this real time application. The minimum latency can be ensured for rescue and emergency management application with 1.25 ms slot size while satisfying the PRR and throughput demands. Finally, for precise athlete monitoring application, a slight compromise in latency is observed since only 2.5 ms slot can support the required throughput.

Table 3. Latency (ms) for low, medium and high data rate use-cases.

Safety and fall monitoring (low-data rate)		
$L_{slot} = 1/T_{slot} = \mathbf{0.625}$ ms	$L_{slot} = 2/T_{slot} = \mathbf{1.25}$ ms	$L_{slot} = 4/T_{slot} = \mathbf{2.5}$ ms
2.5	5	10
Rescue and emergency management (medium-data rate)		
$L_{slot} = 1/T_{slot} = \mathbf{0.625}$ ms	$L_{slot} = 2/T_{slot} = \mathbf{1.25}$ ms	$L_{slot} = 4/T_{slot} = \mathbf{2.5}$ ms
3.8	7.5	15
Precise athlete monitoring (high-data rate)		
$L_{slot} = 1/T_{slot} = \mathbf{0.625}$ ms	$L_{slot} = 2/T_{slot} = \mathbf{1.25}$ ms	$L_{slot} = 4/T_{slot} = \mathbf{2.5}$ ms
3.1	6.3	12.5

5   Conclusion and Future Work

The paper evaluates the SmartBAN PHY and MAC layer performance to support the low, medium and high data rate applications in terms of PRR, aggregated throughput and latency. Smaller slot durations are more suitable for low data rate real-time applications as they provide improved PRR, reduced latency while satisfying the throughput requirements. While for high data rate applications, longer slot durations should be considered since they help achieving better throughput results with a slight trade-off in latency constraints. As a future work, we aim to perform these evaluations with multi-use channel access mode and coded transmissions in SmartBAN.

References

1. Movassaghi, S., Abolhasan, M., Lipman, J., Smith, D., Jamalipour, A.: Wireless body area networks: a survey. IEEE Commun. Surv. Tutorials **16**(3), 1658–1686 (2014)
2. Scazzoli, D., Kumar, A., Sharma, N., Magarini, M., Verticale, G.: Fault recovery in time-synchronized mission critical ZigBee-based wireless sensor networks. Int. J. Wirel. Inf. Netw. **24**(3), 268–277 (2017)
3. Scazzoli, D., Kumar, A., Sharma, N., Magarini, M., Verticale, G.: A novel technique for ZigBee coordinator failure recovery and its impact on timing synchronization. In: Proceedings of IEEE 27th Annual International Symposium on Personal, Indoor, and Mobile Radio Communication (PIMRC), pp. 1–5. IEEE, Valencia (2016)
4. IEEE Standard for Local and metropolitan area networks - Part 15.6: Wireless Body Area Networks. https://ieeexplore.ieee.org/document/6161600. Accessed 25 July 2019

5. Smart Body Area Networks (SmartBAN): System Description. http://www.etsi. org/deliver/etsi_tr/103300_103399/103394/01.01.01_60/tr_103394v010101p.pdf. Accessed 25 July 2019
6. Smith, D.B., Hanlen, L.W.: Channel modeling for wireless body area networks. In: Mercier, P.P., Chandrakasan, A.P. (eds.) Ultra-Low-Power Short-Range Radios. ICS, pp. 25–55. Springer, Cham (2015). https://doi.org/10.1007/978-3-319-14714-7_2
7. Alam, M. M., Hamida, E. B.: Performance evaluation of IEEE 802.15.6 MAC for wearable body sensor networks using a space-time dependent radio link model. In: Proceedings of IEEE/ACS 11th International Conference on Computer Systems and Applications (AICCSA), pp. 441–448. IEEE, Qatar (2014)
8. Smart Body Area Network (SmartBAN): Enhanced Ultra-Low Power Physical Layer. http://www.etsi.org/deliver/etsi_ts/103300_103399/103326/01.01.01_60/ts_103326v010101p.pdf. Accessed 26 May 2018
9. Smart Body Area Network (SmartBAN): Low Complexity Medium Access Control (MAC) for SmartBAN. http://www.etsi.org/deliver/etsi_ts/103300_103399/103325/01.01.01_60/ts_103325v010101p.pdf. Accessed 26 May 2018
10. Khan, R., Alam, M. M.: Joint PHY-MAC realistic performance evaluation of body-to-body communication in IEEE 802.15.6 and SmartBAN. In: Proceedings of IEEE 12th International Symposium on Medical Information & Communication Technology. IEEE, Australia (2018)
11. Simon, M.K., Alouini, M.S.: Digital Communication over Fading Channel, 2nd edn. Wiley, New York (2005)
12. Arnon, S., Bhastekar, D., Kedar, D., Tauber, A.: A comparative study of wireless communication network configurations for medical applications. IEEE Wirel. Commun. **10**(1), 56–61 (2003)
13. Chakraborty, C., Gupta, B., Ghosh, S.: A review on telemedicine-based WBAN framework for patient monitoring. Telemedicine J. E-health: Official J. Am. Telemedicine Assoc. **19** (2013)

Cybersecurity Assessment of the Polar Bluetooth Low Energy Heart-Rate Sensor

S. Soderi$^{(\boxtimes)}$

Florence, Italy
soderi@ieee.org

Abstract. Wireless communications among wearable and implantable devices implement the information exchange around the human body. Wireless body area network (WBAN) technology enables non-invasive applications in our daily lives. Wireless connected devices improve the quality of many services, and they make procedures easier. On the other hand, they open up large attack surfaces and introduces potential security vulnerabilities. Bluetooth low energy (BLE) is a low-power protocol widely used in wireless personal area networks (WPANs). This paper analyzes the security vulnerabilities of a BLE heart-rate sensor. By observing the received signal strength indicator (RSSI) variations, it is possible to detect anomalies in the BLE connection. The case-study shows that an attacker can easily intercept and manipulate the data transmitted between the mobile app and the BLE device. With this research, the author would raise awareness about the security of the heart-rate information that we can receive from our wireless body sensors.

Keywords: Bluetooth · BLE · Security · Sensor · MitM · Heart-rate · WBAN · Privacy

1 Introduction

In the last two decades, Bluetooth became very popular in the short-range communications. Every smartphone, tablet and personal computer embeds this technology. At the same time, many wireless sensors such as fitness sensors, smartwatches, headsets, wireless medical devices (WMDs) rely on Bluetooth to exchange data with the user's smartphone or tablet. Today, wireless body area networks (WBANs) collect humans' information through Bluetooth low energy (BLE) sensors nodes. BLE is thus becoming de-facto a key wireless technology and users leave that interface always enabled on their devices. BLE was introduced as *Wibree* by Nokia in 2006 [23]. Today, BLE is the dominant technology to convey efficiently data in body networks using coin cell battery-powered devices.

Though the advantages offered by any WBAN are substantial, it makes one of the prime targets for security threats and more particularly for users' privacy. WBANs are commonly used to track health and fitness data and it raises the interest of cyber-criminals to this kind of information.

© ICST Institute for Computer Sciences, Social Informatics and Telecommunications Engineering 2019
Published by Springer Nature Switzerland AG 2019. All Rights Reserved
L. Mucchi et al. (Eds.): BODYNETS 2019, LNICST 297, pp. 252–265, 2019.
https://doi.org/10.1007/978-3-030-34833-5_20

Fitness wearable devices collect human's information, and they are designed to be worn all day. The user reads these data through his smartphone, tablet or even by his smartwatch. Historically, these fitness trackers have numerous security vulnerabilities and the wireless sensor or even the software application may disclose users' data. It is clear that it might have important privacy implications [19,20]. In the literature, there are several contributions that deals with security aspects in WBAN health-care applications. Indeed, the security weaknesses of WMDs can lead to a high risk for the patient's safety [25]. On the other hand, standardization bodies have already adopted security solutions. The IEEE802.15.6 defines different levels of security throughout the encryption and authentication of the data [15]. Moreover, the European Telecommunications Standard Institute (ETSI) takes into account the security in the smart body area networks (SmartBANs) [18]. SmartBANs are used for the collection, processing, and transmission of patient's data. It is crucial that the information must be securely treated [24]. The rapid proliferation of wireless implantable medical devices (WIMDs) coupled with their increasing features is raising the risk for patients [26].

The utilization of wireless technology makes the data prone to being eavesdropped, modified and injected. This increases concerns about the privacy of the information managed in WBANs. In this paper, the author is considering man-in-the-middle (MitM) attack in a BLE WBAN fitness scenario. Observing the received signal strength indicator (RSSI) variations, this study proposes a mechanism to detect MitM attacks.

The rest of this paper is organized as follows. Section 2 overviews the BLE specifications. Section 3 describes the security vulnerabilities of a BLE heart-rate sensor and the results of a MitM attack. Then, the paper proposes security countermeasures. Finally, conclusions are presented in Sect. 4.

2 Bluetooth Low Energy (BLE)

2.1 BLE Core Specifications

Bluetooth is an open standard used for short-range communications. This wireless technology operates in the 2.4 GHz ISM band and it is primarily used for consumer, medical and personal devices [8]. With Bluetooth users can create personal ad-hoc networks to transfer any kind of data. Above 5 billion Bluetooth devices are expected to be shipped within 2022 [7]. At the time of writing, Bluetooth 5.0 is the most recent version and it is rapidly adopted in smartphones. Despite the Bluetooth Special Interest Group (SIG) releases newer versions, even older ones are currently in use and is common to find Bluetooth 4.1 and 4.2 in commercial devices [7,9]. The Bluetooth architecture specifies two forms: basic rate/enhanced data rate (BR/EDR) and low energy (LE) [4]. This paper refers to the BLE standard.

Table 1 shows a comparison of the lower layers between BLE and Bluetooth BR/EDR. This comparison indicates a different usage of the radio spectrum.

Table 1. Lower layers comparison between BLE and Bluetooth BR/EDR [8]

Characteristic	Bluetooth LE (BLE)	Bluetooth BR/EDR
Frequency band	2.4 GHz	2.4 GHz
Channels	40 channels with 2 MHz spacing (3 advertising ch./37 data ch.)^a	79 channels with 1 MHz spacing
Channel usage	FHSS	FHSS
Modulation	GFSK	GFSK, $\frac{\pi}{4}$ DQPSK, 8DPSK
Max data-rate	2 Mbps	3 Mbps
Max Tx power	100 mW	100 mW
Power consumption	$(0.01 \div 0.05) \cdot (1)^b$	$(1)^2$
Network topologies	Point-to-Point^c, Broadcast, Mesh	Point-to-Point^c
Connection	Short burst data transmission	Continuous data stream
Typical range	30 m	50 m

^{a}Advertising channels: ch. 37 (2402 MHz), ch. 38 (2426 MHz) and ch. 39 (2480 MHz);
^{b}(1) is the reference value;
^{c}Including piconet.

BLE splits spectrum into 40 channels: 3 advertising channels to establish connections and 37 channels to transmit data. Furthermore, BLE devices are designed to send short bursts of data rather than a continuous data stream. It makes BLE ideal for sensor applications. BLE devices consume very low energy in comparison to other wireless technologies.

BLE is a full protocol stack. It is a combination of hardware parts and software layers [4]. As shown in Fig. 1, BLE architecture is organized in three major blocks: applications, host and controller. The user *application* defines the interface with the Bluetooth stack. *Host* block consists of the upper layers, whereas *controller* includes lower layers. Host and controller communicate through the host controller interface (HCI). This division makes possible to interface many hosts with a single controller by using the HCI.

The generic access profile (GAP) layer controls the role and connection of a BLE device. BLE specifications define GAP roles as follows [4].

– **Broadcaster:** a device that only sends advertising events;
– **Observer:** a device that only receives advertising events;
– **Peripheral:** a device that accepts the establishment of a LE physical link using the connection establishment procedure;
– **Central:** a device that initiates the establishment of a physical connection.

The logical link control and adaptation protocol (L2CAP) layer plays a central role in Bluetooth stack. It takes multiple protocols from the upper layers and encapsulates them into the standard BLE packet format and vice-versa. L2CAP layer is in charge or routing two main protocols: the attribute protocol (ATTP) and the security manager (SM).

Figure 2 shows the connections flow between master and slave BLE devices. In a fitness scenario, the central device, e.g. a smartphone, scans the frequencies

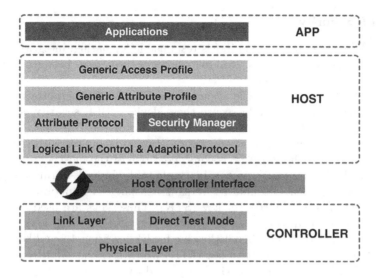

Fig. 1. Architecture of BLE.

for connectable advertising packets. The peripheral devices, e.g. the heart-rate sensor sends connectable advertising packets periodically and accepts incoming connections. Once a connection is established master and slave use generic attribute (GATT) profiles to exchange data. GATT is a simple structured list. Indeed, the data in GATT is organized in services and each service contains one or more characteristics. Each characteristic consists of a universally unique identifier (UUID), a value and a set of properties. Bluetooth SIG defined UUIDs to identify BLE manufacturers as well [3]. By reading UUIDs data, the hacker might gather useful information to plan his attack.

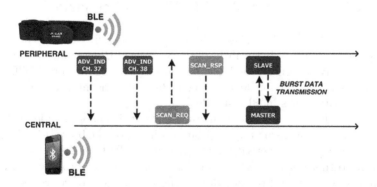

Fig. 2. BLE connection flow.

2.2 BLE Security

In the BLE architecture (Fig. 1) SM is responsible for paring, integrity, authentication, and encryption [23,27]. SM distributes security keys between peers and provides cryptographic functionalities.

NIST 800-121-R2 details the security capabilities of Bluetooth and makes recommendations to effectively secure these devices. BLE security is different from Bluetooth BR/EDR. Since the introduction of the BLE 4.0, the protocol supports a 128-bit advanced encryption standard–counter with CBC-MAC (AES-CCM) [27]. Although AES is considered one of the most secure forms of encryption, the key exchange protocol is exploitable. Indeed, during the *pairing* process devices in BLE 4.0 and 4.1 versions exchange a temporary key (TK) and use it to create a short-term key (STK). These keys are used to encrypt the communication. In this case, an attacker can eavesdrop the keys and then decrypt the connection. This is not the case for BLE version 4.2 and beyond due to the introduction of a long-term key (LTK) which uses the elliptic curve Diffie Hellman (ECDH) key exchange, which is proved to be secure under this type of attack [21,27].

BLE 4.0 and 4.1 devices use the secure simple pairing (SSP) model, in which devices based on their input/output (I/O) capabilities, choose one method from

- **Just Works:** TK is all zeros;
- **Passkey:** TK is a six-digit number combination inserted by the user;
- **Out-of-Band (OOB):** TK is exchanged through a different medium.

The SM can protect the connection from MitM when the operating system (OS) selects Passkey or OOB as paring method. On the other hand, Just Works method does not provide any protection against MitM, that can be exploited by potential hackers.

3 Cybersecurity in a WBAN Fitness Scenario

Despite the Bluetooth SIG released the new Bluetooth 5.0, there is still a huge number of devices in use that utilizes older versions of Bluetooth, such as version 4.1 and 4.2 [7]. Based on a recent estimation last year there were 4 billion BLE enabled devices using version 4.0 or 4.1 [21]. Based on this information, the paper addresses security issues in BLE 4.1 devices.

As shown in Fig. 3, the scenario investigated in this paper includes a Polar H7 heart-rate BLE sensor worn at appropriate positions on the body [12]. The device communicates a person's activity data through the BLE protocol to the smartphone. Due to their nature, WBAN might experience eavesdropping attacks. In this scenario, security and privacy are among major areas of concerns.

Once the author described the BLE protocol in the previous sections, the system analysis must be completed by describing the interfaces present in each device. Figure 4 shows the interfaces between the person, the Polar heart-rate sensor and the smartphone which runs the app to perform the synchronization.

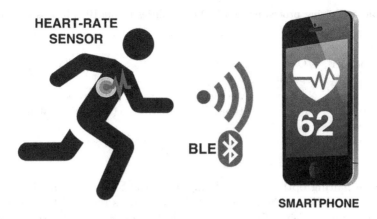

Fig. 3. WBAN fitness scenario.

In particular, by using a SysML internal block diagram (IBD) [14], the author highlighted only those interfaces that might have a key role in this analysis.

The author has already discussed herein how the pairing procedure in BLE 4.1 makes these devices prone to eavesdropping attacks. The use of each association model is based on the I/O capabilities of the device. Considering that the smartphone, i.e. the *initiator*, is equipped with a display and a keyboard display that can be used for pairing by the user. Whereas, the heart-rate sensor, i.e. the *responder*, does not have any I/O capability. Thus, in the scenario under investigation and by analyzing the available interfaces, Table 2 represents

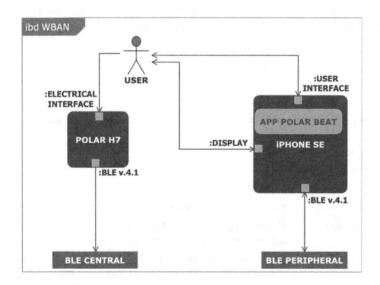

Fig. 4. WBAN fitness interfaces representation with SysML.

Table 2. Pairing procedure and I/O capabilities in the BLE fitness scenario

		Initiator[a]	
Responder[b]	I/O capabilities	Display only	Keyboard display
	No input no output	Just works (unauthenticated)	Just works (unauthenticated)

[a]Smartphone;
[b]Heart-rate BLE sensor;

all possible pairing options. Accordingly, with the SSP model in this scenario, only the Just Works method can be used. The user is required to accept a connection without verifying TK value on both devices, so Just Works provides no MitM protection because it is an *unauthenticated* pairing.

The common type of attacks against BLE communications are

- **MitM** in which an attacker has the ability to both monitor and alter or inject messages into a communication channel;
- **Passive Eavesdropping** in which the attacker is secretly listening (by using a sniffing device) to the private communication of others without consent.

3.1   BLE 4.1 Assessment

This section describes the *cybersecurity assessment* of BLE 4.1 devices in a fitness scenario as shown in Fig. 3. The assessment combined multiple methodologies to best fit the investigation needs. The author selected NIST 800 series to evaluate threats and vulnerabilities of BLE sensors [16,27]. Furthermore, the OWASP guideline is adopted to rate the risk associated with each vulnerability [17].

Table 3. BLE 4.1 vulnerability n.1

Vulnerability n.1	
Vulnerability	Low energy legacy pairing provides no passive eavesdropping protection
Likelihood	High
Technical Impact	High
Risk	Critical
Threat Event	Passive Eavesdropping
Description	Eavesdroppers can capture secret keys (i.e., LTK) distributed during low energy pairing
Mitigation	BLE devices should be paired by using an algorithm that provides a mechanism to exchange keys over an unsecured channel. For instance the ECDH

Table 4. BLE 4.1 vulnerability n.2

Vulnerability n.2	
Vulnerability	The Just Works pairing method provides no MITM protection
Likelihood	High
Technical Impact	High
Risk	Critical
Threat Event	MitM attack
Description	MITM attackers can capture and manipulate data transmitted between trusted devices
Mitigation	Low energy devices should be paired in a secure environment to minimize the risk of eavesdropping and MITM attacks. Just Works pairing should not be used for low energy

Table 5. BLE 4.1 vulnerability n.3

Vulnerability n.3	
Vulnerability	No user authentication exists
Likelihood	Medium
Technical Impact	High
Risk	High
Threat Event	Pairing Eavesdropping
Description	Only device authentication is provided by the specification
Mitigation	Application-level security, including user authentication, can be added via overlay by the application developer

Tables 3, 4, 5, 6 and 7 report found vulnerabilities for the scenario under investigation. By following the methodology selected each table ties together concepts such as likelihood, technical impact, risk and threat events that could exploit the vulnerability. Moreover, for each vulnerability, the author provides a description and possible mitigation. Since these vulnerabilities have a risk mainly rated between *high* and *critical*, it should raise some concerns about the security of the heart-rate information transmitted by the sensor.

3.2 Experiment with MitM Attack

Based on the cybersecurity assessment, in this section, the author proposes an active MitM attack for testing the BLE WBAN in a fitness scenario.

MitM usually involves three actors: Alice, Bob and Eve. In BLE networks this attacks changes its architecture. Indeed, the attacker, i.e. Eve, cannot act simultaneously as a sensor and as a mobile app. Therefore, a BLE MitM needs to make use of two BLE components capable of acting together: one connects

Table 6. BLE 4.1 vulnerability n.4

Vulnerability n.4	
Vulnerability	End-to-end security is not performed
Likelihood	Medium
Technical Impact	Medium
Risk	Medium
Threat Event	MitM attack
Description	Only individual links are encrypted and authenticated. Data is decrypted at intermediate points
Mitigation	End-to-end security on top of the Bluetooth stack can be provided by use of additional security controls

Table 7. BLE 4.1 vulnerability n.5

Vulnerability n.5	
Vulnerability	Discoverable and/or connectable devices are prone to attack
Likelihood	Medium
Technical Impact	High
Risk	High
Threat Event	Passive Eavesdropping, MitM attack
Description	A hacker can try to take over any discoverable and/or connectable BLE device, and then he can get access to all the information
Mitigation	Any device that must go into discoverable or connectable mode to pair or connect should only do so for a minimal amount of time. A device should not be in discoverable or connectable mode all the time

to the mobile app acting as the smartphone, while the other connects to the smartphone acting as the mobile app [23].

The WBAN experiment setup consisted of a Polar H7 heart-rate sensor, i.e. Alice, and an Apple iPhone SE [2], i.e. Bob. The synchronization between the sensor and the smartphone is performed over BLE 4.1. The smartphone ran the Polar Beat mobile app for real-time heart-rate monitoring [13]. As shown in Fig. 5, Eve consists of a laptop that runs Linux Ubuntu 18.10 and two CSR 8510-based USB dongles that support BLE 4.1. These two dongles are connected to the laptop and communicate with each other using the *BtleJuice* web-based software [11].

BtleJuice is a framework to perform MitM attacks on BLE devices. This framework consists of two parts which run on two virtual machines hosted by the same laptop. These parts named *interception core* and *proxy*, and they implement

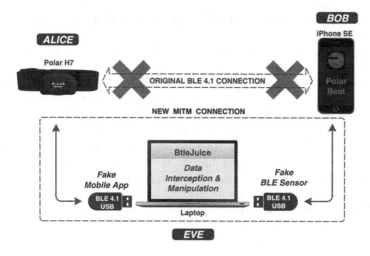

Fig. 5. Active MitM architecture for BLE fitness scenario.

the MitM architecture shown in Fig. 5. And to do this, each virtual machine manages one USB dongle.

BtleJuice acts as a proxy between the mobile app and the BLE heart-rate sensor. Any command sent to the sensor is captured by BtleJuice and relayed to the sensor. In particular, the interception proxy interacts with BLE peripherals and the interception core generates the fake devices with a fake BLE address. Then, the attacker from the web user interface (UI) can control the interception core. He can select the BLE target and intercept GATT operations. From the

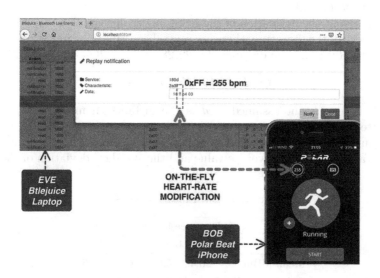

Fig. 6. Heart-rate on-the-fly modification by using replay feature in Btlejuice.

UI, it is possible to replay any GATT operation, but it allows also on-the-fly (OTF) data modification.

In WBAN BLE fitness scenario, Polar H7 heart-rate sensor communicates with the Polar Beat. Since the pairing process is completed, the author started the experiment by attempting to actively sniff BLE traffic. Figure 6 shows how Eve, by using BtleJuice, can intercept the BLE information exchanged between the peripheral and the mobile app and manipulate data OTF.

Once Btlejuice is initialized, the UI allows Eve the selection and the connection of the Polar H7 BLE sensor. In this way, Bob rather than connect to its peripheral, he connects his mobile app to the fake device. As shown in Fig. 6, the attacker by using the replay function in Btlejuice can modify the heart-rate measurement, i.e. characteristics 0x2A37 [5], inside the heart-rate service, i.e. 0x180D [6]. As proof of concept (POC), Eve pushes 255 beats per minute (bpm) in the Polar Beat app.

3.3   Discussion About Security Countermeasures

As pointed out during the cybersecurity assessment (Sect. 3.1), BLE specifications do not offer defenses against MitM attacks. Although the experiment is limited to the WBAN fitness scenario described in this paper, these security leaks can give an advantage to the attacker.

On the L2CAP layer, there is the possibility to request an echo from the BLE sensor to measure round trip time (RTT) on the established link by using the *l2ping* command. It is included in the BlueZ utils [10]. The author assumes that the RTT of the MitM connection in Fig. 5 is greater than the one in the BLE original connection. The evaluation of the RTT might offer a mechanism to detect the MitM. Unfortunately, the *l2ping* command is not supported in most of the BLE peripherals.

Alternatively, the evaluation of the RSSI might offer another way to detect a MitM attack. In the literature, there are several contributions to the relationship between the RSSI and the distance. In [22, 28], RSSI is described as follows

$$RSSI = -10 \cdot N \cdot log(d) + a, \tag{1}$$

where N is a constant assumed 1, d is the distance in meters and a is the transmitted power at 1-m distance.

The author measured the RSSI by using the iPhone and the Bluefruit mobile app [1]. Table 8 shows the average value and the standard deviation of the RSSI

Table 8. RSSI measurements

RSSI	Distance [m]			
	0	0.5	1	3
Mean [dBm]	−26.4	−52.8	−60.8	−66
Std. Dev. [dB]	1.2	3.3	2.6	3

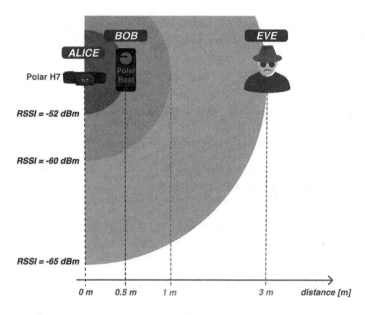

Fig. 7. RSSI .

over 10 measurements for each distance. These measurements validate the RSSI model in (1). Although the indoor environment and layout settings have a direct effect on the RSSI variability, the author assumes that Eve's RSSI can be greater than Bob's RSSI. Figure 7 and Table 8 confirm the assumption. In this scenario, by monitoring the RSSI value Bob can have a mechanism to detect the attack. Indeed, if the RSSI increased unexpectedly then the mobile app might alert the user about a possible attack.

4   Conclusions

This paper aims to raise a concern about the need to be aware on the use of BLE devices. The author analyzed the security issues of BLE 4.1. based sensors. Using the NIST classified threats, the author has identified a list of attacks which apply to BLE devices.

The WBAN scenario under test consists of a Polar H7 heart-rate sensor that communicates with the Polar Beat mobile app using the BLE technology. Being Polar Electro a top player in the wearable smart health devices, its BLE-based sensors are spread worldwide. With this research, the author would raise awareness about the security of the heart-rate information that we can receive from our wireless body sensors.

The case study shows that an attacker can easily intercept and manipulate the data transmitted between the mobile app and the BLE device. Btlejuice was used to implement an active MitM attack, an operation that can result in the

OTF modification of the data. The author remarks the importance to detect this kind of attack that might modify sensitive information such as the heart-rate.

References

1. Adafruit Bluefruit LE Connect. https://itunes.apple.com/it/app/adafruit-bluefruit-le-connect/id830125974?mt=8
2. Apple iPhone SE - Technical Specifications. https://support.apple.com/kb/sp738?locale=en_GB
3. Bluetooth 16 Bit UUIDs For Members. https://www.bluetooth.com/specifications/assigned-numbers/16-bit-uuids-for-members
4. Bluetooth Core Specifications. https://www.bluetooth.com/specifications/bluetooth-core-specification
5. Bluetooth GATT Characteristics. https://www.bluetooth.com/specifications/gatt/characteristics/
6. Bluetooth GATT Services. https://www.bluetooth.com/specifications/gatt/services/
7. Bluetooth Market Update 2018. https://www.bluetooth.com/markets/market-report
8. Bluetooth Radio Versions. https://www.bluetooth.com/bluetooth-technology/radio-versions
9. Bluetooth SIG. https://www.bluetooth.com
10. BlueZ: An Official Linux Bluetooth protocol stack. http://www.bluez.org
11. BtleJuice Bluetooth Smart (LE) Man-in-the-Middle framework. https://github.com/DigitalSecurity/BtleJuice
12. Polar. https://www.polar.com/en
13. Polar Beat Free Fitness and Training App. https://www.polar.com/en/products/polar_beat
14. SysML Open Source Project - What is SysML? https://sysml.org
15. IEEE Standard for Local and metropolitan area networks - Part 15.6: Wireless Body Area Networks, February 2012. https://doi.org/10.1109/IEEESTD.2012.6161600
16. NIST 800–30. Guide for Conducting Risk Assessments Revision 1 (2012)
17. OWASP Testing Guide v4 (2014). https://www.owasp.org/index.php/OWASP_Testing_Project
18. Smart body area networks (smartban): system description, January 2018. http://www.etsi.org/deliver/etsi_tr/103300_103399/103394/01.01.01_60/tr_103394v010101p.pdf
19. Cyr, B.S., Horn, W., Miao, D., Specter, M.: Security analysis of wearable fitness devices (fitbit) (2014). https://pdfs.semanticscholar.org/f4ab/ebef4e39791f358618294cd8d040d7024399.pdf
20. Das, A.K., Pathak, P.H., Chuah, C.N., Mohapatra, P.: Uncovering privacy leakage in BLE network traffic of wearable fitness trackers. In: Proceedings of the 17th International Workshop on Mobile Computing Systems and Applications, Hot-Mobile 2016, pp. 99–104. ACM, New York (2016). http://doi.acm.org/10.1145/2873587.2873594
21. Filizzola, D., Fraser, S., Samsonau, N.: Security analysis of Bluetooth technology (2018). https://courses.csail.mit.edu/6.857/2018/project/Filizzola-Fraser-Samsonau-Bluetooth.pdf

22. Karani, R., Dhote, S., Khanduri, N., Srinivasan, A., Sawant, R., Gore, G., Joshi, J.: Implementation and design issues for using Bluetooth low energy in passive keyless entry systems. In: 2016 IEEE Annual India Conference (INDICON), pp. 1–6, December 2016. https://doi.org/10.1109/INDICON.2016.7838978

23. Melamed, T.: An active man-in-the-middle attack on Bluetooth smart devices. Int. J. Saf. Secur. Eng. **8**, 200–211 (2018). https://doi.org/10.2495/SAFE-V8-N2-200-211

24. Mucchi, L., Jayousi, S., Martinelli, A., Caputo, S., Marcocci, P.: An overview of security threats, solutions and challenges in WBANs for healthcare. In: 2019 13th International Symposium on Medical Information and Communication Technology (ISMICT), pp. 1–6, May 2019. https://doi.org/10.1109/ISMICT.2019.8743798

25. Partala, J., et al.: Security threats against the transmission chain of a medical health monitoring system. In: 2013 IEEE 15th International Conference on e-Health Networking, Applications Services (Healthcom), pp. 243–248, October 2013. https://doi.org/10.1109/HealthCom.2013.6720675

26. Pycroft, L., Aziz, T.Z.: Security of implantable medical devices with wireless connections: the dangers of cyber-attacks. Expert Rev. Med. Devices **15**(6), 403–406 (2018). https://doi.org/10.1080/17434440.2018.1483235. pMID: 29860880

27. Scarfone, K.A., Padgette, J.: NIST SP 800-121. Guide to Bluetooth Security (2008)

28. Tosi, J., Taffoni, F., Santacatterina, M., Sannino, R., Formica, D.: Performance evaluation of bluetooth low energy: a systematic review. Sensors **17**, 2898 (2017). https://doi.org/10.3390/s17122898

User's Authentication Using Information Collected by Smart-Shoes

Luca Brombin, Margherita Gambini, Pietro Gronchi, Roberto Magherini,
Lorenzo Nannini, Amedeo Pochiero, Alessandro Sieni,
and Alessio Vecchio(✉)

University of Pisa, Pisa, Italy
alessio.vecchio@unipi.it

Abstract. In the last years, smart-shoes moved from the medical domain, where they are used to collect gait-related data during rehabilitation or in case of pathologies, to the every-day life of an increasing number of people. In this paper, a method useful to effortlessly authenticate the user during gait periods is proposed. The method relies on the information collected by shoe-mounted accelerometers and gyroscopes, and on the distance between feet collected by Ultra-WideBand (UWB) transceivers. Experimental results show that a balanced accuracy equal to 97% can be achieved even when information about the possible impostors is not known in advance. The contribution of the different information sources, accelerometer, gyroscope, and UWB, is also evaluated.

Keywords: Gait · Authentication · Biometrics · Wearable device · Smart-shoe

1 Introduction

Wearable devices gained widespread popularity during the last years. Smart-watches and smart-wristbands are daily used by a large fraction of people to track their activities, estimate the amount of burnt calories, and as an unobtrusive means for receiving notifications [2,20]. More recently, also smart-shoes started being adopted by the general public. In fact, smart-shoes were initially used in the e-health domain, to collect data about gait-related pathologies [7,9]. Now, they are increasingly used by sports professionals and amateur athletes to track their sessions and obtain detailed information about their performance. Several major brands operating in the footwear sector now include smart-shoes in their catalogs.

Smart-shoes are generally equipped with an Inertial Measurement Unit (IMU) and a transceiver. The former is used to capture the movements of the user, the latter to transmit the data to an external device, such as a smartphone. In some cases, pressure sensors may be available as well [18]. Data collected by means of smart-shoes are not only highly informative about the running/walking

© ICST Institute for Computer Sciences, Social Informatics and Telecommunications Engineering 2019
Published by Springer Nature Switzerland AG 2019. All Rights Reserved
L. Mucchi et al. (Eds.): BODYNETS 2019, LNICST 297, pp. 266–277, 2019.
https://doi.org/10.1007/978-3-030-34833-5_21

style of the user, they are also able to provide abundant information about the identity of the user himself. Several studies demonstrated that accelerometric information collected during gait periods can be used to identify or authenticate the user [8,14,16]. In authentication, the goal is to automatically understand if the current user is the legitimate one or not. In identification, the goal is to automatically recognize the current user among a set of known ones [5,25]. Both possibilities can be extremely useful: authentication, to reduce the burden required from the user of mobile devices, who is frequently asked to confirm his/her identity through pins and/or passwords; identification, to customize the parameters of operations of devices shared among a set of people.

In this paper, we focus on an authentication method based on smart-shoes. Information provided by accelerometers and gyroscopes is used to understand if the user is the legitimate one or not. Besides the information provided by IMUs, the method also relies on distance information collected by means of Ultra-WideBand (UWB) transceivers. The possibility of collecting distance information via UWB was considered because of the increasing diffusion of IEEE 802.15.4-2011 in the wearable domain [23,24]. IEEE 802.15.4-2011 is a standard for low-rate personal area networks that also includes a UWB physical layer. Results demonstrate that reliable authentication of the legitimate user is possible also when the learning phase does not make use of other users' gait samples.

2   Related Work

The limited input interfaces of wearable devices and their personal nature gave rise to new challenges in the security domain. For this reason, the possibility of using a person's gait as an authentication behavioral biometrics has been explored in recent years [17].

Some gait-based authentication methods relied on the acceleration signal collected by a smartphone attached to the hip [6,15,16]. In other cases, acceleration was collected using a wrist-worn device, as this position can be more comfortable for the end users [4,10]. The security strength of a smartphone-based authentication system against zero-effort and impersonator attacks was studied in [13], where professional actors tried to mimic the gait style of other users. Results show that mimicking does not increase the chances of obtaining a false positive, i.e. the erroneous recognition of another user as the legitimate one.

More recently, Fangmin et al. [21] proposed a speed-adaptive gait cycle segmentation method and an individualized method for setting the threshold used to distinguish the legitimate user from possible impostors. These mechanisms make easier to identify gait cycles even in the presence of changes in gait speed. In addition, adapting the threshold contributes to reducing the authentication error. Finally, the proposed adaptive methods were compared with the ones obtained by other state-of-the-art techniques. Results show improvements both in gait recognition and user authentication.

Other authors studied the possibility of using One-Class Classification (OCCs) to achieve biometrics-based continuous authentication [12]. Consistently with the OCC philosophy, the approach relies on the availability of a sufficient

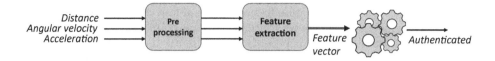

Fig. 1. Overview of the authentication method.

number of positive (genuine) behavioral samples only, while ruling out the negative (impostor) ones. Four methods – Elliptic Envelope (EE), Vector Machine (SV1C), Local Outlier Factor (LOF), and Isolation Forest (IF) – along with their fusions were investigated. The performance was assessed on four distinct behaviometric datasets, which comprised both motion and touch gesture patterns. SV1C and LOF achieved the best results in terms of error rates. The performance of OCC methods was also compared with the performance of eight well-known multi-class classifiers. SV1C and LOF outperformed half of the investigated more traditional classifiers, therefore proving the feasibility of OCC for continuous authentication.

Identification by means of inertial sensors attached to users' feet was studied in [11]. Gait data were collected in terms of 3-axial acceleration and 3-axial angular velocity at both feet. Features were extracted using discrete cosine transform restricted to the low frequencies. Then, identification was carried out by means of a random forest classifier, with a group of eight users.

Besides user's authentication and identification, gait has been proposed as a method for sharing a secret between devices worn by the same subject. In particular, BANDANA is an authentication scheme that allows two wearable devices, placed at random body location, to pair in a secure way through a fresh secure shared secret extracted from user's gait [19]. First, the data produced by each sensor is rotated so that each z-axis is oriented in the opposite direction to gravity, then the signal is denoised by a bandpass filter. A quantization process produces fingerprint bits evaluating the energy difference between Z_i and A, where Z_i is the ith gait cycle and A is the average gait cycle. The higher is this difference, the more reliable the related bit is, then the least reliable ones are discarded. Each device is then able to reach the same key using fuzzy cryptography. Being the gait style unique, only devices on the same body are authenticated.

Differently from most of the above-mentioned works, we study the effectiveness of gait-based authentication using information collected by means of smart-shoes. We believe that this category of wearable devices will be even more popular in the next future. In addition, our study does not only consider data generated by IMUs, but also includes the distance between feet collected by means of UWB. Finally, the proposed method does not rely on the availability of possible impostors' gait samples, but operates according to a realistic usage scenario where only the data produced by the legitimate user is available during the training phase.

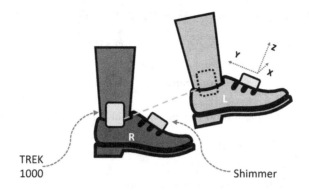

Fig. 2. Position of devices on users' feet and orientation of axes of Shimmer devices.

Table 1. Volunteers' physical characteristics.

ID	Age	Gender	Height (cm)	Weight (kg)
1	24	M	180	95
2	24	M	174	63
3	24	M	165	58
4	27	M	183	85
5	25	M	180	90
6	24	M	186	78
7	25	F	159	57
8	24	M	180	65
9	28	F	165	59
10	23	M	178	75

3 Method

Users' gait is observed in terms of acceleration and angular velocity of feet, and distance between feet. Data are segmented into non-overlapping windows and pre-processed. Then, from each window, a set of features is extracted. A one-class classifier is trained using only the data originated from the legitimate owner. The trained system is evaluated against previously unseen users (the possible impostors). An overview of the proposed method is depicted in Fig. 1.

3.1 Data Acquisition and Pre-processing

Data were collected from ten volunteers, two females and eight males, having the physical characteristics shown in Table 1. The equipment consisted of two Shimmer3 IMU devices - used to acquire inertial data from each foot - and two devices from the DecaWave TREK1000 kit - used to acquire the distance

Table 2. Configuration parameters of the Shimmer devices.

Sampling rate	102.4 Hz
Accelerometer range	±8 g
Gyroscope range	±500 dps

Table 3. Configuration parameters of the TREK1000 devices.

Sampling rate	10 Hz
Data rate	6.8 Mbps
Power source	Tag: battery powered
	Anchor: connected to portable PC via USB

between feet. Shimmer devices were configured to collect acceleration and angular velocity according to the parameters shown in Table 2. The four devices were attached to volunteers' feet and ankles as shown in Fig. 2. The orientation of the axes of the accelerometer and of the gyroscope, with respect to the device case, are also shown in Fig. 2. TREK1000 devices are equipped with a transceiver compatible with the IEEE 802.15.4-2011 UWB standard. Each device is able to estimate the distance towards other devices by using a technique based on two-way ranging time-of-arrival. One of the devices from the DecaWave TREK1000 kit was configured as an anchor (right foot) and the other one as a tag (left foot). Table 3 provides the other operational parameters.

Volunteers were asked to walk for five minutes keeping their normal pace. For each volunteer, thirteen signals were collected: the acceleration and the angular velocity along the three axes for each foot, and the distance between feet. An example of such signals - acceleration and gyroscope for just one foot and the distance between feet - is shown in Fig. 3.

The dataset is available at:
http://vecchio.iet.unipi.it/vecchio/data/.

The traces produced by the Shimmer and TREK devices were first synchronized and trimmed. This last step was carried out to remove non-walking data at the beginning and at the end of each trace. Signals were then filtered by applying a low-pass Butterworth filter with a cut-off frequency of 15 Hz for inertial signals and 4.9 Hz for the distance signal. In the end, 4 min and 30 s of clean, filtered walking data were available for each user.

3.2 Feature Extraction

Traces were divided into fixed-duration windows. For each window, a set of features commonly used in similar domains was extracted from all the thirteen signals. The set of features is: *mean, standard deviation, max-min, median absolute deviation, average absolute variation* [1], and *mean crossing rate.*

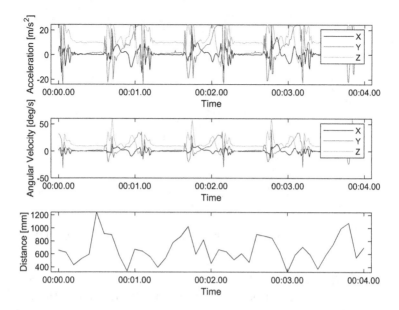

Fig. 3. Acceleration, angular velocity, and distance data when walking.

A vector containing 78 features is then produced for each window (the above-indicated six features computed on the 13 signals). Feature vectors are used to train the one-class classifier and for its evaluation, as described later. Figure 4 shows the gait samples of one of the volunteers in the feature space, restricted to two dimensions to make the image readable, against the other volunteers. The user's model produced by a trained OCC method is represented too. The training phase was performed by using the samples coming from the examined user only (the samples of the genuine/target user); the samples collected from the other users (i.e. the impostors' samples) were added to the scatterplot only later.

4   Results

The performance of the proposed approach was evaluated by training an OCC method using a portion of the data of one of the volunteers and then testing the trained system on previously unseen data (produced by the same user, to test the capability of the model to recognize the legitimate owner, and produced by other volunteers, to test the capability of the model to reject the possible impostors).

4.1   Impact of Window Size on Authentication Accuracy

As previously mentioned, gait data were divided into fixed-duration windows. To understand the influence of the duration of windows on authentication results,

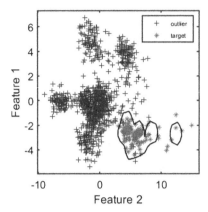

Fig. 4. A user's model in a two-dimensional space, and gait instances of other users.

window sizes in the range from 1 s to 6 s were evaluated. Figure 5 shows the Balanced Accuracy (BA) - a performance index which works well with imbalanced data [3] - when varying the window size. In particular, the BA values depicted in Fig. 5 are the average of the BA values obtained when using five different OCC methods, operating according to different principles (to better understand how this parameter impacts the classification accuracy in general, i.e. not relatively to a single OCC method). The five considered methods are the OCC version of the following classifiers: Gaussian, Minimum Spanning Tree (MST), k-Means, k-Nearest Neighbors (kNN), and Auto Encoder [22]. The Gaussian OCC method models the target class according to a Gaussian distribution; in MST, the distance from a minimum spanning tree derived from the training instances is used as an indicator of distance from the class to be recognized; in k-Means, the class to be recognized is modeled as k clusters; in kNN, the distance from the k nearest neighbors is used to classify new instances; Auto Encoders are neural networks trained to reconstruct the input at the output, then the difference between the input and the output is used to identify the target class.

The performance was evaluated under the assumption that the gait model of the legitimate user is learned automatically during the initial 2 min of walk. The remaining part of the user's trace (2.5 min) was used for testing the performance of the trained classifier on previously unseen data. The capability of the trained classifier to reject impostors was evaluated using the same amount of data (2.5 min) extracted from every other user's trace. Finally, results were averaged across all users.

The best result is obtained when using windows with a duration of 3 s. Therefore, this value is used for computing the results presented in the next sections.

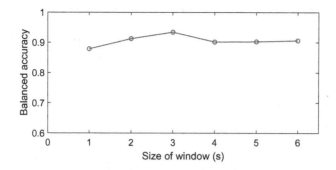

Fig. 5. Balanced accuracy when varying the windows size.

Table 4. Average balanced accuracy of five OCC methods when varying the number of dimensions.

# features	BA
5	90%
10	93%
15	92%
20	88%

4.2 Reduction of the Feature Space

As mentioned, the number of features used to describe the gait style of users is 78. The feature space was reduced to a smaller number of dimensions in order to avoid overfitting and improve the efficiency of the classification model. Reduction of dimensionality was obtained using Principal Component Analysis (PCA). This method maps the entire features space in a new space that has a smaller number of dimensions.

Table 4 shows how the BA varies when the number of dimensions of the PCA space is changed. The BA value is the average of the BA obtained by the same five OCC methods. The best results are obtained when setting the PCA space to 10–15 dimensions.

4.3 Techniques for One-Class Classification

The accuracy that can be achieved by some popular OCC techniques was evaluated. In particular, besides the already introduced five OCC methods, also the following classifiers were assessed: MCD Gaussian, where a minimum covariance determinant density is fit onto the data; Naive Parzen, where Gaussian kernels are centered on training instances and used for estimating the probability density [22].

For each classifier, the evaluation was carried out again using 2 min of walking for training and 2.5 min for the evaluation, with a preliminary reduction to a

Table 5. Balanced accuracy obtained with different OCC methods.

Method	BA (%, *mean ± std.dev.*)	FPR (%)	FNR (%)
Gaussian	93.0 ± 4.6	~0	14.0
MCD Gaussian	94.1 ± 3.6	5.2	6.6
k-NN	90.1 ± 9.2	16.9	3.0
MST	97.0 ± 1.4	2.4	3.6
k-Means	92.3 ± 5.7	9.0	6.4
Naive Parzen	92.4 ± 3.4	6.3	9.0
Auto Encoder	93.8 ± 2.8	0.4	12.0

Table 6. Balanced accuracy obtained by MST when using the different sources of information.

Sensor	BA
Accelerometer	92.8%
Gyroscope	89.7%
UWB	77.8%

feature space with 10 and 15 dimensions. In addition to BA, the OCC methods were evaluated also in terms of False Positive Rate (FPR) - an impostor being incorrectly classified as the legitimate user - and False Negative Rate (FNR) - the legitimate user being incorrectly classified as an impostor.

Table 5 reports the BA values obtained by averaging the results across all the users in the dataset. For every user, the remaining ones were used as possible impostors. Only the best BA value obtained with 10 and 15 dimensions is reported.

MST is the method that provides the best results, with a BA of 97%. Also, the standard deviation of BA is small, this means that the method operates consistently across all users.

4.4   Contribution of the Different Sensors

As stated in Sect. 3, data were acquired from three different typologies of sensors: accelerometers (both feet), gyroscopes (both feet), and UWB transceivers (to estimate the distance between feet).

We evaluated the contribution of the different information sources to the authentication process. To this purpose, the best OCC method found in the previous section - MST - was evaluated again on data originated from a single information source at a time. PCA feature selection was applied to the set of accelerometric features to reduce the number of dimensions from 36 to 10. The same was done to the features extracted from the data produced by the gyroscope. For UWB, all 6 features were used. Results are shown in Table 6.

A BA of 92.8% can be achieved - by an MST classifier - when using the data produced by the accelerometers only. The BA that can be obtained when using information produced by the gyroscopes is relatively close. Distance collected via UWB seems to be less useful as, in the absence of the two other information sources, is able to reach a BA value of 77.8%. However, it is important to note that distance is collected at 10 Hz (the maximum frequency allowed by the adopted hardware solution), whereas acceleration and angular velocity are collected at a much higher rate (102.4 Hz). It is thus possible that the limited sampling rate is unable to capture all the details of an individual's gait style.

5   Conclusion

Smart-shoes, which are increasingly used by common users, can be extremely useful to achieve passive, effortless authentication. Experimental results show that a balanced accuracy as high as 97% can be reached when using IMUs and UWB transceivers as sources of information and adopting a one-class classification approach.

It is important to note that, differently from most of the existing literature on authentication based on smart-shoes, the training phase of the system has been carried out using only the data of the legitimate user. This makes the training phase simpler, as there is no need for other users' data to create a model of the possible impostors.

Of the three considered sensors, accelerometers proved to be the most useful information sources for authentication purposes. However, the contribution of gyroscopes and UWB transceivers is not negligible, as they make possible to increase the balanced accuracy from 92.8% to 97%. This highlights the benefits achieved by approaches based on sensor fusion.

Our study considered only users walking at a normal pace, but it would be interesting to evaluate the performance of the proposed technique when varying the walking speed or in case of changes in the physical condition of the user (for example after intense fatigue).

Acknowledgment. This work was partially funded by the Italian Ministry of Education and Research (MIUR) in the framework of the CrossLab project (Departments of Excellence).

References

1. Abbate, S., Avvenuti, M., Cola, G., Corsini, P., Light, J., Vecchio, A.: Recognition of false alarms in fall detection systems. In: Proceedings of the IEEE Consumer Communications and Networking Conference (CCNC), pp. 23–28, January 2011. https://doi.org/10.1109/CCNC.2011.5766464
2. Avila, L., Bailey, M.: The wearable revolution. IEEE Comput. Graph. Appl. **35**(2), 104–104 (2015). https://doi.org/10.1109/MCG.2015.44

3. Brodersen, K.H., Ong, C.S., Stephan, K.E., Buhmann, J.M.: The balanced accuracy and its posterior distribution. In: Proceedings of the 20th International Conference on Pattern Recognition, pp. 3121–3124. IEEE (2010)

4. Cola, G., Avvenuti, M., Musso, F., Vecchio, A.: Gait-based authentication using a wrist-worn device. In: Proceedings of the 13th International Conference on Mobile and Ubiquitous Systems: Computing, Networking and Services, MOBIQUITOUS 2016, pp. 208–217. ACM, New York (2016). https://doi.org/10.1145/2994374.2994393

5. Cola, G., Avvenuti, M., Vecchio, A.: Real-time identification using gait pattern analysis on a standalone wearable accelerometer. Comput. J. **60**(8), 1173–1186 (2017). https://doi.org/10.1093/comjnl/bxw111

6. Derawi, M.O., Nickel, C., Bours, P., Busch, C.: Unobtrusive user-authentication on mobile phones using biometric gait recognition. In: Proceedings of the Sixth International Conference on Intelligent Information Hiding and Multimedia Signal Processing, pp. 306–311, October 2010. https://doi.org/10.1109/IIHMSP.2010.83

7. Eskofier, B.M., et al.: An overview of smart shoes in the Internet of health things: gait and mobility assessment in health promotion and disease monitoring. Appl. Sci. **7**(10) (2017). https://doi.org/10.3390/app7100986, http://www.mdpi.com/2076-3417/7/10/986

8. Gafurov, D., Snekkenes, E., Bours, P.: Gait authentication and identification using wearable accelerometer sensor. In: Proceedings of the IEEE Workshop on Automatic Identification Advanced Technologies, pp. 220–225, June 2007. https://doi.org/10.1109/AUTOID.2007.380623

9. Howell, A.M., Kobayashi, T., Hayes, H.A., Foreman, K.B., Bamberg, S.J.M.: Kinetic gait analysis using a low-cost insole. IEEE Trans. Biomed. Eng. **60**(12), 3284–3290 (2013). https://doi.org/10.1109/TBME.2013.2250972

10. Johnston, A.H., Weiss, G.M.: Smartwatch-based biometric gait recognition. In: Proceedings of the IEEE International Conference on Biometrics Theory, Applications and Systems (BTAS), pp. 1–6, September 2015. https://doi.org/10.1109/BTAS.2015.7358794

11. Kim, J., Lee, K.B., Hong, S.G.: Random forest based-biometric identification using smart shoes. In: Proceedings of the Eleventh International Conference on Sensing Technology (ICST), pp. 1–4. IEEE (2017)

12. Kumar, R., Kundu, P.P., Phoha, V.V.: Continuous authentication using one-class classifiers and their fusion. In: Proceedings of the IEEE International Conference on Identity, Security, and Behavior Analysis (ISBA), pp. 1–8. IEEE (2018)

13. Muaaz, M., Mayrhofer, R.: Smartphone-based gait recognition: from authentication to imitation. IEEE Trans. Mob. Comput. **16**(11), 3209–3221 (2017). https://doi.org/10.1109/TMC.2017.2686855

14. Ngo, T.T., Makihara, Y., Nagahara, H., Mukaigawa, Y., Yagi, Y.: The largest inertial sensor-based gait database and performance evaluation of gait-based personal authentication. Pattern Recogn. **47**(1), 228–237 (2014)

15. Nickel, C., Busch, C.: Classifying accelerometer data via Hidden Markov Models to authenticate people by the way they walk. IEEE Aerosp. Electron. Syst. Mag. **28**(10), 29–35 (2013). https://doi.org/10.1109/MAES.2013.6642829

16. Nickel, C., Wirtl, T., Busch, C.: Authentication of smartphone users based on the way they walk using k-NN algorithm. In: Proceedings of the Eighth International Conference on Intelligent Information Hiding and Multimedia Signal Processing, pp. 16–20, July 2012. https://doi.org/10.1109/IIH-MSP.2012.11

17. Oak, R.: A literature survey on authentication using behavioural biometric techniques. In: Bhalla, S., Bhateja, V., Chandavale, A.A., Hiwale, A.S., Satapathy, S.C. (eds.) Intelligent Computing and Information and Communication. AISC, vol. 673, pp. 173–181. Springer, Singapore (2018). https://doi.org/10.1007/978-981-10-7245-1_18

18. Ramirez-Bautista, J.A., Huerta-Ruelas, J.A., Chaparro-Cárdenas, S.L., Hernández-Zavala, A.: A review in detection and monitoring gait disorders using in-shoe plantar measurement systems. IEEE Rev. Biomed. Eng. **10**, 299–309 (2017). https://doi.org/10.1109/RBME.2017.2747402

19. Schürmann, D., Brüsch, A., Sigg, S., Wolf, L.: BANDANA - body area network device-to-device authentication using natural gait. In: Proceedings of the IEEE International Conference on Pervasive Computing and Communications (PerCom), pp. 190–196. IEEE (2017)

20. Seneviratne, S., et al.: A survey of wearable devices and challenges. IEEE Commun. Surv. Tutorials **19**(4), 2573–2620 (2017). https://doi.org/10.1109/COMST.2017.2731979

21. Sun, F., Mao, C., Fan, X., Li, Y.: Accelerometer-based speed-adaptive gait authentication method for wearable iot devices. IEEE Internet Things J. **6**(1), 820–830 (2019)

22. Tax, D.: DDtools, the Data Description Toolbox for Matlab, January 2018, version 2.1.3

23. Vecchio, A., Cola, G.: Fall detection using ultra-wideband positioning. In: 2016 IEEE Sensors, pp. 1–3, October 2016. https://doi.org/10.1109/ICSENS.2016.7808527

24. Vecchio, A., Mulas, F., Cola, G.: Posture recognition using the interdistances between wearable devices. IEEE Sens. Lett. **1**(4), 1–4 (2017). https://doi.org/10.1109/LSENS.2017.2726759

25. Vecchio, A., Cola, G.: A method based on UWB for user identification during gait periods. Healthcare Technol. Lett. (2019). https://digital-library.theiet.org/content/journals/10.1049/htl.2018.5050

ICT Solutions for Diagnosis and Social Inclusion

Social Inclusion for Children with Disabilities: The Role of ICT in Play and Entertainment Activities

Paolo Lucattini[1], Sara Jayousi[2], Alessio Martinelli[2],
Lorenzo Mucchi[2(✉)], and Grazia Lombardi[3]

[1] Agazzi Rehabilitation Centre "Madre Divina Provvidenza" of Passionisti,
52100 Arezzo, Italy
plucattini@istitutoagazzi.it
[2] Department of Information Engineering, University of Florence,
50139 Florence, Italy
{sara.jayousi,alessio.martinelli,
lorenzo.mucchi}@unifi.it
[3] Department of Primary Educational Science, University of Campobasso,
Campobasso, Italy
Grazia.lombardi@unimol.it

Abstract. Family associations, educational and university institutions, political and health systems, companies and local agencies, and third sector organizations are involved in and committed to consolidate the historical and cultural path of children's right to play, including children with disabilities. The objective of this paper is to explore the potential role of Information and Communication Technologies (ICT) and in particular of the digital games to create opportunities for social inclusion through playful and entertainment activities for children with disabilities. Starting from the analysis on the role of "play" in the life of children, the main goals and requirements of entertainment are presented with the aim to highlight how the adoption of digital technological solutions can enable social inclusion for disabled children. Guidelines for digital game design are presented together with advanced digital solutions for engaging children with disabilities and increasing their participation and communication capabilities. Robotics, interactive platforms and devices and artificial intelligence algorithms are considered in this analysis. Finally, ICT challenges, innovative approaches and future applications in the context of social inclusion are reported.

Keywords: Information and Communication Technologies · ICT · Play · Children with disabilities · Social inclusion · Digital games · Rights

1 Introduction

Globally, more than 1,000 million people with disabilities (15% of the world population) live worldwide, including around 93 million children (moderate or severe disability). 80% of people with disabilities live in developing countries where, compared

© ICST Institute for Computer Sciences, Social Informatics and Telecommunications Engineering 2019
Published by Springer Nature Switzerland AG 2019. All Rights Reserved
L. Mucchi et al. (Eds.): BODYNETS 2019, LNICST 297, pp. 281–300, 2019.
https://doi.org/10.1007/978-3-030-34833-5_22

to people without disabilities, they encounter more difficulties in accessing education, employment and services [1].

As an example, [2] provided an in-depth assessment of epilepsy, intellectual disability, hearing loss, vision loss, autism spectrum disorder, attention deficit disorder and hyperactivity in 195 countries. In particular, the total number of children under the age of 5 with one of the abovementioned conditions is approximately 53 million. It should be emphasized that 95% of those children live in low and middle-income countries and that vision loss is the most common type of disability, followed by hearing loss, intellectual disability and autism spectrum disorder.

It is worth highlighting that estimation of data on children with disabilities is strongly influenced by adopted assessment methods, as well as cultural and linguistic difficulties [3].

On the other hand, considering the need of extending particular care to the rights of children, several documents testify this constantly evolving historical process. In this framework, the *Geneva Declaration of the Rights of the Child* (1924) [4], the *Universal Declaration of Human Rights* (1948) [5], the *Declaration of the Rights of the Child adopted by the General Assembly* (1959) [6], the *International Covenant on Civil and Political Rights* (1966) [7], the *International Covenant on Economic, Social and Cultural Rights* (1966) [8] and the *Convention on the Rights of the Child* (1989) [9] represent significant achievements. In particular, issues connected to play and entertainment activities receive notable attention in [9]. Children have the right to rest, to engage in leisure and recreational activities appropriate to their age, to participate freely and fully in cultural life and the arts. States must "encourage the provision of appropriate and equal opportunities for cultural, artistic, recreational and leisure activities" (Article 31).

Moreover, considering children with disabilities, [9], in addition to emphasizing the importance of active community participation of disabled children, invites the States to ensure that children have access to recreational activities to achieve full "social integration and individual development" (Article 23). The *Convention on the Rights of Persons with Disabilities* (2006) [10], besides underlining "that children with disabilities have the right to express their views freely on all matters affecting them, their views being given due weight in accordance with their age and maturity, on an equal basis with other children" (Article 7), dedicates a detailed article to questions related to participation in cultural life, recreation, leisure and sport (Article 30). The concepts of equality with others, accessibility of communication formats, participation in leisure time within as well as outside educational institutions, represent commitments recognized by the States and at the same time serve as an enrichment of the society.

Starting from these considerations and focusing on the need of providing new opportunities to facilitate social inclusion, particularly, for children with disabilities, the adoption of ICT in this context shall be analyzed.

"ICT" is defined as all the technologies that enable the transmission, reception and processing of data and information. It primarily focuses on communication technologies (such us Internet, wireless communication networks and systems, etc.) and includes all the mechanisms to access information (communication access technologies, protocols and interfaces), but also digital technological solutions.

In the framework of digital solutions, *digital games* defined as any interactive electronically mediated game, either online or stand-alone, are considered part of ICT.

The objective of this paper is to explore the potential role of ICT and in particular of the digital games to create opportunities for social inclusion through playful and entertainment activities for children with disabilities.

To introduce the application context of this study and identify the benefits of ICT for improving inclusion of people with disabilities trough entertainment experience, it is important: (i) to clarify the meaning of *social inclusion* and to know what results are linked to *inclusive education* and (ii) to highlight the need of technological tools for supporting play activities by creating different opportunities of social inclusion.

1.1   Social Inclusion

As proposed by Simplican, Leader, Kosciulek and Leahy [11] "[…] social inclusion is a broad term which includes social interaction and community participation". With social interaction, the authors refer to relatives, colleagues, friends, acquaintances and intimate partners (with or without disability). With community participation, they refer to leisure activities (hobbies, art and sport), productive activities (employment or education, consumption or access to goods and services, etc.).

Research conducted by the *European Agency for Special Needs and Inclusive Education* [12] highlights that Inclusive Education facilitates significant friendships between students, with and without disabilities, promoting social interactions and supporting networks both throughout the school period and immediately after obtaining the diploma. However, with the passing of time and the subsequent aging of a person with disability, these positive tendencies, together with the sustainability of the previous results, gradually diminish. This underlines a need to encourage projects that further explore the experiences of students during their school life, paying particular attention to those activities, contexts and programs that ensure functional transitions between Inclusive Education and employment as well as between Inclusive Education and community living.

1.2   Play for Children with Disabilities: The Need of Technological Support

In the last decades, the theme of play and entertainment activities for children with disabilities has been the focus of many studies. Most works are focused on single topics, on specific disabilities, or seem to address defined actors engaged in educational activities, rehabilitation services and/or research.

Among the reviewed material, the *COST Action TD1309—Play for Children with Disabilities* (LUDI) [13] is one of the clearest example of a project born with an inclusive perspective. It is a joint effort of researchers, professionals and users, with the aim of creating a new and autonomous field of research and application on play for children with disabilities. In addition to collecting and systematizing all existing educational research, clinical initiatives, and know-how on resource centers and users' associations, in order to develop new knowledge related to contexts, tools and methodologies associated with the play of children with disabilities, LUDI (2014–

2018) is also an important cultural and scientific milestone thanks to the numerous information dissemination activities (participation in international conferences, organization of two annual plenary meetings, exchanges between over 100 researchers and professional operators in the sector from 32 countries and involved in different scientific areas) and the production of 7 books, 1 special publication and 2 Training Schools.

LUDI adopts as a central scientific issue the crossing of three autonomous research areas [14]. The first relates to the types and functioning characteristics of the disability. The second focuses on features, development and evaluation of play and on the right to play. The third observes environmental factors, such as technologies, contexts, and game situations.

Among the 7 books produced, [15] provides guidelines for supporting children with disabilities' play. It highlights the importance of play for every child, and furthermore includes a detailed analysis on the importance of play for children with disabilities, on the barriers that children must overcome in order to play and on the possible roles of the adult as a facilitator. These guidelines host references on the different types of assistive technologies needed for children with disabilities to take part in the game. Finally, insights on various types of games (including digital games), environments, contexts and toys most appropriate for children with disabilities are reported.

Through cultural references and application examples, it emerges how ICT allows children with disabilities to participate in play. ICT generally contribute to the reduction of the gap between the requirements of the game (including relationships with other children and environmental characteristics) and the skills of children, providing support to their functional areas or adapting the proposed activity.

1.3   Our Contribution

This paper is the result of an interdisciplinary work that gathered the knowledge and skills of various professionals (university professors, researchers and third sector operators), engaged in the areas of Information Engineering, Special Education and Physical Education.

It is motivated by these professionals' recognition of the need to conceptualize, design and create products and services with an inclusive perspective, understood as discovery, enhancement and promotion of the meaning of diversity and of acting together to build together products and services useful to all [16].

Starting from the review of the state of the art on social inclusion for children, this paper aims at analyzing how ICT can provide advanced solutions to reduce barriers and increase facilitators by creating *inclusive* opportunities through play and entertainment activities for children with disabilities.

The paper is organized as follows: the application context of the proposed study (inclusive entertainment) is introduced in Sect. 2 by providing an overview of the concepts of barriers and facilitators and the benefit of the adoption of ICT in playing activities and social inclusion for children with disabilities; Sect. 3 focuses on ICT solutions for social inclusion, highlighting the requirements in designing digital games based on a specific disability and reporting some achievements in robotics, interactive platforms and artificial intelligence; ICT challenges and future applications for improving social inclusion are considered in Sect. 4; finally conclusions are drawn in Sect. 5.

2 Inclusive Entertainment: Requirements and ICT Role in Contexts, Rights and Goals

2.1 Context and Requirements

In 2013, the United Nations Committee on the Rights of the Child examined Article 31 of the Convention on the Rights of the Child (1989) through the General Comment No. 17 (GC17) [17]. In addition to underlining the scarce recognition by the States of the rights contained in the Article, the consequent lack of investments and dedicated legislation, the absence of themes related to children in local and national policies, the Committee expresses a series of concerns for the difficulties faced by particular categories of young people, such as girls, poor children, children with disabilities, indigenous children, children belonging to minorities. Within the GC17, play and recreational experiences are considered fundamental for the health and well-being of children. These experiences increase self-confidence and self-efficacy, and develop cognitive, emotional, physical and social skills. Playing teaches children to negotiate, resolve conflicts and make decisions. Playing allows children to explore and experience the world around them. Playing leads children to experiment with ideas and roles. The concerns expressed in the Introduction are transformed into an invitation to trigger changes to cultures, policies and inclusive practices [18] by the States, organizations, family members and professionals. All children must have the opportunity to realize the rights expressed in Article 31 without discrimination of any kind, including situations of disability (Article 2). Environments and facilities must be accessible and inclusive, to allow also children with disabilities to enjoy the rights set forth in Article 31. The value of inclusive play as a mean of achieving optimal development must be recognized by family members, health professionals, school staff, and in general by all professionals. In this process of enhancing inclusive play, the States must compete by promoting opportunities for children with disabilities, as equal and active participants, through awareness-raising actions in the community and by providing adequate support (Article 23). Programs that are overly structured and decided by adults, such as mandatory sporting activities, rehabilitation activities for children with disabilities, household chores in particular for girls, must be limited because they negatively affect the development of young persons' self-determination skills [19]. Likewise, government investments that focus on recreational activities with predetermined and specific purposes, or the choices of adults relating to youth organizations to be attended by children must be limited.

Starting from the awareness that concentrating all the free time of children in planned or performing activities can be harmful for his physical, emotional, cognitive and social well-being, it is worth highlighting that free time slots, where children have the right also to do nothing (if they wish), must be favored. An absence of activity that becomes functional in activating forms of creativity (Article 42).

The GC17 reveals the presence of multiple barriers that separate children with disabilities from the rights stated in Article 31. These barriers are present in the school as well as in informal and social contexts, in places where friendships are formed, where games and recreational activities are held. Barriers exist in communities, where there are negative and hostile cultural attitudes and stereotypes, and sometimes a source of refusal towards children with disabilities. Further examples include: physical barriers in public spaces, parks, playgrounds with equipment, cinemas, theaters, concert halls, sports facilities; political-decision-making barriers that for security reasons on some occasions exclude children with disabilities from sports or cultural venues; and communication barriers, due to inability to interpret or lack of adaptive technology. Finally, barriers can be witnessed in transport.

2.2 Barriers and Facilitators

The concepts of Barriers and Facilitators were introduced by the International Classification of Functioning, Disability and Health (ICF), considered as the "framework for organizing and documenting information on functioning and disability" [20] within which the functioning is perceived as a "dynamic interaction between a person's health condition, environmental factors and personal factors" [21]. In using classifiers and codes, a neutral and standard language, and a conceptual basis for defining disabilities, the ICF has the value of integrating the medical model and the social model, and reaching synthesis with the bio-psycho-social model, in which environmental factors become a dimension that can generate conditions of disability. "Functioning and disability are understood as umbrella terms denoting the positive and negative aspects of functioning from a biological, individual and social perspective [...]. ICF is a multi-dimensional model that covers the entire life span and shifts attention away from the conditions of health to the functioning of the person[...]. ICF is not associated with specific health problems or diseases; it describes the associated functioning dimensions in multiple perspectives at body, person and social levels". The interactions between the elements of the ICF model are outlined in Fig. 1, which draws inspiration from [20].

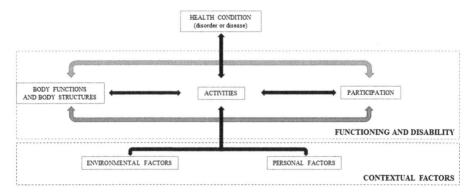

Fig. 1. Interaction between the different parts of ICF model

As shown in Fig. 1, the information is organized in two parts: the part of Functioning and Disability, which includes the Body Functions and Body Structures, Activities, and Participation components, and the part of Contextual Factors, which includes the Environmental Factors and Personal Factors components. The Environmental Factors interacting with the person in a specific health condition determine the level and extent of the person's functioning. In other words, the Environmental Factors can represent barriers or facilitators for the functioning of the person. The attitude of a school group towards inclusive play, as well as the communication of rules within a digital game, are external environmental factors with respect to children with disabilities and play a key role in its inclusive processes.

Focusing on children, in 2007 WHO developed the International Classification of Functioning, Disability and Health: Children & Youth Version ICF-CY, thus responding to the need of defining a specific and universally recognized document for children, in the health, education and social sectors [22].

The ICF-CY has paid particular attention to the issue of participation, understood as involving the person in life situations. In the early part of childhood, opportunities for participation are determined by those people in close connection to the children (family members, babysitters, educators). Social interactions develop substantially in the environment closest to children and involve parents, siblings and peers. The nature and complexity of social interactions change in the transition from early childhood to adolescence and together with them environments change as well. These changes are associated in particular with the development of skills and independence.

Environmental factors, defined as "the physical, social and attitudinal environment in which people live and conduct their lives" can be viewed as a series of successive systems that differentiate and expand according to the age and level of development of children. Environmental factors have a significant impact on the developing children and play a key role in its functioning: "intervention and prevention efforts to promote children's health and well-being focus on modification or enhancement of the physical, social or psychological environment" [22].

Within the ICF-CY, information about play can be found in chapters 8 and 9 of the Activities and Participation components. Chapter 8, entitled Major life areas, contains the alphanumeric codes d 880 Engagement in play, d 8800 Solitary play, d 8801 Onlooker play, d 8802 Parallel play and d 8803 Shared cooperative play. In Chap. 9, entitled Community, social and civic life, there are alphanumeric codes d 920 Recreation and leisure and d 9200 Play. Information on technological devices used during game situations can be found in Chap. 1 of the Environmental Factors component. In Chap. 1 entitled Products and technology, there are the alphanumeric codes and 1152 Products and technologies used for play and 140 Products and technology for culture, recreation and sport.

2.3 Benefits of Adopting ICT Solutions

"Play" is a key factor in the life of children with disabilities and its benefits may be fostered by the usage of technological solutions.

Participating in play and entertainment activities becomes an essential condition for achieving full social integration and complete individual development for children with disabilities [9].

In this framework, ICT can first contribute to facilitate children's relationships either within intimate contexts (family, schoolmates, group of friends) or external contexts (public parks, entertainment venues, community initiatives). ICT can also reduce distances between the needs of the game (environmental characteristics, relationships with other participants, etc.) and the abilities of the children with disabilities, through supports for the functional areas involved at certain moments of the game as well as through appropriate adaptations to the single activities present in the game [15].

In order to know, identify and monitor the frequencies, intensities and types of these supports and adaptations, the use of ICF-CY, an international language shared by different professionals, can help in understanding the functioning of children with disabilities, placing their skills and performances in the spotlight [23].

Based on these considerations, the adoption of ICT is widely recognized to have a high potential of providing opportunities of social inclusion [24]. Specifically addressing to children with disabilities, technological tools can be used for different purposes, ranging from education (school e-inclusion) [25] and rehabilitation [26] to playful and entertainment activities [27]. Table 1 lists some of the main skills that can be improved through play and entertainment and the corresponding benefit the technology can provide.

Table 1. Skill-Technology benefit matrix.

Skill	Technology benefit
Motor	Improve movement skill including coordination (physical rehabilitation)
Cognitive	Improve cognitive skills (cognitive rehabilitation)
Sensory	Improve sensory skills
Communicative	Support inclusive practice
Learning	Assist and enable learning
Social	Improve social interactions and enhancing acceptance
Leisure	Support for playing and engagement in play and recreation

Focusing on playing activities and social inclusion and on the role of digital technologies in this context, the improvement of children skills may rely on three main functionalities of the technology solutions. These are:

1. *Communication Function.* Speech-generating devices capable of producing voice output from a written text, as well as Augmentative and Alternative Communication (AAC) software, allow children to communicate with other participants during various stages of play. Communication can also be facilitated by simple switches connected to devices with pre-recorded voice messages. In the presence of children with sensory disabilities, other forms of communication such as different textures,

Braille text, tactile/auditory/visual feedback, symbols of sign language, etc. can be incorporated into toys [15].

2. *Computer or Tablet Accessibility Function.* Devices such as keyboards (standard or modified), mice (standard or modified), ocular/vocal tracking systems and head pointers can facilitate direct selection when using a computer or a tablet. Similarly, specific switches (mechanical, electromagnetic, electrical control, proximity, phonation, etc.) can support the choice of the desired element among those that run on the screen, in cases where direct selection is impossible [15].

3. *Assistive Sensory Function.* Devices for displaying an enlarged image of a subject captured by a video camera can increase the visual capacity of visually impaired children (*seeing capability*). Tactile computer displays, screen readers, devices that concentrate, amplify and modulate sound, can increase the hearing ability of children with hearing problems (*hearing capability*). Sound indicators as well as voice to text software represent an alternative to sensory pathways for deaf children during game situations. Moreover, operating and controlling devices, such as buttons or switches, allow children to manage an electronic toy (*manipulation capability*) [15].

3 ICT Solutions for Social Inclusion

Different digital technologies are proposed to improve lives of children with disabilities in terms of autonomy, goal achievements, entertainment and social inclusion. Focusing on ICT for social inclusion, [24] explores which types of ICT applications and/or digital services have been suggested to facilitate the social integration of people with different types of disabilities. The authors highlight that while all of the revised works consider beneficial the adoption of technologies to increase the active participation of these people in society, the analysis of any potential infrastructural, socio-technical, cultural, or legal obstacles is missing.

3.1 The Design of a Digital Game

Digital games have gained a considerable role in children's daily experiences and this brings an emerging need for adults to take on a role of control and support. The choice of any new game should be guided, taking into account the element of fun, interests, motivations and preferences of children. In order to make a game to become a pleasant and meaningful moment, it is necessary to analyze the communicative, motor and visual abilities of children, as well as the possibility of accessing and activating the game with ease [15].

The adult as a facilitator should try the game first, with the aim of assessing whether or not it will be suitable for the children and possibly making adaptations to the environment or to some characteristics of the game itself. Within the gaming practice, the adult should however limit her/himself to provide support only if necessary, respecting the children's preferences and leaving them the possibility to explore the different application methods of the game.

As reported in Sect. 1, we consider *digital game* any interactive and electronically mediated game, either online or live. In order to highlight how digital games can be an opportunity for social inclusion for people with disabilities, the main features that should be considered in the definition and design of digital games are analyzed in the following. Moreover, to better detail the main requirements, they are grouped based on the different and specific disability contexts.

Visual Impairments. In the presence of mild or medium visual disabilities, games should have a simple background with relevant visual information. The contrast between background and foreground should be high both in terms of color and in terms of brightness. Controls and actions should also provide auditory feedback. From one screen to another, the various game controls should maintain the same position. In the presence of important or total visual disabilities, it is necessary to rely only on tactile and auditory feedback [15].

Motor Impairments. In the presence of motor disability, games should take into consideration which gestures are necessary in order to interact within the different game phases - for example, whether movements with a finger, such as touching, holding, scrolling, dragging, etc., or with two fingers like rotating, moving, etc. are required. Extensions that allow the game to tolerate involuntary touches, the possibility of returning to the previous action in case of error, the size of buttons and the distances between them should also be assessed. In case of need, it should be possible to use alternative inputs such as voice controls, eye tracking and single switches [15].

Hearing Impairments. In the presence of hearing impairments, games should accommodate the possibility of associating visual feedback with audio rewards and directions provided during the game phases, with the aim of generating pleasure in the children. In case of mild or moderate hearing difficulties, it becomes important to assess the presence of background sounds that could somehow disturb the children [15].

Autism Spectrum Disorders. In the presence of autism spectrum disorders, it is important to evaluate the possibility of adjusting the game sound and using headphones to support concentration on individual game actions. It is important that there is consistency in the position of the various game controls during the succession of screens as well as in the effect produced by a certain action during different phases of the game. Being able to personalize content with images and symbolic representations allows the children amplifies the children's involvement and enjoyment, just as it is useful to be able to return with ease to a familiar screen after a random and rapid exploration of the game [15].

Intellectual Disabilities. In the presence of intellectual disabilities, it is important to be able to access the game and interact throughout the different phases of the game in a way that is intuitive and easy to remember. The on-screen scenarios, the possibility of recovering from errors, as well as the overall flow of the game, must be linear and simple. The various levels of difficulty generally expected within a game must be determined by the children and not automatically by completing the previous level [15].

To design an effective digital game for children with disabilities, besides following the previous recommendations, it is worth highlighting the importance of participatory approaches in the definition of the system interactivity, including the user interface with the involved technologies.

The field of Human-Computer Interaction as a whole relies on a participatory design to satisfy the needs of the end user and improve their quality of experience. Focusing on children with disabilities, the adoption of the participatory design (PD) concept raises specific challenges and poses more fundamental questions about the limits of PD. In [28], the principles of deep engagement, interdisciplinary, individuality, and practicality are discussed, while [29] reviews the design methods and techniques that have been used to involve children with special educational needs and/or disabilities in the technology design process.

3.2 Robotics and Interactive Devices/Platforms

In the framework of digital games, both robotics and interactive devices/platforms play a key role in the context of advanced solutions for engaging children with disabilities. In the following, for each category, some examples of existing systems, mainly focused on increasing participation and communication capabilities, are reported.

Robotics. Robotic technological solutions are widely diffused and represent a key element to support play activities with children with severe disabilities.

Assistive robotics (AR), socially interactive robotics (SIR) and socially assistive robotics (SAR) are some examples. Differently from SIR, which aims at developing close and effective interactions for the sake of interaction itself, SAR combines the concepts of AR and SIR, providing assistance to users through social interactions in order to achieve a measurable progress in some activities (e.g. rehabilitation, learning, etc.) [27].

Starting from the assumption that play-like activities and play for play's sake are very important for children with special needs, some robots developed for rehabilitation and education are presented below (Fig. 2), highlighting their potentialities in supporting play activities.

IROMEC (Interactive RObotic Social MEdiator as Companions) is a mobile robotic platform developed with the aim to help children in discovering different play styles. It acts as a social mediator and it is addressed to children with autism spectrum disorder, children with severe motor impairments and children with cognitive disabilities [27]. It is equipped with sensors, camera, touchscreen, screen (face), wheels, moving lights and wireless interfaces and can be used in several scenarios such as collaborative turn taking activities, follow me, get in contact (tactile, fear and communicative mode [30]).

ZORA is a 58 cm high humanoid robot with seven senses for natural interaction: moving, feeling, hearing and speaking, seeing, connecting and thinking [31]. In order to interact with users or dance, pre-programmed scenarios can be used; moreover, ZORA behavior can be created by pre-programming sensors (e.g. to react on the user's touch). Its appearance and the capability of creating different interactions and communication situations, makes ZORA suitable both for achieving therapy and educational goals and for playful sessions. The qualitative and quantitative study reported in [27] identifies three main domains where ZORA represents a promising solution: movement, communication and cognitive skills. However, ZORA also contributes towards eliciting motivation, concentration, taking initiative and improving the attention span of the children.

ZORA is a commercially available robot as NAO [32], which is the same robot including simplified software developed for ZORA and focused on application in the rehabilitation and care sector.

In the context of "robot assisted playing" for severe physically disabled children, robots should assist in manipulation of standard toys and thus allow autonomous playing. PlayROB [33] is a remote controlled robot system helping the user to handle LEGO bricks. To demonstrate the potentialities of the robot and its learning effects, a long-term multicenter study is carried out [34]. Results show that children's concentration and fun increase while playing also over a longer period of time and no significant reduction of interest is seen. Using the robot is recognized as "learning with great fun" and PlayROB is attractive also for children who were normally able to play with bricks.

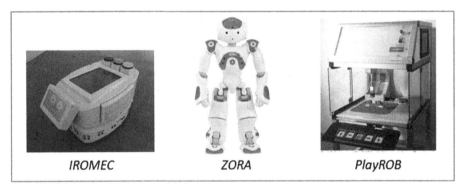

IROMEC   ZORA   PlayROB

Fig. 2. IROMEC, ZORA and PlayROB robots.

Interactive Devices and Platforms. Besides assisting children in setting goals, interactive platforms including video games, enhance and stimulate interactivity through fun activities, helping the development of social skills even in children with severe cognitive disabilities and developmental problems (e.g. autism). Providing skills in psychomotor coordination and in simulations of real-life events, training aids in classrooms and therapeutic settings are some of the main potential of video games.

Some studies are carried out to investigate the potentialities of the Nintendo Wii both as solution to support disabled children in education and as a platform for improving motor skills. [35] describes the achieved results on the evaluation of Wii and commercially available games: (i) to assist in the development of key skills; (ii) to provide students with an adequate simulation of real-life events; and (iii) to help in the areas of health and therapy. Thanks to new engagement mechanisms, such us the Wii Remote Controller, a wireless controller including sensors which can detect motion and rotation in three dimensions, physical interaction may engage different groups in individual and collaborative activities ranging from simulating real life events to sports. Results show that with any game even students who had more difficulties are able to play at least one game on the Wii console and improve over time. Wii provides a platform, which is engaging, motivating and interesting to the learners, and therefore suitable for therapeutic setting and social interactions (e.g. those students who were watching encouraged those who were playing).

In this context, it is worth mentioning the Xbox Adaptive Controller [36], which is a customizable controller designed primarily to meet the needs of gamers with limited mobility. It consists of large programmable buttons and connects to external switches, buttons, mounts and joysticks to make gaming more accessible. The high customization feature of the controller allows the creation of multiple controller profiles (e.g. button remapping) and an easy switch among them. Its design, functionality and packaging are the results of inputs coming from strong partnerships with The Able Gamers Foundation, The Cerebral Palsy Foundation, Special Effect, War Fighter Engaged and many community members.

Other interactive platforms consisting in touch-sensitive screen, voice recognition systems, screen magnification programs and specific assistive software programs have been developed to support children with disabilities especially for educational purposes (e.g. TAPit platform [37]).

3.3   The Role of Artificial Intelligence

Artificial Intelligence (AI) is a branch of computer science that deals with the definition and development of algorithms and systems able to make a machine imitating intelligent human behavior. It allows computers to perform tasks normally requiring human intelligence, such as visual perception, speech recognition, decision-making, and translation between languages.

This technology is becoming part of our daily lives (e.g. Siri, Alexa, Cortana and other similar services). In particular, many companies have been investing in inclusive designs of their products, making them simpler for everyone to use, including disabled people (accessibility and inclusive design).

AI is behind robotic and interactive platforms and devices. An interesting application of the AI in the context of games for children affected by autism is presented in [38]. The authors proposed a method called Dynamic AI Difficulty of the game. It consists of a fuzzy logic that allows the game to identify the adequate game-difficulty to be dynamically proposed to the player according to his/her level of skills. This is performed by recording some relevant parameters shown by the player during playtime and by processing them to measure the player location within the autism spectrum. Social skills in autistic people are improved by the dynamic evaluation procedure which enables the tuning of the game challenges based on the player's communication level.

In the framework of serious game (SG), [39] proposes a SG, Antonyms, for enhancing inhibition mechanisms in children with Attention Deficit/Hyperactivity Disorder (ADHD) by promoting learning and autonomous management of impulsive behaviors and inhibiting irrelevant thoughts. Antonyms focuses on a cognitive mechanism (inhibition), prompts self-regulation, and stimulates metacognition and provides multi-modal, detailed, and immediate feedbacks (visual and auditory messages); moreover, it is capable of monitoring the player's behavior during the game by saving different types of errors (e.g. errors in waiting, wrong answers, etc.) and playing time.

4   The ICT Challenges in the Context of Social Inclusion

4.1   ICT Limits and Main Challenges

In general, people with disabilities encounter barriers due to: (i) inadequate funding, legislation and strategies; ii) the lack of services provided; (iii) negative attitudes and discrimination; (iv) the lack of accessibility, awareness and understanding of disability situations; and (v) the lack of participation in decisions that directly affect their lives. Many of the barriers are avoidable and the disadvantage associated with disability can be overcome [3].

ICT is deeply impacting on multiple aspects of the society and may convey a great potential in facilitating the social inclusion of everyone. However, even if many possibilities can be fostered by ICT, there are some key challenges that remain to be addressed if we expect people with disabilities to fully benefit from the use of ICT.

An important challenge refers to the cost of the assistive technologies, in particular their assessment, training in the use and related support services. When considering people with disabilities living in developing countries, the aforementioned issue becomes a tough barrier into the ecosystem of the technologies. Typically, one of the primary channels supporting the assistive technologies is the education system, which is often underfunded in most of the countries. This may lead to the absence of programs promoting the use of assistive technologies.

In the lifelong education area, the main challenge can be identified in the lack of policies to foster widespread availability of accessible ICT, the lack of an effective implementation of the aforementioned policies, and the lack in the awareness by people with disabilities of what ICT could do for facilitating their social inclusion. At the moment, only 36 percent of countries have a definition of accessibility which includes ICT or electronic media in their lows of regulations compliant with the definition of accessibility in UNCRPD (Article 9) [40].

The remaining part of this Section addresses the challenges and points at the solutions to enhance social inclusion through the use of digital games [41]. The latter suffer from a negative consideration among target users, intermediaries and policy makers. There is the perception that digital games lead people to be unsocial, less human, less empathic, and sometimes they are looked at harming to children. Cultural aspects can also reveal barriers in both public and private sectors, in particular with middle management who opposes in including games in programmes and organizational practices. Informing the general public, decision makers and politicians of the potential benefits of digital games can help to overcome these stereotypes.

A considerable part of the value of digital games is realized through organizations that address social inclusion, developing game-based approaches and incorporating them into professional practice where appropriate. Challenges to achieving this can be found at the level of individuals, organizations, and more generally in policy. Digital games can adapt particularly well to the informal and non-formal learning approaches. With respect to the formal context generally used in school environment, the informal and non-formal ones are commonly preferred within initiatives related to social inclusion and fostered by third-sector intermediary associations. The lack of resources invested towards innovative interventions for people with disabilities causes barriers to an effective involvement of developers, intermediary organizations and users in order to define stable practices. These challenges can be addressed by promoting digital games as a mean of inclusion and empowerment between intermediary organizations. Digital games are often criticized for having low levels of quality and sustainability of game-based inclusion projects. Many research projects produce little lasting impact and implementation projects do not last past the initial funded stages. In order to overcome these issues and building sustainability by ensuring the achievement of the results, clear requirements should be defined and satisfied. The interest and requirements of inter-mediary organizations and target user groups are fundamental to a successful devel-opment of digital game-based approaches. Moreover, multi-stakeholder alignment and the role of innovation intermediaries can facilitate interactions and social learning processes. It is also important to define assessable targets, either qualitative or quan-titative. Programmes and projects need to take place within longer term strategies, considering how they will sustain the initiative and approach the market and the user community after the development and testing phases. Projects need well organized and financed studies on marketing researches and dissemination plan adapted to the needs and requirements of intermediaries and target groups.

4.2   Innovative Approaches and Future Applications

The massive overall number of children with disabilities along with the characteristics of their countries highlighted in [42], must be taken into account in defining proposals for future applications and innovative approaches. These proposals orientate towards two directions and originate from two international documents.

In accepting the definitions present in Article 2 of the *Convention on the Rights of Persons with Disabilities* (UN, 2006) [10], the concepts of *Reasonable accommodation* and *Universal design* represent respectively the starting point and the arrival point of a cultural and evolutionary path. *Reasonable accommodation* refers to changes that are perceived as necessary and not particularly burdensome, but at the same time are useful for guaranteeing rights and freedoms to people with disabilities. Meanwhile, *Universal design* can be defined as "the design of products, environments, programs and services to be usable by people, to the greatest possible extent, without the need for adaptation or specialized design. [...] ".

In reference to play and entertainment activities, the conception, planning and realization of an animated children's cartoon in an inclusive perspective (for example CuerdaS [43], Ian [44], The Present [45], etc.) can be considered as an example of *Universal design*. Through the characters presented and the stories told, an animation can bring participants closer to the themes of selflessness, prosocial behaviors, respect and appreciation of diversity. Taking inspiration from the *Charter to change the lives of people with disabilities* [46], an animated cartoon can include interactive moments in which the participant finds himself making decisions to guide the continuation of the story, developing capacity for self-determination. Or, taking inspiration from the *Special Olympics Young Athletes* program [47], a cartoon can contain scenes where children with and without disabilities experiment with motor games on various levels of ability, and develop cooperative learning skills, being aware of their fundamental and indispensable role in the success of the game (positive interdependence).

In accepting the invitation expressed by the United Nations through the *Transforming our world: the 2030 Agenda for sustainable development* [48] with its 17 sustainable development goals (SDGs), Goals 3, 4, 5, 8, 10, 11 and 16 become elements of reference and global development. Just like implementing the agenda and reaching its SDGs requires a strong involvement of all the components of the society, the realization of ICT in a manner that is functional to the promotion of inclusive processes through play and entertainment activities similarly calls for the involvement of public and private organizations, philanthropic and political institutions, universities and research centers, information and culture professionals. Within this participatory planning, children with disabilities must have a central position together with their families, friends, interests and motivations. An example of participatory planning linked to play and entertainment activities can be the conception, design and implementation of an mobile application in an inclusive perspective (for example Jooay [49], Yoocan [50], Patient Innovation [51], etc.) through which children with disabilities and their families can identify opportunities for free time, adapted to age and skill levels. In addition to facilitate the participation of children with disabilities in community contexts, such mobile applications represent an enrichment for society, triggering connections between scholastic and extra-scholastic realities. Thanks to the contribution of individuals as well as organizations, these types of mobile applications can become functional transitions of information and learning, fun and useful also for children without disabilities, their families and their friends.

5 Concluding Remarks

The aim of this paper is to describe the role of ICT in the processes of social inclusion of children with disabilities through play and recreational activities. Children remain children, regardless of their disability or discomfort. The desire for play is always the same, even in the presence of diseases or difficult living conditions.

As widely described by international documents and as evidenced by the activities promoted globally by the International Play Association and the World Leisure Organization, play is an inalienable right of the children. Play for children becomes a fundamental element for the construction of their personality and well-being. Play can foster the children's self-confidence and their sense of self-efficacy, knowledge of the world, conflict resolution together with the creation of meaningful relationships. During childhood, play is that bridge that connects fantasy to reality and favors the development of resilience in times of difficulties. The game also has the advantage of being a transcultural language and achieving full social inclusion and the participation of all children, especially those with disabilities, is a gradual process that cuts across all countries. First, it is important that family members, professionals and politicians who have the power to change laws and culture recognize the children's right for play.

In the last ten years, the international debate, through the creation of the bio-psycho-social model (as the ICF-CY), has underlined the importance of the context and of everything to prevent or facilitate the participation of all (in this case of children) to social and community life. As reported in [52]: "In fact, in order to make an environment "inclusive", it is required that every activity presented within it is accessible also to children with disabilities".

Functional limitations such as the presence of motor, cognitive or sensorial deficits and environmental barriers, such as the lack of adequate contexts and accessible game materials and not least the presence of cultural prejudices, even on the use of technologies, contribute to the generation of situations of "playful deprivation" and "non-participation". Several studies have shown that the adoption of ICT can greatly enhance children's communication and interactions with other children, with objects and with spaces, in a completely different and unexpected way. Many times the children themselves have shown creative solutions involving the use of technological tools [53]. Although, new technologies can also reduce barriers due to movement in space, shorten the time and become the extension of certain persons' functions, in the last years, the focus of studies on disability and technology has shown that including these tools in living environments is not enough.

In fact, the approach to the adoption of technologies has evolved over time: the focus has shifted from the mere "assistive function" or compensatory function to the "inclusive function", supporting sharing and relationship in the contexts where the technologies are used. Within play and entertainment activities, in addition to facilitating educational and rehabilitative learning, ICT become functional to support children in the need for play for the sake of play [14].

The achievement of this "inclusive function" relies on a dialogue and on an interdisciplinary involvement among the different entities included in the processes of social inclusion: educators, motor science experts, psychologists, engineers, teachers, speech therapists, technicians of rehabilitation, health figures, animators and not least the family and the children themselves. Recent studies have shown that it is important to focus on the objectives before designing.

To this end, the involved adults should know or be trained on the use of new technologies to be able to mediate in a truly inclusive perspective. It is essential to identify the most suitable technology for the selected purpose and to experiment the effects on all the involved variables. Every action shall be individualized and personalized, based on the context and its protagonists.

It is important to understand together with the experts, what to adapt or modify to ensure maximum accessibility, but above all to know the point of view of the children, and to experiment with them the most attractive or amusing tools. Finally, it is worth checking how technologies are really contributing to the creation of an inclusive environment and to the improvement of the quality of children's relationships and lives.

References

1. World Health Organization: WHO global disability action plan 2014–2021: better health for all people with disability. WHO Press, World Health Organization, 20 Avenue Appia, 1211 Geneva 27, Switzerland (2015). ISBN 9789241509619
2. Global Research on Developmental Disabilities Collaborators: Developmental disabilities among children younger than 5 years in 195 countries and territories, 1990–2016: a systematic analysis for the Global Burden of Disease Study 2016Lancet Glob Health20186e1100210.1016/S2214-109X(18)30309-7 Vol. 6, no. 10, Pe1100-e1121 (2018)
3. World Health Organization: World report on disability 2011 WHO Library Cataloguing-in-Publication Data (2001). ISBN 978 92 4 068636 6 (ePUB)
4. Geneva Declaration of the Rights of the Child, adopted 26 September 1924, League of Nations, O.J. Spec. Supp. 21 at 43 (1924)
5. UN General Assembly: Universal Declaration of Human Right. 217 A (III) (1948). https://www.refworld.org/docid/3ae6b3712c.html. Accessed 25 June 2019
6. Declaration of the Rights of the Child G.A. res. 1386 (XIV), 14 U.N. GAOR Supp. (No. 16) at 19, U.N. Doc. A/4354 (1959). Reference The United Nations and Human Rights, 1945–1995, Department of Public Information, United Nations, New York (1995). ISBN 92-1-100560-4
7. International Covenant on Civil and Political Rights Adopted and opened for signature, ratification and accession by General Assembly resolution 2200A (XXI) of 16 December 1966, entry into force 23 March 1976. in accordance with Article 49
8. International Covenant on Economic, Social and Cultural Rights Adopted and opened for signature, ratification and accession by General Assembly resolution 2200A (XXI) of 16 December 1966 entry into force 3 January 1976. in accordance with article 27
9. Convention on the Rights of the Child: London EC1 V 0DU Adopted and opened for signature, ratification and accession by General Assembly Resolution 44/25 of 20 November 1989 entry into force 2 September 1990. in accordance with Article 49
10. UN General Assembly: Convention on the Rights of Persons with Disabilities and its Optional Protocol (A/RES/61/106), New York, USA (2006)
11. Simplican, S.C., Leader, G., Kosciulek, J., Leahy, M.: Defining social inclusion of people with intellectual and developmental disabilities: an ecological model of social networks and community participation. Res. Dev. Disabil. **38**, 18–29 (2015)
12. European Agency for Special Needs and Inclusive Education: Evidence of the Link Between Inclusive Education and Social Inclusion: A Review of the Literature. In: Symeonidou, S. ed. Odense, Denmark (2018)
13. COST Action TD1309—Play for Children with Disabilities (LUDI). https://www.ludi-network.eu/. Accessed 25 June 2019
14. Besio, S., Bulgarelli, D. and Stancheva-Popkostadinova, V.: Play development in children with disabilities. Published by De Gruyter Open Ltd., Warsaw/Berlin Part of Walter de Gruyter GmbH, Berlin/Boston. The book is published with open access (2017). www.degruyter.com. e-ISBN (PDF) 978-3-11-052214-3
15. Encarnação, P., Ray-Kaeser, S., Bianquin, N.: Guidelines for supporting children with disabilities' play. Methodologies, tools, and contexts. Published by De Gruyter Poland Ltd, Warsaw/Berlin Part of Walter de Gruyter GmbH, Berlin/Boston. The book is published with open access (2018). www.degruyter.com e-ISBN (PDF) 978-3-11-061344-5
16. Lucattini, P.: Il diritto ad un applauso. In: Costantini, E., et al. (eds.) Pedagogia e Vita: Rivista di problemi pedagogici educativi e didattici, Sport e Educazione. Edizioni STUDIUM S.r.l, pp. 208–222, Anno 75, January 2017

17. United Nations Committee on the Rights of the Child General Comment No. 17 on the right of the child to rest, leisure, play, recreational activities, cultural life and the arts (art. 31) (2013)

18. Booth, T., Ainscow, M.: Index for inclusion: developing learning and participation in schools (revised edition 2002). Editing and production for CSIE by Mark Vaughan, New Redland Building, Coldharbour Lane, Frenchay, Bristol BS16 1QU, UK (2002)

19. Wehmeyer, M.L., Metzler, C.A.: How self-determined are people with mental retardation? the national consumer survey. Mental Retard. vol. 33, no. 2, pp. 111–119 (1995)

20. World Health Organization: International classification of functioning, disability and health, ICF: short version (2001). http://www.who.int/iris/handle/10665/42417 ISBN 9788879466288, (1995)

21. World Health Organization WHO: How to use the ICF. A practical manual for using the International Classification of Functioning, Disability and Health (ICF), Exposure draft for comment. Geneva, Switzerland (2013). http://www.who.int/classifications/drafticfpracticalmanual2.pdf?ua=1. Accessed 25 June 2019

22. World Health Organization: International Classification of Functioning, Disability and Health: Children & Youth Version: ICF-CY. WHO Press, World Health Organization, 20 Avenue Appia, 1211 Geneva 27, Switzerland ISBN 9789241547321, 2007

23. World Health Organization: International Classification of Functioning, Disability and Health: Children & Youth Version: ICF-CY. WHO Press, World Health Organization, 20 Avenue Appia, 1211 Geneva 27, Switzerland (2007). ISBN 9789241547321

24. Manzoor, M., Vimarlund, V.: Digital technologies for social inclusion of individuals with disabilities, Health Technol. 8, 377 (2018). https://doi.org/10.1007/s12553-018-0239-1

25. Ott, M., Pozzi, F.: Inclusive education and ICT: reflecting on tools and methods. In: Emiliani, P.L. et al. (ed.), Proceedings of AATE 2009-Assistive Technology from Adapted Equipment to Inclusive Environments (2009)

26. Shalash, W.M., AlTamimi, S., Abdu, E., Barom, A.: No limit: a down syndrome children educational game. In: IEEE Games, Entertainment, Media Conference (GEM), pp. 352–358, Galway (2018). https://doi.org/10.1109/gem.2018.8516519

27. Van Den Heuvel, R.J.F.: The next generation of play: robots to support play in rehabilitation and special education for children with physical disabilities. Maastricht, Datawyse/Universitaire Pers Maastricht (2018). https://doi.org/10.26481/dis.20180704rh

28. Frauenberger, C., Good, J., Alcorn, A.: Challenges, opportunities and future perspectives in including children with disabilities in the design of interactive technology. In: Proceedings of 11th International Conference on Interaction Design and Children. ACM, Bremen, Germany, pp. 367–370 (2012)

29. Benton, L., Johnson, H.: Widening participation in technology design: a review of the involvement of children with special educational needs and disabilities. Int. J. Child-Comput. Interact, 3–4, 23–40 (2015). https://doi.org/10.1016/j.ijcci.2015.07.001. ISSN 2212-8689

30. Van Den Heuvel, R.J.F., Lexis, M.A.S., Janssens, R.M.L., Marti, P., De Witte, L.P.: Robots supporting play for children with physical disabilities: exploring the potential of IROMEC. Technol. Disabil. 29(3), 109–120 (2017). https://doi.org/10.3233/TAD-160166

31. Njoki, M., Wabwoba, F.: The Role of ICT in Social Inclusion: A Review of Literature (2015)

32. Mwangi, E., Barakova, E.I., Díaz, M., Mallofré, A.C., Rauterberg, M.: Dyadic gaze patterns during child-robot collaborative gameplay in a tutoring interaction. In: 27th IEEE International Symposium on Robot and Human Interactive Communication (RO-MAN), pp. 856–861 Nanjing (2018). https://doi.org/10.1109/roman.2018.8525799

33. Kronreif, G., Prazak, B., Mina, S., Kornfeld, M., Meindl, M., Furst, M.: PlayROB - robot-assisted playing for children with severe physical disabilities. In: 9th International Conference on Rehabilitation Robotics, 2005. ICORR 2005, pp. 193–196, Chicago, IL (2005). https://doi.org/10.1109/icorr.2005.1501082

34. Kronreif, G., Prazak, B., Kornfeld, M., Hochgatterer A., Furst, M.: Robot assistant "PlayROB" - user trials and results. In: The 16th IEEE International Symposium on Robot and Human Interactive Communication, pp. 113–117, Jeju. (2017). https://doi.org/10.1109/roman.2007.4415063

35. Pearson, E., Bailey, C.: Evaluating the potential of the Nintendo Wii to support disabled students in education. In: Proceedings of ASCILITE ASCILITE - Australian Society for Computers in Learning in Tertiary Education Annual Conference, pp. 833–836 (2007). https://www.learntechlib.org/p/46150/. Accessed 12 June 2019

36. XBOX. https://www.xbox.com/it-IT/xbox-one/accessories/controllers/xbox-adaptive-controller. Accessed 25 June 2019

37. TeachSmart. https://www.teachsmart.org/. Accessed 25 June 2019

38. Khabbaz, A.H., Pouyan, A.A., Fateh, M., Abolghasemi, V.: An adaptive RL based fuzzy game for autistic children. In: 2017 Artificial Intelligence and Signal Processing Conference (AISP), pp. 47–52, Shiraz, (2017) https://doi.org/10.1109/aisp.2017.8324105

39. Colombo, V., Baldassini, D., Mottura, S., Sacco, M., Crepaldi, M., Antonietti, A.: Antonyms: a serious game for enhancing inhibition mechanisms in children with attention deficit/hyperactivity disorder (ADHD). In: 2017 International Conference on Virtual Rehabilitation (ICVR), Montreal, QC, pp. 1–2 (2017). https://doi.org/10.1109/icvr.2017.8007457

40. The Global Initiative for Inclusive ICTs (G3ict), CRPD 2012 ICT Accessibility Progress Report (2012)

41. Stewart, J., et al: Digital Games for Empowerment and Inclusion (DGEI) The Potential of Digital Games for Empowerment and Social Inclusion of Groups at Risk of Social and Economic Exclusion?: Evidence and Opportunity for Policy. Scientific and Policy Report by the Joint Research Centre of the European Commission (2013)

42. Global Research on Developmental Disabilities Collaborators 2018 Developmental disabilities among children younger than 5 years in 195 countries and territories, 1990–2016: a systematic analysis for the Global Burden of Disease Study 2016 Lancet Glob Health, vol. 6, ISSUE 10, Pe1100-e112. https://doi.org/10.1016/S2214-109X(18)30309-7

43. Cuerda, S.: https://www.youtube.com/watch?v=4INwx_tmTKw&t=467s. Accessed 25 June 2019

44. IAN. https://www.youtube.com/watch?v=Hz_d-cikWmI&t=3s. Accessed 25 June 2019

45. The Present. https://www.youtube.com/watch?v=WjqiU5FgsYc. Accessed 25 June 2019

46. Global disability summit charter to change the lives of people with disabilities. https://www.gov.uk/government/publications/global-disability-summit-charter-for-change. Accessed 25 June 2019

47. Special Olympics Young Athletes. https://www.specialolympics.org/our-work/young-athletes. Accessed 25 June 2019

48. UN General Assembly: Transforming our world: the 2030 Agenda for Sustainable Development (A/RES/70/1). New York, USA (2015)

49. Jooay. http://jooay.com/. Accessed 25 June 2019

50. Yoocan. https://yoocanfind.com/. Accessed 25 June 2019

51. Patient Innovation. https://patient-innovation.com/. Accessed 25 June 2019

52. Pennazio, V.: Disabilità, gioco e robotica nella scuola dell'infanzia. TD Tecnologie Didattiche, **23**(3), 155–163 (2015). Accessed 25 June 2019

53. Italian Journal of Special Education for Inclusion anno vol. 1 (2017)

Digital Resources Aiding Opportunities for Affiliation and Practical Reasoning Among People with Dementia: A Scoping Review

C. Melander[1], M. Olsson[1], S. Jayousi[2], A. Martinelli[2],
and L. Mucchi[2(✉)]

[1] Department of Health Science, Luleå University of Technology,
97187 Luleå, Sweden
{catharina.melander,malin.olsson}@ltu.se
[2] Department of Information Engineering, University of Florence,
50139 Florence, Italy
{sara.jayousi,alessio.martinelli,
lorenzo.mucchi}@unifi.it

Abstract. Persons with dementia face several challenges in daily life and the consequences of the disease can be a threat to live a dignified life. Martha Nussbaum has developed the concept of dignified life for people with dementia and suggests the capability approach focusing on what people are able to do and to be in certain agreed-upon areas. Particularly, affiliation and practical reasoning are crucial to preserve a dignified life. For people with dementia the consequences of the disease may affect their opportunities to achieve these vital human capabilities. Digital resources have been shown to have potential to support people in their everyday life and provide them with the means necessary to participate in all aspects of life. In this study, our purpose is to describe digital resources aimed at supporting opportunities for affiliation and practical reasoning among people with dementia. Specifically, we wanted to give an overview of the existing digital resources used to support affiliation and practical reasoning and how such resources affect opportunities for people with dementia. A framework for scoping reviews was used and literature searches were conducted in PubMed and Scopus. The results, by providing a deep analysis of digital resources for affiliation and practical reasoning, highlight the need for a clearer direction towards the very core of vital aspects in a dignified life. Hence, there is a need for a framework that can guide attention towards crucial aspects for supporting a dignified life when developing and evaluating digital resources.

Keywords: Digital resources · Dementia · Affiliation · Practical reasoning · Social interaction · Decision making · Independence

1 Introduction

1.1 Dementia: Needs and Challenges

Dementia is known to cause both disability and dependence among older people. It impairs cognitive functioning and impacts memory, thinking, orientation, and learning

© ICST Institute for Computer Sciences, Social Informatics and Telecommunications Engineering 2019
Published by Springer Nature Switzerland AG 2019. All Rights Reserved
L. Mucchi et al. (Eds.): BODYNETS 2019, LNICST 297, pp. 301–314, 2019.
https://doi.org/10.1007/978-3-030-34833-5_23

ability [1], causing challenges in the daily living activities. Both people who live with dementia and their families need to face with multiple challenges to cope with the illness, as well as to live their everyday lives despite changes that the illness causes [2, 3].

For persons who lives with dementia Kitwood [4] stated the need for a subjective insight on what it is actually like to live with dementia. The advantages of this insight and understanding come when considering each person's experiences as unique. Persons who lives with dementia have described comfort, attachment, and inclusion as phenomena of importance to feel involved in everyday living. Nevertheless, they often have worries regarding loss of life as familiar, loss of abilities and anxiety of becoming a burden to others. Losses of familiarity in daily living is a phenomenon closely linked to dignity [5]. For persons with dementia, the support of a dignified life has been shown to be a challenging task; still the importance of a dignified life is crucial for quality care despite context. Living with dementia dignity as phenomenon can be understood as threatened in a twofold manner, both by the illness itself, and from external views and perceptions of what dementia means [6].

Dementia does not singularly imply disability and dependence; it has additionally been shown to constitute a threat to living a dignified life for the persons affected. The reduced cognitive ability caused by the illness affects the individuals own ability to preserve dignity and live a dignified human life [7]. It is therefore crucial that all support is planned and provided with an outset aiming to sensitively guiding the persons living with dementia towards vital human capabilities of importance to live a dignified life [8]. Livingston et al. [9] described how close relatives caring for people with dementia experience a huge responsibility of hard decision-making during the entire course of the disease. Further, the main troubling areas of decision-making involved areas such as accessing dementia related health and social services, and to be prepared with a plan for the person with dementia if the close relatives became unable to adequately support the person. These two areas imply uncertainty in the everyday lives of close relatives who care for a person with dementia.

For people living with dementia Cohen-Mansfield et al. [10] have shown that the most common and also unmet needs among people with dementia concern aspects such as boredom/sensory deprivation, loneliness and lack of social interaction. Social stimulation and meaningful activities were shown to promote quality of life among people with dementia. Martin and Younger [11] highlighted the importance of empowering persons who live with dementia and showed that it was crucial to be given choices around aspects of everyday life. The health of close relatives when caring for a person with dementia is to be seen as strongly related to how the needs of the person with dementia are being met and the assurance of preserving the dignity of the person with dementia is of crucial importance in everyday living [9].

1.2 Human Dignity in the Context of People with Dementia: Nussbaum's Approach

Human dignity can be understood in a variety of ways; for example, Nordenfelt [12] stated that all human beings are equal by virtue of their humanity. Nussbaum [13] provides an outlook of dignity that focuses on what a dignified life should include. To live a dignified life, Martha Nussbaum [13] suggests a capability approach that focuses on what people are able to do and to be in certain agreed-upon areas that are thought to be central to the quality of the human life. Nussbaum suggests that a dignified human life comprises ten human capabilities: life, bodily health, bodily integrity, senses, imagination, and thought, emotions, practical reasoning, affiliation, other species, play, and control over one's environment. Even though Nussbaum emphasizes that all capabilities are important, the pursuit of affiliation and practical reasoning is crucial since they permeate all other capabilities. Affiliation includes opportunities to live with and for others, to recognize and show concern for other human people, and to engage in various forms of social interaction. It also entails to be treated as a dignified being whose worth is equal to that of others. Practical reasoning concerns opportunities of being able to form a conception of the good and to engage in critical reflection about the planning of one's life. However, for people living with dementia the consequences of the disease may affect their opportunities to engage in social interactions [14] and achieve the human capability of affiliation. There might also be challenging for them to participate in the planning of their lives and attain the human capability of practical reasoning [7]. A dignified life for individuals with dementia requires adapted and sufficient support that targets these vital human capabilities.

1.3 Digital Resources Supporting People with Dementia

Digital resources are today used in several ways with the goal of supporting the daily life of people with dementia leading them to become more independent and to participate in all aspects of life [15]. Additionally, digital resources have been described as useful ways to discover, communicate and give meaningful feedback on situations and conditions with relevance for the person who lives with dementia, families and carers. Martínez-Alcalá et al. [16] showed that digital resources could be used to strengthen the quality of life among people with dementia as well as their close relatives. When it comes to the everyday dependency, that is common in persons who live with dementia, the use of digital resources can provide attention towards improving the well-being of the person and also to decrease stress among families. Using technological resources for people with dementia has previously mainly focused on safety and monitoring, and has now evolved to include empowering the person with dementia and promoting independence through the completion of daily physical and psychosocial activities [17]. The most frequently adopted digital resources are tele-assistance, information systems and internet, while geolocation and robotics were less commonly used as support in everyday living related to dementia. Digital resources have the potential to support the individuals to maintain their capabilities and hence, preserve dignity. Sharkey [18] discussed the need for an ethical approach on studies in the area of digitalization and older people, and highlighted that the capability approach of Nussbaum [13] has some advantages over other accounts of dignity, but that further research is needed.

2 Aim

This paper aims to describe digital resources that support opportunities for affiliation and practical reasoning among people with dementia. Specifically, we provide an overview of the kind of existing digital resources used to support affiliation and practical reasoning and how such resources affect the opportunities for persons with dementia.

3 Methodology

In this study, we used a framework described by Arksey and O'Malley [19] concerning scoping reviews. With this framework, we could apply a broader approach and include studies regardless of study design, such as research articles, and reviews, as well as grey literature. Since we focused on gaining an in-depth and broad view concerning the aim of the study, we undertook an iterative process to ensure that the literature was covered in a comprehensive manner. To undertake the scoping we worked in five stages built on reflexivity. In the first stage, we formulated one research question with a wide approach to enable a breadth coverage of the topic. After achieving a sense of volume and general scope of the field we decided on the parameters related to the term "digital resources", as well as what could be included in the terms "affiliation" and "practical reasoning", to let these parameters guide our literature search. For example, social, communication, and engagement were deemed as appropriate parameters for searches concerning affiliation, while decision, empower, and independence were used for searches concerning practical reasoning. The inclusion criterion was papers written in English between the years of 2014–2019.

The second and third stage involved identifying and selecting relevant studies, which in this study implied searching for literature in the electronic databases PubMed and Scopus. To enhance the comprehensiveness in data collection, we also performed a manual search in reference lists. The selection of relevant studies was performed in several steps, starting with reading the title of the studies, followed by reading the abstract. If the article seemed to fit the scope of this study after these initial steps, or if the relevance of an article was unclear from the abstract, the full article was read. After reading the materials in full 38 papers (30 focusing on affiliation, and 17 papers focusing on practical reasoning), were selected for final inclusion. Meaning that some papers were included in both domains.

In the fourth stage, a narrative review of the articles was undertaken, applying a broad view on extraction of textual units from the included articles. This approach allowed to include information (e.g. the description of a system utilized for a digital resource) in order to contextualize and make the outcome understandable. We recorded information concerning author(s), year of publication, study location, type of digital utilized resource(s), important results related to the parameters set for affiliation, and practical reasoning. Together, these data formed the basis of the analysis. The extracted data were then sorted into domains based on the type of digital resource described in the article. At the last stage, we collated and summarized the results in order to provide a narrative account of the existing literature. The results are reported as a running text for affiliation and practical reasoning, respectively, and are divided into domains for presenting the digital resources.

4 Results

4.1 Characteristics of Included Studies

The 38 included papers (30 focusing on affiliation, and 17 papers included for practical reasoning) mostly took part in Western countries.

4.2 Digital Resources for Affiliation

Robotics

Robotic Animals. One study described the usage of pet-robots [20], and three studies focused on the Paro robotic seal [21–23]. Paro is a socially responsive robot with moving parts. It makes authentic baby seal sounds and recognizes voices. Paro had a clear positive impact on social interactions and connections. Pet-robots are suggested to stimulate persons with dementia's interaction with the robot, as well as with other people. However, people might lose interest due to the limited behavioral repertoire of the robot [20].

Robotic Telepresence System. A review by Blackman et al. [24] outlined a robotic telepresence system that remotely connects carers to individuals and their homes. The impact was not presented. Moyle et al. [25] deployed the Giraffe telepresence robot, which provides opportunities for families to 'virtually' visit people with dementia by videoconferencing. The Giraffe can be moved by the user and driven to chosen places in the environment. The Giraffe was viewed as having the potential to decrease social isolation and increase connection by enabling persons with dementia, families and friends to "visit" each other.

Assistive and Social Robots. Wang et al. [26] utilized a custom-designed robot to provide stepwise prompting and complete activities at home. A trained tele-operator remotely controlled movements, speech, and prompting functions. The robot was viewed as having the potential to improve interactions and relationships between the person with dementia and families. Chu et al. [27] studied social robots designed specifically for emotional and intentional communication and interaction purposes. The robots had baby-face-like appearances and features such as face and emotion change recognition, voice vocalization and emotive expressions, singing, and dancing. Social interaction increased with the robots. Similarly, in [28] a social robot with human attributes, such as baby-face-like appearance, human voices, facial expressions, gestures, and body movements was used. The robot affected engagement in general, and specifically verbal engagement with others was observed. However, it was not clear if the robot helped persons to make more friends. In [29] a robot that could move autonomously within predefined areas was deployed. It addressed by-passers asking if they liked to interact with it via voice output. Interested persons could then click through some information about the robot and the research project on the screen, or had the information read out aloud. Even though people were interested in the robot, it was viewed as never being able to replace humans.

Multimedia Digital Tools for Reminiscence. The review by Holthe et al. [30] outlined a tablet with photos, music, and video clips used for reminiscence. The tablet increased the interaction between carers and persons with dementia. A tablet with a reminiscence conversation aid was also utilized in a study by Purves et al. [31], which provided a strong sense of shared history within a group when discussing something that all participants had been a part of, or by having different perspectives on a shared topic. In [32] a digital photo diary was used. It automatically took photographs and annotated them with geolocations using global positioning systems diary using a wearable camera. The digital photo diary created a shared connection between the persons with dementia and their partner having shared memories to discuss. Subramaniam and Woods [33] utilized multimedia digital life storybooks, which were experienced as encouraging communication and interaction between the persons with dementia and their families, as well as with carers. Samuelsson and Ekström [34] and Davis and Shenk [35] studied a multimedia digital tool in which personalized and generic material were created using videos and other visual stimuli. The tablets supported finding things to talk about. In [36] online reminiscence tools, which allowed the storing of photos and music and enabled connection with family and friends, were described. The impact of these tools was not outlined. Another multimedia digital tool for reminiscence was studied by Garlinghouse et al. [37]: a 3D printing to create small-scale models that individuals with dementia could recognize and relate to their personal past was investigated. The models influenced the person with dementia to talk to family members about both old and new topics and encouraged carers to interact more with the person with dementia.

Smart Home Environment. In [38] a smart home environment, in which a person's location could be detected, and lost objects could be located, is outlined. Development of this environment included technologies enabling the possibility to identify person's activities, such as watching TV, and preparing a meal. The impact of this smart home environment was not described.

Touchscreen Technologies/Apps/Social Media. Ekström et al. [39] utilized a touchscreen tablet with a communication application with individually designed pages consisting of for example personal pictures and films with accompanying speech. The number of communicative initiatives made by the person with dementia was not affected, but this system facilitated topics to talk about. In [24] a care management system was developed. The impact of this system was not described. Cutler et al. [40] conducted technology sessions using a range of software, games, and apps for the Apple iPads, Nintendo Wii, and Nintendo DS. Digital gaming promoted social interaction among persons with dementia, as well as the development of group cohesion.

Four studies [30, 41–43] described the usage of tablets for leisure activities, to assist in daily living, and social contact. The tablets were used to carry out a range of different activities, such as playing music, games, art and drawing, use of Skype, emailing, and playing videos. The tablets supported social connections between residents and provided opportunities to interact with a wider community than without this technology, for example to stay in touch with families and friends by using Skype for remote contact [41, 43]. The tablets also changed the way family members spent time together, with improvement in their relationships and the possibility of bringing people from different generations closer together by providing shared activities [42, 43]. The activities carried out with the tablet facilitate conversational topics [41, 43], and supported communication for the person with dementia [41]. In addition, the balance in conversations became more equal when using the tablet, making the person with dementia initiate significantly more interactions [42]. The tablets strengthened carers' interpersonal connection with persons with dementia by getting to know them better [42, 43]. Djabelkhir et al. [44] deployed a tablet with a cognitive engagement program, which facilitated creation of social ties between the persons participating. The usage of tablets for simple video chat with relatives and the possibility to join interest-based groups was described in the study by Nauha et al. [45]. The tablet was considered useful and provided opportunities for persons with dementia to communicate with their family. In [46] a videophone mock-up with a touch screen provided the possibility to receive a call and make a call to a person on the contact list. The videophone was perceived as useful and easy to use after understanding the basic functions. Lazar et al. [47] deployed a commercially available computer system with touch screen that provided activities, such as video calling, emailing, and Facebook, games, videos, and music. The system promoted interaction and communication between the person with dementia, families and carers. In [36] distance communication via mobile phone or Internet applications was described as common means for social interaction and networking. Social media and the internet were also described as ways to share experiences, engage with others, and receive support.

4.3 Digital Resources for Practical Reasoning

Smart Environment. Braley et al. [48] utilized smart home auto-prompting to increase the functional independence of people with dementia. A smart home testbed equipped with sensors, cameras, and a prompting system was used. The impact of this technology related to practical reasoning was not described. In [49] smart homes with pattern-analysis were described, such as electronic calendars, registering water taps, gas and water sensors and mobile phones. These technologies were emphasized as supportive, especially in tasks that require learning and decision-making, facilitating independence. Another smart home technology, which focused on secure communication between different sensors for localization and presence identification, was described in [38]. The system included a user interface designed to provide the persons with dementia with support to promote their independence. Impact of the system was not described.

Audio/Visual Prompts/Reminders. Burleson et al. [50] investigated a dressing prototype to guide the person with dementia through dressing processes to promote independence. The impact of the prototype related to practical reasoning was not described. [51] and [52] outlined different audio/visual prompts to support people with dementia in daily activities (e.g. audio/visual prompts applied to everyday activities and prompts to promote activity performance). In sum, the impact of these prompts was positive, with fewer interactions needed from carers, higher correct activity performance, and better completion of activities. In similarity, reviews by Holthe et al. [30] and Siegel and Dorner [49] described a range of assistive technologies for cognitive aid to support the person with dementia to perform daily activities by, for example, providing step-wise audio prompts. This kind of technologies may promote independence and autonomy by reminding persons with dementia about the steps in a given task, and hence, making them recapture the performance. van der Cammen et al. [53] described augmented reality glasses to guide the person with dementia in daily routine activities. The impact of these glasses was not described. In [54] sensors were utilized to provide individualized prerecorded voice reminders if the person with dementia had not carried out activities at certain times. The sensors supported the person with dementia, provided a sense of security and independence and allowed to establish daily routines and create the life they wanted. Still, some sensors were deemed as reducing the sense of being in control by being told what to do, and technological problems were considered as a threat to be independent. Reminders were also described in [49] and outlined that reminders to support the persons to perform daily activities may enable them to act more independently. Fleming and Sum [51] described technologies to aid memory and increase independence, such as night-and-day calendar, remote day planner, pre programmable telephone, a picture gramophone, and medicine reminder. Holthe et al. [55] conducted a study focusing on a range of technological devices to support people with young onset dementia, e.g. object locators, visual and verbal reminders, remote digital calendar, and memory clock. Technology that promoted independence and freedom was deemed important.

Every Day Assistive Technologies. Every day assistive technologies were described in [30, 55] and comprised, for example, a simple remote control to TV, mobile phones [55], computers, coffee maker, microwave ovens, cash machines, and flat-iron [30]. Technologies that supported meaningful and safe activities, especially when the person with dementia was alone, were considered important.

Positioning System/GPS. GPS was outlined in [45, 52, 55] either as part of mobile devices or in bracelets. The GPS device enabled the person with dementia to go out alone and take independent walks. In [53] GPS tracking to provide outdoor guidance was described, and Magnusson et al. [56] studied the usage of mobile phones with emergency response, GPS and geofencing. Independence related to outdoor activities increased, with the person with dementia being able to take walks by himself or herself.

Decision-Making Support. [57] outlined an interactive web tool aiding shared decision-making for people with dementia. The web tool had a chat function that facilitate communication among users, a step-by-step guide for decision-making, and a function that supports the users to give their individual opinions based on their own situation. This technology was deemed important by persons with dementia. It enabled them to do the things they wanted without asking for permission or support from others.

Touchscreen Technologies/Games. In a study by Swan et al. [43], touchscreen tablets with applications were deployed to provide individualized activities to the person with dementia. For example, music, sensory stimulation, email, games, joining the local library, searching information, and writing life stories were some of the utilized applications. The impact related to practical reasoning was not outlined. Tablets were also used in a study by Evans et al. [41] to carry out different activities, such as playing music, videos and games, and using Skype. This facilitated opportunities for persons with dementia to share their thoughts with others on their own terms. In [40] technology sessions with software, games, and apps for the Nintendo DS, Nintendo Wii, and Apple iPad were performed with people with dementia. The games promoted independence for the persons with dementia, as it enabled them to explore games, and equipment independently in absence of carers.

5   Discussion and Concluding Remarks

The objective of this study was to describe digital resources aimed at supporting opportunities for affiliation and practical reasoning among people with dementia. Specifically, we wanted to provide an overview of the typology of existing digital resources adopted and their impact in supporting affiliation and practical reasoning for people with dementia. The achieved results on affiliation showed that social stimulation and interaction were encouraged by digital resources. For example, digital resources affected carers to spend more time with the person living with dementia due to finding topics to talk about and sharing experiences. This social interaction was said to strengthen the relationship between staff members and the person with dementia. Social interaction is important to strengthen and support a dignified life for people who live with dementia; still there is a risk of missing out on creating deep and meaningful relations that are a core in the concept of affiliation. Affiliation as concept refers not only to relating to others in general, instead it is important to grasp the very notion of the concept as being able to live with and towards others, and to be able to show and express concern for others [13]. The results show that some studies on digital resources supported the maintenance of relations to close relatives, which can be understood as supporting meaningful relationships, and hence, promoting affiliation.

Moreover, the existing research related to practical reasoning is mainly focused on phenomena such as security, independence and empowerment of the person who lives with dementia. Whilst research tends to focus on independence there is very sparse research on what supports the person with dementia to actually exercise the ability to be involved in daily matters that concerns decision making in one's own life. Very few studies focused on digital resources that supported the person with dementia to make decisions to be able to do the things they wanted and live a life in line with their wishes and desires. To be involved in decision making and to critically reflect when planning one's own life are the core of practical reasoning [7, 13].

Therefore, this study highlights the need for a framework that can guide attention towards key aspects to support a dignified life when developing and evaluating digital resources. To ensure a dignified life for the person who lives with dementia the capability of affiliation and practical reasoning needs to be supported [7, 13]. This means that the person needs support that creates opportunities to live with and for others, to recognize and show concern for other human people, and to engage in various forms of social interaction and opportunities to form a conception of the good and to engage in critical reflection concerning the own life.

The existing research tends to miss out on essential aspects of what a dignified life ought to contain if it is to be called dignified. For example, it is evident that social interaction and independence are important areas that the development of digital resources strive to support. Still, it is not clear what actually is regarded as a meaningful social interaction or independence and how it relates to core values in a dignified life. The support towards leading a dignified life despite living with dementia is well known as crucial for a society that aims to create equal opportunities for all, despite decline in functions and cognitive ability [58]. Nussbaum's approach on human capabilities could offer future development of digital resources guidance by directing the attention towards vital aspects important to support to preserve a dignified life for people with dementia. The capability approach could also be of benefit when considering the evaluation of digital resources aiming to support the lives of people with dementia.

Taking into account the previous considerations, our suggestion is that future research on digital resources should focus on developing resources that can aid and nourish the capabilities of affiliation and practical reasoning. By using the capability approach as a foundation, future research on digital resources could more specifically target a dignified life for persons who live with dementia. Practical reasoning and affiliation are to be seen as crucial when it comes to ensuring a dignified life, and according to Nussbaum [13] these two human capabilities permeates all other human capabilities.

Upcoming 5G technologies can furtherly improve the possibility to help people with dementia. Features like ultra-low latency and anytime anywhere real-time ultra-high definition video can lead to the development of new applications/services to help people with dementia to be more autonomous. Moreover, the accurate positioning that 5G technologies can provide, even without GPS, can provide additional location-based services and alerts that help carers to even better monitor people with dementia.

References

1. World Health Organization: Dementia (2019). https://www.who.int/news-room/fact-sheets/detail/dementia. Accessed 8 June
2. Ferri, C.P., et al.: Global prevalence of dementia: a Delphi consensus study. Lancet **366** (9503), 2112–2117 (2005). https://doi.org/10.1016/s0140-6736(05)67889-0
3. Zwaanswijk, M., Peeters, J.M., van Beek, A.P.A., Francke, A.L., Meerveld, J.C.H.M.: Informal caregivers of people with dementia: problems, needs and support in the initial stage and in subsequent stages of dementia: a questionnaire survey. Open Nurs. J. **7**(1), 6–13 (2013). https://doi.org/10.2174/1874434601307010006
4. Kitwood, T.: The experience of dementia. Aging Ment. Health **1**(1), 13–22 (1997). http://search.ebscohost.com.proxy.lib.ltu.se/login.aspx?direct=true&db=c8h&AN=107259597&lang=sv&site=eds-live&scope=site. Accessed 8 June 2019
5. Toombs, S.K.: The Meaning of Illness: A Phenomenological Account of the Different Perspectives of Physician and Patient. Kluwer Academic, Dordrecht (1993)
6. Tranvåg, O., Petersen, K.A., Nåden, D.: Dignity-preserving dementia care: a metasynthesis. Nurs. Ethics **20**(8), 861–880 (2013). https://doi.org/10.1177/0969733013485110

7. Melander, C., Sävenstedt, S., Wälivaara, B.-M., Olsson, M.: Human capabilities in advanced dementia: Nussbaum's approach. Int. J. Older People Nurs. **13**(2), e12178 (2018). https://doi.org/10.1111/opn.12178

8. Nussbaum, M.: The capabilities of people with cognitive disabilities. Metaphilosophy **40**(3–4), 331–351 (2009). https://doi.org/10.1111/j.1467-9973.2009.01606.x

9. Livingston, G., et al.: Making decisions for people with dementia who lack capacity: qualitative study of family carers in UK. BMJ (Clin. Res. Ed.) **341**, c4184 (2010). https://doi.org/10.1136/bmj.c4184

10. Cohen-Mansfield, J., Dakheel-Ali, M., Marx, M.S., Thein, K., Regier, N.G.: Which unmet needs contribute to behavior problems in persons with advanced dementia? Psychiatry Res. **228**(1), 59–64 (2015). https://doi.org/10.1016/j.psychres.2015.03.043

11. Martin, G.W., Younger, D.: Anti oppressive practice: a route to the empowerment of people with dementia through communication and choice. J. Psychiatric Ment. Health Nurs. **7**(1), 59–67 (2000). http://search.ebscohost.com/login.aspx?direct=true&db=cmedm&AN=11022512&lang=sv&site=eds-live&scope=site. Accessed 8 June 2019

12. Nordenfelt, L.: Dignity and the care of the elderly. Med. Health Care Philos. **6**(2), 103–110 (2003). https://doi.org/10.1023/a:1024110810373

13. Nussbaum, M.: Creating Capabilities: The Human Development Approach. Harvard University Press, Cambridge (2011)

14. Eggers, T., Norberg, A., Ekman, S.: Counteracting fragmentation in the care of people with moderate and severe dementia. Clin. Nurs. Res. **14**(4), 343–369 (2005). https://doi.org/10.1177/1054773805277957

15. Bennett, B., et al.: Assistive technologies for people with dementia: Ethical considerations. Bull. World Health Organ. **95**(11), 749–755 (2017). https://doi.org/10.2471/blt.16.187484

16. Martínez-Alcalá, C.I., Pliego-Pastrana, P., Rosales-Lagarde, A., Lopez-Noguerola, J.S., Molina-Trinidad, E.M.: Information and communication technologies in the care of the elderly: systematic review of applications aimed at patients with dementia and caregivers. JMIR Rehabil. Assist. Technol. **3**(1), e6 (2016). https://doi.org/10.2196/rehab.5226

17. Ienca, M., et al.: Intelligent assistive technology for Alzheimer's disease and other dementias: a systematic review. J. Alzheimer's Dis. **56**(4), 1301–1340 (2017). https://doi.org/10.3233/jad-161037

18. Sharkey, A.: Robots and human dignity: a consideration of the effects of robot care on the dignity of older people. Ethics Inform. Technol. **16**, 63–75 (2014). https://doi.org/10.1007/s10676-018-9494-0

19. Arksey, H., O'Malley, L.: Scoping studies: Towards a methodological framework. Int. J. Soc. Res. Methodol. **8**(1), 19–32 (2005). https://doi.org/10.1080/1364557032000119616

20. Preuß, D., Legal, F.: Living with the animals: animal or robotic companions for the elderly in smart homes? J. Med. Ethics **43**(6), 407–410 (2017). https://doi.org/10.1136/medethics-2016-103603

21. Birks, M., Bodak, M., Barlas, J., Harwood, J., Pether, M.: Robotic seals as therapeutic tools in an aged care facility: a qualitative study. J. Aging Res. 1–7 (2016). https://doi.org/10.1155/2016/8569602

22. Joranson, N., Pedersen, I., Rokstad, A.M.M., Aamodt, G., Olsen, C., Ihlebaek, C.: Group activity with Paro in nursing homes: systematic investigation of behaviors in participants. Int. Psychogeriatr. **28**(8), 1345–1354 (2016). https://doi.org/10.1017/s1041610216000120

23. Moyle, W., et al.: Use of a robotic seal as a therapeutic tool to improve dementia symptoms: a cluster-randomized controlled trial. J. Am. Med. Direct. Assoc. **18**(9), 766–773 (2017). https://doi.org/10.1016/j.jamda.2017.03.018

24. Blackman, S., et al.: Ambient assisted living technologies for aging well: a scoping review. J. Intell. Syst. **25**(1), 55–69 (2016). https://doi.org/10.1515/jisys-2014-0136

25. Moyle, W., Jones, C., Cooke, M., O'Dwyer, S., Sung, B., Drummond, S.: Connecting the person with dementia and family: a feasibility study of a telepresence robot. BMC Geriatr. **14**, 7 (2014). https://doi.org/10.1186/1471-2318-14-7
26. Wang, R.H., Mihailidis, A., Sudhama, A., Begum, M., Huq, R.: Robots to assist daily activities: views of older adults with Alzheimer's disease and their caregivers. Int. Psychogeriatr. **29**(1), 67–79 (2017). https://doi.org/10.1017/s1041610216001435
27. Chu, M.-T., Khosla, R., Khaksar, S.M.S., Nguyen, K.: Service innovation through social robot engagement to improve dementia care quality. Assist. Technol. **29**(1), 8–18 (2017). https://doi.org/10.1080/10400435.2016.1171807
28. Khosla, R., Nguyen, K., Chu, M.-T.: Human robot engagement and acceptability in residential aged care. Int. J. Hum.-Comput. Interact. **33**(6), 510–522 (2017). https://doi.org/10.1080/10447318.2016.1275435
29. Hebesberger, D., Koertner, T., Gisinger, C., Pripfl, J.: A long-term autonomous robot at a care hospital: a mixed methods study on social acceptance and experiences of staff and older adults. Int. J. Soc. Robot. **9**(3), 417–429 (2017). https://doi.org/10.1007/s12369-016-0391-6
30. Holthe, T., Halvorsrud, L., Karterud, D., Hoel, K.-A., Lund, A.: Usability and acceptability of technology for community-dwelling older adults with mild cognitive impairment and dementia: a systematic literature review. Clin. Intervent. Aging **13**, 863–886 (2018). https://doi.org/10.2147/cia.s154717
31. Purves, B.A., Phinney, A., Hulko, W., Puurveen, G., Astell, A.J.: Developing CIRCA-BC and exploring the role of the computer as a third participant in conversation. Am. J. Alzheimer's Dis. Other Dement. **30**(1), 101–107 (2015). https://doi.org/10.1177/1533317514539031
32. Karlsson, E., Zingmark, K., Axelsson, K., Sävenstedt, S.: Aspects of self and identity in narrations about recent events communication with individuals with Alzheimer's disease enabled by a digital photograph diary. J. Gerontol. Nurs. **43**(6), 25–31 (2017). https://doi.org/10.3928/00989134-20170126-02
33. Subramaniam, P., Woods, B.: Digital life storybooks for people with dementia living in care homes: an evaluation. Clin. Intervent. Aging **11**, 1263–1276 (2016). https://doi.org/10.2147/cia.s111097
34. Samuelsson, C., Ekström, A.: Digital communication support in interaction involving people with dementia. Logop. Phoniatr. Vocol. **44**(1), 41–50 (2019). https://doi.org/10.1080/14015439.2019.1554856
35. Davis, B.H., Shenk, D.: Beyond reminiscence: using generic video to elicit conversational language. Am. J. Alzheimers Dis. Other Dement. **30**(1), 61–68 (2015). https://doi.org/10.1177/1533317514534759
36. Lorenz, K., Freddolino, P.P., Comas-Herrera, A., Knapp, M., Damant, J.: Technology-based tools and services for people with dementia and carers: mapping technology onto the dementia care pathway. Dement. Int. J. Soc. Res. Pract. **18**(2), 725–741 (2019). https://doi.org/10.1177/1471301217691617
37. Garlinghouse, A., et al.: Creating objects with 3D printers to stimulate reminiscence in memory loss: a mixed-method feasibility study. Inform. Health Soc. Care **43**(4), 362–378 (2018). https://doi.org/10.1080/17538157.2017.1290640
38. Al-Shaiq, R., Mourshed, M., Rezgui, Y.: Progress in ambient assisted systems for independent living by the elderly. SpringerPlus **5**(1), 624 (2016). https://doi.org/10.1186/s40064-016-2272-8
39. Ekström, A., Ferm, U., Samuelsson, C.: Digital communication support and Alzheimer's disease. Dement. Int. J. Soc. Res. Pract. **16**(6), 711–731 (2017). https://doi.org/10.1177/1471301215615456

40. Cutler, C., Hicks, B., Innes, A.: Does digital gaming enable healthy aging for community-dwelling people with dementia? Games Cult. **11**(1–2), 104–129 (2016). https://doi.org/10.1177/1555412015600580

41. Evans, S.B., Bray, J., Evans, S.C.: The iPad project: introducing iPads into care homes in the UK to support digital inclusion. Gerontechnology **16**(2), 91–100 (2017). https://doi.org/10.4017/gt.2017.16.2.004.00

42. Tyack, C., Camic, P.M.: Touchscreen interventions and the well-being of people with dementia and caregivers: a systematic review. Int. Psychogeriatr. **29**(8), 1261–1280 (2017). https://doi.org/10.1017/s1041610217000667

43. Swan, J., et al.: Meaningful occupation with iPads: experiences of residents and staff in an older person's mental health setting. Br. J. Occup. Ther. **81**(11), 649–656 (2018). https://doi.org/10.1177/0308022618767620

44. Djabelkhir, L., et al.: Computerized cognitive stimulation and engagement programs in older adults with mild cognitive impairment: comparing feasibility, acceptability, and cognitive and psychosocial effects. Clin. Intervent. Aging **12**, 1967–1975 (2017). https://doi.org/10.2147/cia.s145769

45. Nauha, L., Keränen, N.S., Kangas, M., Jämsä, T., Reponen, J.: Assistive technologies at home for people with a memory disorder. Dementia **17**(7), 909–923 (2018). https://doi.org/10.1177/1471301216674816. (14713012)

46. Boman, I.-L., Lundberg, S., Starkhammar, S., Nygård, L.: Exploring the usability of a videophone mock-up for persons with dementia and their significant others. BMC Geriatr. **14**, 49 (2014). https://doi.org/10.1186/1471-2318-14-49

47. Lazar, A., Demiris, G., Thompson, H.J.: Evaluation of a multifunctional technology system in a memory care unit: opportunities for innovation in dementia care. Inform. Health Soc. Care **41**(4), 373–386 (2016). https://doi.org/10.3109/17538157.2015.1064428

48. Braley, R., Schmitter-Edgecombe, M., Fritz, R., Van Son, C.R.: Prompting technology and persons with dementia: the significance of context and communication. The Gerontol. **59**(1), 101–111 (2019). https://doi.org/10.1093/geront/gny071

49. Siegel, C., Dorner, T.E.: Information technologies for active and assisted living-influences to the quality of life of an ageing society. Int. J. Med. Inform. **100**, 32–45 (2017). https://doi.org/10.1016/j.ijmedinf.2017.01.012

50. Burleson, W., Lozano, C., Ravishankar, V., Lee, J., Mahoney, D.: An assistive technology system that provides personalized dressing support for people living with dementia: capability study. JMIR Med. Inform. **6**(2), 321–335 (2018). https://doi.org/10.2196/medinform.5587

51. Fleming, R., Sum, S.: Empirical studies on the effectiveness of assistive technology in the care of people with dementia: a systematic review. J. Assist. Technol. **8**(1), 14–34 (2014). https://doi.org/10.1108/jat-09-2012-0021

52. Kim, K., Gollamudi, S.S., Steinhubl, S.: Digital technology to enable aging in place. Exp. Gerontol. **88**, 25–31 (2017). https://doi.org/10.1016/j.exger.2016.11.013

53. van der Cammen, T.J.M., Albayrak, A., Voute, E., Molenbroek, J.F.M.: New horizons in design for autonomous ageing. Age Ageing **46**(1), 11–17 (2017). https://doi.org/10.1093/ageing/afw181

54. Olsson, A., Persson, A.-C., Bartfai, A., Boman, I.-L.: Sensor technology more than a support. Scand. J. Occup. Ther. **25**(2), 79–87 (2018). https://doi.org/10.1080/11038128.2017.1293155

55. Holthe, T., Jentoft, R., Arntzen, C., Thorsen, K.: Benefits and burdens: family caregivers' experiences of assistive technology (AT) in everyday life with persons with young-onset dementia (YOD). Disabil. Rehabil.: Assist. Technol. **13**(8), 754–762 (2018). https://doi.org/10.1080/17483107.2017.1373151

56. Magnusson, L., Hanson, E., Sandman, L., Rosén, K.G.: Extended safety and support systems for people with dementia living at home. J. Assist. Technol. **8**(4), 188–206 (2014). https://doi.org/10.1108/jat-10-2014-0021

57. Span, M., et al.: Involving people with dementia in developing an interactive web tool for shared decision-making: experiences with a participatory design approach. Disabil. Rehabil. **40**(12), 1410–1420 (2018). https://doi.org/10.1080/09638288.2017.1298162

58. Agenda 2030. https://www.regeringen.se/regeringens-politik/globala-malen-och-agenda-2030/. Accessed 26 January 2019

The Relationship Between Diagnosed Burnout and Sleep Measured by Activity Trackers: Four Longitudinal Case Studies

Elizabeth C. Nelson[1(⊠)], Rosanne de Keijzer[1],
Miriam M. R. Vollenbroek-Hutten[1,2], Tibert Verhagen[3],
and Matthijs L. Noordzij[1]

[1] University of Twente, 7522 NB Enschede, The Netherlands
elizabeth@learnadaptbuild.com
[2] Ziekenhuis Groep Twente, 7555 DL Hengelo, The Netherlands
[3] Amsterdam University of Applied Sciences, 1097 DZ Amsterdam
The Netherlands

Abstract. Employee burnout is an increasing global problem. Some countries, such as The Netherlands, diagnose and treat burnout as a medical condition. While deficient sleep has been implicated as the primary risk factor for burnout, the longest current sleep measurement of burnout individuals is 4 weeks; and no studies have measured sleep throughout the burnout process (i.e.: pre-burnout, burnout diagnosis, recovery time, and returning to work). During a 7 month longitudinal study on wearable technology use, 4 participants were diagnosed with (pre)burnout by their company doctor using the Maslach's Burnout Inventory (MBI). Our study captured the participants' sleep data including: sleep quality, number of awakenings, sleep duration, time awake, and amount of light sleep during the burnout and recovery process. One participant experienced a burnout diagnosis, recovery at home, and returning to work within the 7 months providing the first look at sleep trends during the entire burnout process. Our results show that the burnout participants experienced decreased sleep quality (n = 2), sleep duration (n = 2), and light sleep (n = 3). In contrast, a sample of 3 non-burnout participants sleep remained stable on all measures except for time awake for one participant. The results of this study answer past calls for longer analysis of sleep's influence on burnout and highlight the vast opportunity to extend burnout research using the millions of active devices currently in use.

Keywords: eHealth · Wearable technology · Sleep quality · Quantified self · Digital health · Self-tracking

1 Introduction

The identification of burnout as an increasing global problem has significant implications for individuals, organizations, and healthcare systems [1–4]. Few countries diagnose and treat burnout as a medical disorder. In The Netherlands the number of individuals medically diagnosed with burnout per year has increased from 11% in 2007

© ICST Institute for Computer Sciences, Social Informatics and Telecommunications Engineering 2019
Published by Springer Nature Switzerland AG 2019. All Rights Reserved
L. Mucchi et al. (Eds.): BODYNETS 2019, LNICST 297, pp. 315–331, 2019.
https://doi.org/10.1007/978-3-030-34833-5_24

to 14% in 2014 [5] and employees reporting mental exhaustion increased from 13% in 2015 to 16% in 2017 [6]. Burnout is a slow progressive loss of energy and enthusiasm, resulting from chronic stress [7]. It contributes to a general decline in health [8], including depression, anxiety, and sleep impairment [9–11]. Poor sleep, too little sleep, or regular deviation from 7 to 9 h of sleep can negatively affect health and put individuals at risk for burnout [9, 12–16]. While sleep problems are an indicator of burnout they are also a symptom of burnout. So insufficient sleep can lead to burnout and burnout can lead to insufficient sleep. One reason for sleep's impact on burnout may be sleep's restorative role in facilitating appropriate emotional reactivity and prominence discrimination; individuals are more sensitive to stressful stimuli without proper sleep [17], and more vulnerable to misinterpretation or overreaction [18]. One study found that individuals with burnout reported subjectively less cognitive recovery after a night of sleep compared to healthy individuals [19]. The suggested correlation between sleep and burnout along with the gradual progression and regression of burnout highlights the value of longitudinal measurement of sleep quality and duration. The current popularity of wearable technology and self-tracking trends enable a unique opportunity to gather deeper understanding of the relationships between sleep and burnout over the long term and on a large scale. The aim of the current study is to explore how sleep quality, including number of awakening's during sleep, sleep duration, time awake, and amount of light sleep fluctuate over time for individuals in a (pre)burnout state.

To obtain deeper understanding of the ways in which sleep is impaired in individuals with burnout, it is important to understand the accuracy and flexibility of different sleep measurement tools. Polysomnography (PSG), a multi-parameter test analyzing changes during sleep, is considered the most accurate in reporting different sleeping phases [20, 21]. However, polysomnography involves studying patients in an artificial sleep environment (i.e.: laboratory) [22], which is impractical, invasive and expensive for longitudinal studies. A less intrusive process of measuring sleep is via actigraphy, which measures rest/activity cycles through the person's movement (i.e.: accelerometry) [23]. Actigraphy trackers are worn on the body and are usually small, cordless, easy to wear, require no lifestyle changes, and consequently are suitable for longitudinal research [21, 24, 25]. One study compared five different actigraphy activity trackers with (PSG): Basis Health Tracker, Misfit Shine, Fitbit Flex, Withings Pulse O2, and Actiwatch Spectrum [20]. The activity trackers gave valid measures of total sleeping time. Time asleep, total time in bed, and total time asleep differed from PSG in all activity trackers except for Actiwatch. Light sleep was consistently underestimated for all activity trackers. Deep sleep was overestimation by 4 out of 5 activity trackers. No differences between PSG and Basis were found. While some actigraphy sleep parameters are not validated, wake time and sleep duration can be accurately measure [20, 21] and have an overall agreement rating of 87.3% to Polysomnography [21]. The relatively high agreement rating to PSG as well as the unobtrusive functionality and affordability suggest that use of actigraphy activity trackers was suitable for this longitudinal study of sleep measurement for some sleep measures.

Previous research on sleep's implications on burnout using activity trackers has been limited to short intervals [26–28], the longest lasting for 4 weeks [27, 28]. This shorter research has identified the need for longitudinal analysis to verify findings [26,

28]. In a 5 night actigraphy study researchers found that sleep duration was not related to burnout symptoms in shift workers [26]. During a 4 week actigraphy study, more sleep was predictive of fewer reported burnout symptoms [28]. Another 4 week actigraphy study revealed that faculty members had higher burnout rates, less total sleep, and more rapid sleep onset compared to residents [27]. During a one week actigraphy study chronic stress in adolescents was shown to positively relate to nocturnal awakenings, lower sleep efficiency and subjective lower sleep quality [29]. Additionally, researchers found a negative relationship between sleep duration and burnout [27, 28] and people with chronic stress report lower sleep quality and more nocturnal awakenings [29]. In long term sleep studies using sleep journals, burnout participants experienced a slow deterioration in sleep [9, 12–16] while sleep trends remained stable in non-burnout individuals, [30, 31]. In summary, decreasing sleep trends have been related to increased burnouts while stable sleep has been consistent with non-burnout individuals; and while sleep journal studies suggest long-term trends of decreasing sleep in burnout individuals, sleep trackers have only measured a 4 week period. This research extends past research from 4 weeks to 7 months and gives insight into the different stages of burnout (pre-burnout, diagnosed, and recovery).

Based on these past research studies an expectation could be that sleep quality and sleep duration as measured with activity trackers would also deteriorate over time for our participants as (pre)burnout becomes more severe. Furthermore, number of awakenings per night might occur more frequently over time as (pre)burnout becomes more severe. Discovering distinctive patterns in the burnout participants would provide ground for analyzing whether this difference is also found in a larger sample that is more representative of the general population. The quantified self movement could enable a large study since this way of looking at health, wellbeing and adaptability fits very well with the current trends that involve monitoring daily activities, including sleep and movement. Data for a large study could become available through eHealth and digital health tools, which are increasingly being used for both personal and medical practice. The present study could provide the incentive and motivation for systematically analyzing sleep data in relation to burn-out, which could lead to identification of early burnout indicators. Finally, these indicators could then guide tool-based interventions designed for prevention and treatment of the different stages of burnout.

2   Methodology

In this study we used sleep data captured during a longitudinal study of wearable technology use (n = 41). Multiple sleep parameters (sleep quality, sleep duration, light sleep, awake time, and frequency of awakenings) were capturing through the activity tracker's actigraphy, which measured movement via the accelerometer in the device. This data was collected over seven months in 41 employees of a consultancy company in the Netherlands. While consultancy covers a wide array of industries it is considered a high stress occupation with a elevated burnout rate in many countries [32] thus making it a representative sample given the aims of this study. Of the 41 participants, 4 individuals were diagnosed with (pre)burnout during the longitudinal study, which gave us the opportunity to look closely at their sleep parameters.

2.1 Participants

Before the start of the data collection, the participants were asked to read and sign an informed consent regarding the use of their biological data for scientific analysis and publication. At the end of the research, it was discovered that 4 individuals were medically diagnosed with (pre)burnout during the 7 months study using the Maslach's Burnout Inventory (MBI) by their company doctor. A second consent form was therefore drafted and signed by the 4 participants to address the highly personal nature of the data in line with General Data Protection Regulation (GDPR) guidelines [33]. This form addressed the use of their sleep data for analysis and scientific publication while keeping their personal details private. The participants were between the ages of 31 and 40, two female and two male. Any further personal details are kept private as agreed upon by the second consent agreement. The initial and additional consent were approved by the ethics committee of the faculty of Behavioral Management and Social Sciences at the University of Twente.

2.2 Measurements

2.2.1 Sleep

In this study, several parameters of sleep were measured with actigraphy including: light sleep, sleep duration, awake time and frequency of awakenings. These measurements were combined within the Jawbone tool to give an overall sleep value called sleep quality. The activity trackers that were used were the Jawbone UP move [34] wristbands (see Fig. 1). Participants had to install an application of the activity tracker and a secondary application [35] on their smartphone prior to the research study to collect the sleep data securely. Data was collected via the Jawbone UP move application and forwarded to the secondary application for collecting, storing and visualizing the data in a structured and secure system.

Sleep quality has been quantified through different measures involving sleep quality and sleep duration [36]. In this case, light sleep, sleep duration, and nocturnal awakenings were measured in hours and minutes through tracking movements of participants while they were sleeping with the help of an accelerometer [23]. Sleep quality

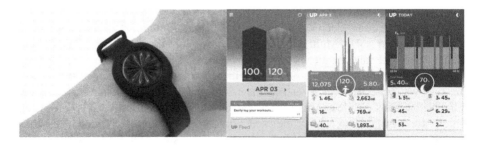

Fig. 1. Jawbone UP move wristband and app

was calculated based on combination of the different sleep measures: light sleep, sleep duration, nocturnal awakenings and was measured in hours and minutes. Light sleep, the REM stage before deep sleep [37], was categorized through smaller unique movement during sleep. Sleep duration was established from the start time of being asleep until the end time. To determine beginning and end of being asleep or awake, participants had to press a button before going to sleep and when they awoke. Manual input of sleep and awake time can help decrease false sleep measures (i.e.: lying still watching TV) and thus can improve the validity of the sleep measurement [20]. Frequency of awakenings were established through nighttime movement consistent with wakefulness.

2.2.2   (pre)Burnout Diagnosis

Burnout is not an official disorder in most countries and does not appear in the Diagnostic and Statistical Manual of Mental Disorders (DSM-V), a tool used by medical practitioners to diagnose mental conditions [38]. However, in the Netherlands, burnout is diagnosed by either a doctor or psychologist who instruct the burned out individual to leave work and rest at home for a period of weeks or months. The Maslach's Burnout Inventory (MBI) is the most commonly used screening tool to detect burnout [39]. The MBI has 22 questions that are used to detect burnout symptoms and severity of symptoms [40]. The MBI includes three different multi-item instruments: depersonalization (5 items), emotional fatigue (9 items), and personal accomplishment (8 items). A sample item from the depersonalization scale is 'I feel burned out from my work'. An example item from the emotional fatigue scale is 'I feel emotionally drained from my work'. An example item from the personal fulfillment scale is 'working with people all day is really a strain for me.' Each item was filled out by the participant on a 7-point Likert scale with 1 indicating never and 7 indicating every day. Each multi-item scale was calculated and placed in categories of high (Emotional exhaustion $\geq$ 27, Depersonalization $\geq$ 14, Personal accomplishment 0–30), moderate (Emotional exhaustion 17–26, Depersonalization 9–13, Personal accomplishment 31–36), and low (Emotional exhaustion 0–16, Depersonalization 0–8, Personal accomplishment $\geq$ 37) to indicate the severity of burnout for each scale with cut-off scores for certain diagnoses (i.e.: pre burnout or burnout). Personal accomplishment is scored in the opposite direction from emotional exhaustion and depersonalization. The doctor used the MBI's scores in conjunction with information taken from sessions with the employees, combined with professional judgment to decide the severity and state of the burnout symptoms [41]. The specific dates of pre-burnout and burnout diagnosis were noted for the 4 participants.

2.3   Procedure

At the start of the data collection, one of the researchers helped participants to install the activity tracker's application on their phone and set up the device. The Jawbone app took the participants through a virtual tour of how to use the functionality of the activity tracker and jawbone app. Sleep analytics and feedback were available on their mobile application as well as some notifications of irregular behavior (i.e.: a shorter or longer period of total sleep often popped up as a notification to alert the participant of a change from the individual's norm). Sleep data was presented each day and trends were represented with multiples days, weeks, or months. The Jawbone application suggested a nightly overall sleep period (including light and deep sleep) of 8 h in total. Most of the individuals reported following this goal, and some adjusted their devices in an effort to strive for a different goal. The participants were asked to behave naturally and engage in their normal daily activities. Wearing the wristband was voluntary and the participants could stop wearing the wristband at any time. One of the researchers was present each week at the company so that participants could ask questions about their wristband or mobile application or discuss any problems related to the devices (i.e.: needing a new battery for the device, trouble with the mobile application, or customizing the functionality/notifications). Data was collected for the 41 participants over 7 months. Multiple sleep measurements were captured each night (sleep quality, sleep duration, light sleep, time awake and frequency of awakenings). The multiple data points were then used for single subject time series measurement and correlation.

2.4   Data Analysis

For execution of the data analysis, the software package *Statistical Package of the Social Sciences* was used [42]. A time series analysis: single subject approach was used to analyze the relationships of the sleep variables to themselves, other sleep variables, and to time in days within a single case study [43]. This approach allowed us to discover the within-person variability of a particular case study. We chose two methods for our time series analysis. To analyze frequency of awakenings, a method was specifically developed for analyzing trends in longitudinal single case studies [44]. With this seven step method we calculated the direction of trends and stability of data points for number of awakenings.

Following this 7 step process [44], the total number of awakenings for every two weeks was calculated using SPSS for the participants. During the first 2 steps, the number of conditions and sessions are determined. During step 3, the mean, median, range and stability envelope are calculated. The median value × 0.25 gives the range of the stability envelope. In step 4 the median of the first half and second half of the sessions are calculated as well as the first value of available data and last value. During step 5, the mid-dates and the mid-rates are calculated to estimate the trend. After creating a visualization of the trend, trend stability is determined by looking at the percent of data points that fall within the stability envelope (step 6). At least 80 percent need to fall within the stability envelope to conclude that the trend is stable. In the last step, three questions are answered: (1) the direction of the trend (accelerating or decelerating) (2) the stability of the trend (either stable or not stable) (3) the number of paths within the trend (singular or multiple) [44].

Pearson correlations were calculated, to analyze the correlation between time in days and: sleep quality, sleep duration, light sleep, awakenings, and awake time in burnout participants. Most of the time series analysis includes all 7 months of available data for each case study. Participant 1 (pre burnout) and participant 2 (full burnout) remained in the same burnout state throughout the study. Participant 4 (pre burnout) only changed states in the last 2 weeks of the study. However, participant 3 experienced multiple states within the burnout process (pre burnout, diagnosis and recovery at home, returning to work part time, and returning to work almost full time). This participant's data was separated to look for differences in awakening during these different stages of burnout.

3   Results

Data were collected for each participant, manually sorted in SPSS, and missing values were noted. Values of 0 for sleep duration, sleep quality, and light sleep were interpreted as missing values and indicated accordingly. Participant 3 frequently napped during the day. The naps could be a confounder and could create a bias in the measurement. Therefore, the nap-data was excluded. Not all participants recorded their sleep every night during the duration or the data collection, which led to some missing data (see Table 2). When data points within a 2 week period did not reach the stability criterion of 80% or more, that time period was excluded.

3.1   Descriptive Statistics

For the burnout participants, means and standard deviations for sleep quality, sleep duration, light sleep, awake time and awakenings were calculated (see Table 1). Total period of measurements with available and missing data-points are presented in Table 2. All burnout participants were individually analyzed using a time series analysis: single subject approach [43] and discussed in the following paragraphs.

Table 1. Means and (Standard Deviations) for sleep quality, sleep duration in hours, light sleep in hours, awake time during sleep in hours, number of awakenings during sleep

Participant number	Sleep quality	Sleep duration	Light sleep	Awake time	Awakenings	(pre) burnout
1	80,4 (17,4)	7,1 (1,7)	3,5 (1,1)	0,3 (0,2)	0,4 (0,6)	Yes
2	77,0 (19,5)	8,5 (1,8)	3,8 (1,3)	0,6 (0,5)	0,8 (1,2)	Yes
3	70,8 (39,0)	7,1 (3,7)	3,7 (2,27)	0,5 (0,5)	1,1 (1,1)	Yes
4	73,1 (26,5)	7,5 (2,1)	2,4 (2,0)	0,6 (0,6)	1,2 (1,4)	Yes

Table 2. Total number of nights of sleep captured: available data-points and missing data-points, measured in nights

Participant number	Total period	Available data-points	Missing data-points
1	108	74	34
2	134	100	34
3	235	310	1
4	77	31	46

3.2   Participant 1: Pre Burnout Diagnosis Throughout 7 Months - Continued Working Full Time

Participant 1 was diagnoses as pre burnout before the start of the research study and remained in that state throughout the 7 month study. However, the individual did not leave work and continued to work full time. The results are consistent with what we would expect from someone developing burnout: sleep quality, light sleep, and sleep duration decreased, while frequency of awakening increased during the 7 months. This individual ranged from waking up 0-3 times per night during the 7 months. Time in days was significantly negatively correlated to: sleep quality r (74) = −0.263, p = 0.02, light sleep $r(74)$ = −0.292, p = 0.01, and sleep duration $r(74)$ = −0.288, p = 0.01. In short, as number of days increased, sleep quality, light sleep, and sleep duration decreased. No significant correlation between time awake and time in days was found (see Fig. 2). The evaluation of level change in frequency of awakenings showed an accelerating trend (see Fig. 2). However, in week 9–13 more than 20% of data was missing so these weeks were excluded. The percentage of data points within the stability envelope is 100%, which is within the stability criterion of 80%. Therefore, we conclude that a stable trend was found.

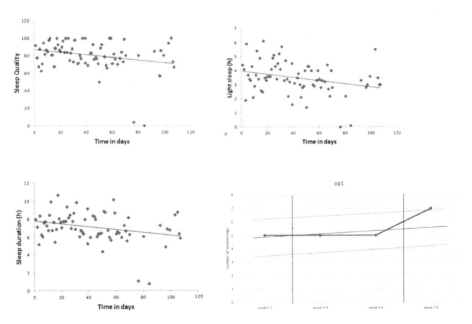

Fig. 2. Sleep quality, light sleep and sleep duration verses time in days. Frequency of awakenings, horizontal accelerating line is the trend line & dotted lines the stability envelope midrates are indicated by the horizontal black lines.

3.3 Participant 2: Burnout Diagnosis- Recovering at Home Throughout Most of Study

Participant 2 was diagnosed as burned out during the beginning of the study and went home to recover, staying there throughout the remainder of the study and remained diagnosed as burned out at the end of the study. This individual's data is consistent with literature stating burnout individuals experience decreased sleep quality. However, their frequency of awakening also went down during their recovering time except for the last weeks (week 11 & 12). This individual had the highest number of awakenings in a single night, ranging from 0–8 awakenings per night. The variables time in days and the variable sleep quality were significantly negatively correlated, $r(100) = -0.207$, $p = 0.04$. When time in days increased, sleep quality deteriorated. No significant correlations between time in days and: light sleep, sleep duration or time awake were found (see Fig. 3). Frequency of awakenings analysis shows a decelerating trend (see Fig. 3). However, The percentage of data points within the stability envelope is below the stability criterion of 80% (66,66%) therefore, no stable trend was found.

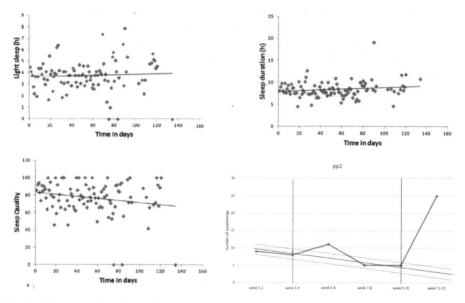

Fig. 3. Sleep quality, light sleep and sleep duration verses time in days. Frequency of awakenings calculated over every two weeks. The horizontal decelerating line is the trend line and dotted lines indicate the stability envelope. (Week 13–16 data was <80% and therefore excluded)

3.4 Participant 3: Pre Burnout, Burnout Diagnosis, Recovery at Home, Return to Work Part Time, Return to Work Almost Full Time

Participant 3 gave us the most comprehensive look at the full spectrum of burnout. This individual experienced pre burnout from day 0–33, full burnout diagnosis recovering at home day 34–107, returned to work part time day 107–216, and returning almost full time to work day 217+. Overall, this participant experienced decreased sleep duration and light sleep and had the second most number of awakenings in a night ranging from 0–6 awakenings per night. No significant correlation was found for time in days: and sleep quality or time awake for the entire period of the study. Time in days and sleep duration, r (234) = −0.192, $p < 0.01$ and light sleep were significantly negatively correlated, r (234) = −0.140, $p = 0.03$. In short, as time passed, amount of light sleep and overall sleep decreased (see Fig. 4).

The data from different burnout states (i.e.: burnout diagnosis/sick leave and recovery from burnout/returning to work) allowed us to separate the different burnout states conducting 3 different analyses for frequency of awakenings. Analysis was conducted over the data (1) in general (including the entire 7 months), (2) within-condition (time recovering at home and returning to work), (3) between-condition analyses (between recovery time at home and returning to work) [44] (see Fig. 5). The frequency of awakenings over the entire time (*general analysis*) indicated a decelerating trend. However, The percentage of data points within the stability envelope was below the stability criterion of 80% (53,33%). Therefore, no distinguishable stable trend was found for the data over the entire time span. Results of the *within-condition analysis* indicated that awakenings were decelerating during burnout and the period returning to work. Data was stable during burnout state (condition A), (100% data within stability envelope), and, returning to work (condition B) (87.5% data within stability envelope). A decelerating stable trend was observed in both conditions. Results of the *between-condition analysis* show no significant difference between conditions, both trends were decelerating.

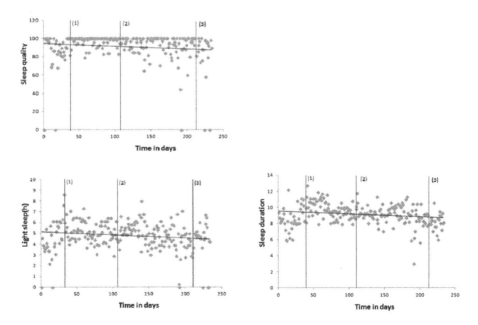

Fig. 4. Sleep duration, Light sleep, & Sleep quality verses time in days. Frequency of awakenings calculated over every two weeks. Line (1) indicates burnout diagnosis, line (2) indicates part time return to work and line (3) indicates almost full time at work.

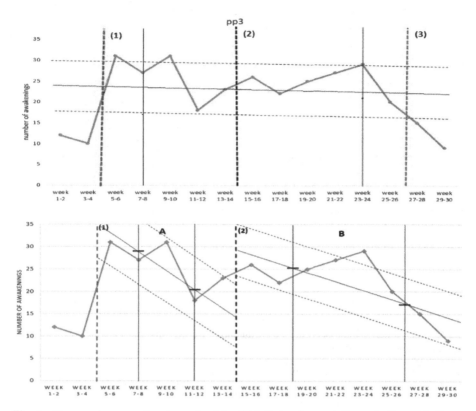

Fig. 5. Time awake verses time in weeks. Line (1) indicates burnout diagnosis, line (2) indicates part time return to work and line. The decelerating horizontal lines display the trend lines and dotted lines indicate the stability envelopes. A = burnout phase & B = returning to work for within-and between-condition analysis

3.5 Participant 4: Pre Burnout Diagnosis Day 74 - Worked Full Time Until Diagnosis

Non-burnout Participants

Three participants of the study without burnout, participant 5, 6 and 7, were randomly selected for comparison. With 1 exception the sleep measures of these participants remained stable for the duration of the study. For participant 7, a significant correlation was found for time in days and time awake, $r(104) = -0.242, p = 0.01$. When time in days progressed, the time awake decreased (See Fig. 6). No other significant correlations were found for the three participants for time in days and sleep quality, sleep duration, light sleep, or awake time (See Fig. 7). Participant 5 and 7 had missing data during some of the 2 - weeks periods of the study which rose above 20%. Therefore, the stability could not be calculated for the entire period. Participant 6 showed an accelerating trend. The percentage of data points within the stability envelope is 100%. This is above the stability criterion of 80% which means that the data is stable. Therefore, a distinguishable stable trend was found. Figure 7 shows participant 8's

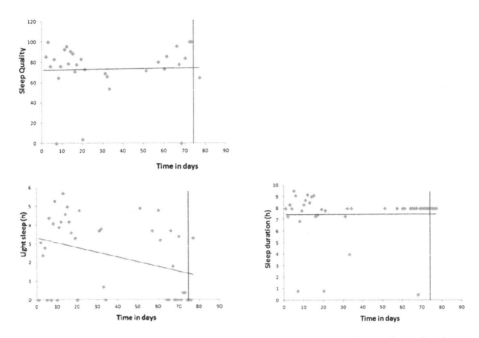

Fig. 6. Sleep quality, light sleep and sleep duration. The red line indicates diagnosis of pre-burnout. (Color figure online)

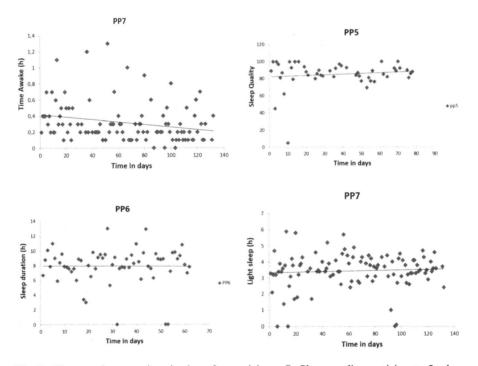

Fig. 7. Time awake over time in days for participant 7, Sleep quality participants 5, sleep duration participant 6 & light sleep participant 7.

decelerating trend in time awake and time in days. It also shows the three separate sleep measures: sleep quality sleep duration and light sleep for the separate participants. Since sleep measures were found to be stable for the 3 non-burnout participants, this figure shows the 3 measures and 3 participants to show the trend across all measures and participants (See Fig. 7).

4   Discussion and Conclusions

In this study we looked at the relationship between sleep and burnout in four longitudinal burnout case studies. Our findings suggest three main outcomes. First, we found a progressive decrease in sleep quality (Participant 1 & 2), sleep duration (Participant 1 & 3), and light sleep (Participant 1, 3, & 4) over the 7 month period. This is consistent with past short term studies on burnout [15, 27, 28]. Burnout is a gradual and progressive decrease in energy, so the decrease in sleep quality and sleep duration would also be expected to progress slowly if the burnout remains stable [7]. We found a possible correlation between light sleep and sleep duration (Participant 1 & 3). It seems logical that when total sleep duration decreases, the amount of sleep of all sleep phases gets shorter, including light sleep [37]. Participant 4, our pre-burnout participant, deviates from this pattern: light sleep decreased over time, but sleep duration did not. For participant 4, it must be noted that considerable data is missing and therefore conclusions are less reliable. Moreover, only data before the pre-burnout state of this participant was available. We are therefore reticent when interpreting the light sleep data of the participants, since some research has concluded that activity trackers are not accurate when measuring some sleep phases including light sleep [20].

Second, we found a decreasing trend in number of awakenings during the burnout state (on sick leave) and after returning to work for participant 3. Participant 3 experienced multiple burnout states including: pre burnout, burnout diagnosis recovering at home, returning to work part time, and returning to work almost full time. The decline in awakenings could be an indication that Participant 3 was recuperating during their time recovering at home. This could also explain why participant 3 did not experience decreased sleep quality during the study.

Third, no changes in sleep parameters were found for healthy participants, except for participant 7 who decreased in time awake during the night and displayed an upward trend for number of awakenings as time progressed. Unchanging sleep patterns are consistent with sleep research on non-burnout participant in both sleep diary studies and laboratory experiments [30, 31]. They found that sleep parameters remain stable for months or even years. The stability of sleep for the healthy participants supports the idea that the trends we found in burnout participants are associated to the burnout process.

Fourth, this study gave an initial indication that activity trackers may be an efficient and viable tool for measuring certain sleep parameters for longitudinal case studies. Past studies have highlighted the validity of certain measurements captured by activity trackers [20, 21]. While no studies could be found specifically on the Jawbone up move's (which was used in the present study) sleep validity and reliability. Other studies have shown that Jawbone wristbands such as the Jawbone up overestimates sleep when compared to PSG [45, 46]. Total sleep time was overestimated by 10 min (p < 0.001), sleep efficiency was overestimated by 1.9% (p < 0.001), and sleep onset latency was overestimated by 1.3 min (p = 0.33), and wake time after sleep onset was overestimated by 10.6 min (p < .001). The affordability, mobility, and popularity of activity trackers makes them an attractive option for large longitudinal studies. Data for a large study could become available through eHealth and digital health tools, which are increasingly being used for both personal and medical practice. Gathering more data could lead to identification of early burnout indicators as well as gained understanding of the different stages of burnout such as pre-burnout, diagnosed burnout, and partial/full recovery. This information could then guide tool-based interventions designed for prevention in the early stages of burnout as well as burnout and post burnout treatment. While the opportunity for measurement and treatment is substantial, careful steps must be taken to protect the privacy of individuals, especially in work settings. In this case extra consent was requested by the researchers and presented to the ethics committee for approval. This approach can be a good example for other researchers who want to further understanding in this area while protecting their participants wishes and privacy. While participants reported the wristbands were comfortable during sleep, the feedback of sleep information to the individual is equally important [47]. For instance, an individual may become anxious after seeing they slept badly which in turn might affect their sleep the following night [48]. eHealth interventions are especially interesting to countries that do not have a structure in place to recover from burnout. This study was done in The Netherlands where burnout is diagnosed, and individuals leave work to recover over weeks or months. In most countries this diagnosis and support does not exist. Burnout prevention could radically reduce the number of employees working during a state of burnout. This insight could also be used by technology developers to enhance certain features of lifelogging tools as well as eHealth interventions to empower those using sleep trackers to avoid or fight burnout.

This study did experience some limitations. First, the sample size is limited (n = 4) given that this data was captured serendipitously during another study. Research with more cases is advised. Including a burnout measurement tool within an eHealth tool or active tracker's mobile application could produce a larger longitudinal sample. Second, the missing data points for the participants could affect the validity of the findings. In future studies we recommend selecting wearable technology which does not require actions from the participants (in this case pressing a button before going to sleep and upon waking up). This could greatly decrease the number of missing data points captured for sleep. However, it should be noted that the current accuracy of automated sleep detection for activity trackers has shown false positives (e.g. sleep state can be falsely identified if a person is very still) [20]. Hopefully, future evolutions of these products decrease this problem. Third, the accuracy of actigraphy sleep measurements is not absolutely known. As discussed earlier in the paper there are many benefits of using wearable technology (actigraphy) to measure longitudinal sleep trends. However, the flexibility of the device decreases some of the precision used in other measurement tools. Also, the tools themselves differ in their measurement between brand. Further research on validity of the specific measurement of actigraphy tools can shed light on which measurements and which brands are best used in future studies.

References

1. Consiglio, C., Borgogni, L., Alessandri, G., Schaufeli, W.B.: Does self-efficacy matter for burnout and sickness absenteeism? The mediating role of demands and resources at the individual and team levels. Work Stress **27**(1), 22–42 (2013)
2. Ahola, K., et al.: Occupational burnout and medically certified sickness absence: A population-based study of Finnish employees. J. Psychosom. Res. **64**(2), 185–193 (2008)
3. Taris, T.W.: Is there a relationship between burnout and objective performance? A critical review of 16 studies. Work Stress **20**(4), 316–334 (2006)
4. Schaufeli, W.B., Bakker, A.B., Van Rhenen, W.: How changes in job demands and resources predict burnout, work engagement, and sickness absenteeism. J. Organ. Behav. **30** (7), 893–917 (2009)
5. Burn-out: de rol van werk en zorg: Central Bureau of Statistics (2013). https://www.cbs.nl/nl-nl/achtergrond/2013/04/burn-out-de-rol-van-werk-en-zorg. Accessed 14 Jun 2018
6. Meer psychische vermoeidheid ervaren door werkL Statistics, Central of Bureau (2018). https://www.cbs.nl/nl-nl/nieuws/2018/46/meer-psychische-vermoeidheid-ervaren-door-werk. Accessed 07 Apr 2019
7. Leiter, C., Maslach, M. P.: Areas of Worklife Survey Manual. Wolfville: Centre for Organizational Research and Development, Acadia University
8. Kim, H., Ji, J., Kao, D.: Burnout and physical health among social workers: a three-year longitudinal study. Soc. Work **56**(3), 258–268 (2011)
9. Ekstedt, M., Söderström, M., Akerstedt, T., Nilsson, J., Søndergaard, H.-P., Aleksander, P.: Disturbed sleep and fatigue in occupational burnout. Scand. J. Work Environ. Health **32**(2), 121–131 (2006)
10. Toker, S., Biron, M.: Job burnout and depression: unraveling their temporal relationship and considering the role of physical activity. J. Appl. Psychol. **97**(3), 699–710 (2012)
11. Peterson, U., Demerouti, E., Bergström, G., Samuelsson, M., Åsberg, M., Nygren, Å.: Burnout and physical and mental health among Swedish healthcare workers. J. Adv. Nurs. **62**(1), 84–95 (2008)
12. Harrison, Y., Horne, J.A.: One night of sleep loss impairs innovative thinking and flexible decision making. Organ. Behav. Hum. Decis. Process. **78**(2), 128–145 (1999)
13. Maislin, G., Dinges, D.F., Van Dongen, H.P.A., Mullington, J.M.: The cumulative cost of additional wakefulness: dose-response effects on neurobehavioral functions and sleep physiology from chronic sleep restriction and total sleep deprivation. Sleep **26**(2), 117–126 (2003)
14. Hirshkowitz, M., et al.: National sleep foundation's sleep time duration recommendations: methodology and results summary. Sleep Heal. **1**(1), 40–43 (2015)
15. Söderström, M., Jeding, K., Ekstedt, M., Perski, A., Åkerstedt, T.: Insufficient sleep predicts clinical burnout. J. Occup. Health Psychol. **17**(2), 175–183 (2012)
16. Nilsson, J.P., et al.: Less effective executive functioning after one night's sleep deprivation. J. Sleep Res. **14**(1), 1–6 (2005)
17. Vandekerckhove, M., Cluydts, R.: The emotional brain and sleep: an intimate relationship. Sleep Med. Rev. **14**(4), 219–226 (2010)
18. Geurts, S.A.E., Sonnentag, S.: Recovery as an explanatory mechanism in the relation between acute stress reactions and chronic health impairment. Scand. J. Work Environ. Health **32**(6), 482–492 (2006)
19. Sonnenschein, M., Sorbi, M.J., van Doornen, L.J.P., Schaufeli, W.B., Maas, C.J.M.: Evidence that impaired sleep recovery may complicate burnout improvement independently of depressive mood. J. Psychosom. Res. **62**(4), 487–494 (2007)

20. Mantua, J., Gravel, N., Spencer, M.R.: Reliability of sleep measures from four personal health monitoring devices compared to research-based actigraphy and polysomnography. Sensors **16**(5), 646 (2016)
21. Kosmadopoulos, A., Sargent, C., Darwent, D., Zhou, X., Roach, G.D.: Alternatives to polysomnography (PSG): a validation of wrist actigraphy and a partial-PSG system. Behav. Res. Methods **46**(4), 1032–1041 (2014)
22. Van de Water, A.T.M., Holmes, A., Hurley, D.A.: Objective measurements of sleep for non-laboratory settings as alternatives to polysomnography – a systematic review. J. Sleep Res. **20**(1pt2), 183–200 (2011)
23. Berry, M.H., Wagner, R.B.: Sleep Medicine Pearls. Elsevier Health Sciences, Amsterdam (2014)
24. Nelson, E.C., Verhagen, T., Noordzij, M.L.: Health empowerment through activity trackers: an empirical smart wristband study. Comput. Hum. Behav. **62**, 364–374 (2016)
25. Nelson, E.C., Verhagen, T., Vollenbroek Hutten, M.M.R., Noordzij, M.L.: Is wearable technology becoming part of us? Developing and validating a measurement scale for wearable technology embodiment. JMIR mHealth uHealth **7**, e12771 (2019)
26. Tzischinsky, O., Zohar, D., Epstein, R., Chillag, N., Lavie, P.: Daily and yearly burnout Symptoms in Israeli shift work residents. J. Hum. Ergol. (Tokyo) **30**(1–2), 357–362 (2001)
27. Tan, M.Y., Low, J.M., See, K.C., Aw, M.M.: Comparison of sleep, fatigue and burnout in Post-Graduate Year 1 (PGY1) residents and faculty members – a prospective cohort study. Asia Pac. Sch. **2**(2), 1–7 (2018)
28. Shea, J.A., et al.: Impact of protected sleep period for internal medicine interns on overnight call on depression, burnout, and empathy. J. Grad. Med. Educ. **6**(2), 256–263 (2014)
29. Astill, R.G., Verhoeven, D., Vijzelaar, R.L., Van Someren, E.J.W.: Chronic stress undermines the compensatory sleep efficiency increase in response to sleep restriction in adolescents. J. Sleep Res. **22**(4), 373–379 (2013)
30. Hoch, C.C., et al.: Longitudinal changes in diary- and laboratory-based sleep measures in healthy 'old old' and 'young old' subjects: a three-year follow-up. Sleep **20**(3), 192–202 (1997)
31. Gaines, J., et al.: Short- and long-term sleep stability in insomniacs and healthy controls. Sleep **38**(11), 1727–1734 (2015)
32. O'Kelly, F., et al.: Rates of self-reported 'burnout' and causative factors amongst urologists in Ireland and the UK: a comparative cross-sectional study. BJU Int. **117**(2), 363–372 (2016)
33. European Union General Data Protection Regulation: EU GDPR.ORG. https://www.eugdpr. org. Accessed 25 Mar 2018
34. Broughall, N.: Jawbone UP Move review. techradar (2014). https://www.techradar.com/ reviews/gadgets/jawbone-up-move-1277383/review
35. Sense Labs: https://www.sense-labs.com/
36. Pirrera, S., De Valck, E., Cluydts, R.: Nocturnal road traffic noise: a review on its assessment and consequences on sleep and health. Environ. Int. **36**(5), 492–498 (2010)
37. Maquet, P., et al.: Brain imaging on passing to sleep. In: The Physiologic Nature of Sleep, pp. 123–137 (2005)
38. American Psychiatric Association: Diagnostic and statistical manual of mental disorders (DSM-5®). American Psychiatric Publishing (2013)
39. Walter, J.M., Van Lunen, B.L., Walker, S.E., Ismaeli, Z.C., Oñate, J.A.: An assessment of burnout in undergraduate athletic training education program directors. J. Athl. Train. **44**(2), 190–196 (2009)
40. Schaufeli, W.B.: Maslach Burnout Inventory-General Survey (MBIGS). In: Maslach Burnout Inventory Manual (1996)

41. Van Rood, Y., van Ravesteijn, H., de Roos, C., Spinhoven, P., Speckens, A.: Protocollaire behandelingen voor volwassenen met psychische klachten. Deel 2. In [Manualized treatments for adults with psychological disorders, part 2], pp. 15–47 (2010)
42. Arbuckle, J.L.: IBM® SPSS® Amos™ 23 User's Guide (2014)
43. Mehl, C.T.S., Matthias, R.: Handbook of Research Methods for Studying Daily Life. Guilford Press, New York (2011)
44. Lane, J.D., Gast, D.L.: Visual analysis in single case experimental design studies: brief review and guidelines. Neuropsychol. Rehabil. **24**(3–4), 445–463 (2014)
45. Evenson, K.R., Goto, M.M., Furberg, R.D.: Systematic review of the validity and reliability of consumer-wearable activity trackers. Int. J. Behav. Nutr. Phys. Act. **12**(1), 159 (2015)
46. de Zambotti, M., Baker, F.C., Colrain, I.M.: Validation of sleep-tracking technology compared with polysomnography in adolescents. Sleep **38**(9), 1461–1468 (2015)
47. Gorman, G.E.: What's missing in the digital world? Access, digital literacy and digital citizenship. Online Inf. Rev. **39**(2) (2015). https://doi.org/10.1108/OIR-02-2015-0053
48. Hsiao, K.-L.: Compulsive mobile application usage and technostress: the role of personality traits. Online Inf. Rev. **41**(2), 272–295 (2017)

Using Distributed Wearable Inertial Sensors to Measure and Evaluate the Motions of Children with Cerebral Palsy in Hippotherapy

Sen Qiu[1], Jie Li[1(✉)], Zhelong Wang[1], Hongyu Zhao[1], Bing Liang[2],
Jiaxin Wang[1], Ning Yang[1], Xin Shi[1], Ruichen Liu[1], Jinxiao Li[1],
and Xiaoyang Li[3]

[1] School of Control Science and Engineering, Dalian University of Technology,
Dalian 116024, China
{qiu,wangzl}@dlut.edu.cn,
{1165530693,wangjx19890828,yangn_Y,sx,Lrichard}@mail.dlut.edu.cn,
zhy.lucy@hotmail.com, kindawnli@163.com
[2] Suzhou Industrial Park Boai School & Clinic, Suzhou 215000, China
jsboai@163.com
[3] Dalian Qiyu Ipony Equestrian Club Co., Ltd., Dalian 116024, China
3188812@qq.com

Abstract. Cerebral palsy (CP) is a group of nonprogressive neuro-developmental conditions occurring in early childhood that causes movement disorders and physical disability. Measuring activity levels and gait patterns is an important aspect of rehabilitation programs for CP. Hippotherapy is a rehabilitation method to improve motor coordination ability of children with CP. However, there is still no practical evidence for the effectiveness of hippotherapy. This paper introduces a method of motor measurement and evaluation for children with CP based on body area sensor network. Our method uses wearable inertial sensors to measure the motor function of children with CP by sensor fusion algorithm, whose accuracy is verified by optical system. In addition, via introducing the control group, the differences of motor coordination ability and gait parameters between CP and healthy children were discussed. Generally speaking, our method can effectively measure the movement posture and gait parameters of children with CP during hippotherapy, which provides a basis for proving the effectiveness of hippotherapy.

Keywords: Body sensor network · Hippotherapy · Gait analysis · Sensor fusion · Rehabilitation therapy

This work was supported by National Natural Science Foundation of China under Grant No. 61873044, No. 61803072 and No. 61903062 Dalian Science and Technology Innovation fund (2018J12SN077, 2019J13SN99), National Defense Pre-Research Foundation under Grant No. 614250607011708, Fundamental Research Funds for the Central Universities (DUT18RC(4)036) and China Postdoctoral Science Foundation No. 2017M621131 and No. 2017M621132.

L. Mucchi et al. (Eds.): BODYNETS 2019, LNICST 297, pp. 332–346, 2019.
https://doi.org/10.1007/978-3-030-34833-5_25

1   Introduction

CP is a group of neurological disorders that occur in early childhood or infancy, and affect muscle coordination, body movement, and balance [1,2]. At present, there are many motion rehabilitation therapies for children with CP, such as hydrotherapy intervention [3], massage therapy [4], surgical intervention [5], etc. Hippotherapy is one kind of the motor rehabilitation therapies for children with CP which grows up in western from the middle of last century. It is a kind of rehabilitation method that uses horse as a therapeutic tool to treat various functional and physical, psychological, cognitive, social and behavioral disorders of neurotic children utilizing the regular motion model of horse and the characteristics of human-horse interaction under the guidance of physical, occupational and speech therapists [6]. It is an important part of the overall rehabilitation training program to achieve the ultimate goal of functional rehabilitation. In hippotherapy, the children does not require learning horseback riding skills, but is based on improving the functional and sensory integration of the nervous system. At present, hippotherapy has been used to treat most neurological diseases, such as autism, cerebral palsy, arthritis, multiple sclerosis, craniocerebral injury, stroke, spinal cord injury, behavioral and mental disorders. For children with CP, after sitting on the horse's back, their muscles naturally relax [7]. As children with CP usually have scissors feet, when sitting on the horse's back, their feet will open naturally. By interacting with the horse, which can improve their perception and muscle coordination.

In previous studies, Lee et al. studied the effect of hippotherapy on the recovery of gait and balance ability of stroke patients [8]. Through statistical analysis of the therapeutic effect of hippotherapy on 30 stroke patients for 8 weeks, the effectiveness of hippotherapy was proved. Lee [9] et al. studied the effects of hippotherapy on brain function and blood-derived neurotrophic factor (BDNF) levels in children with attention deficit hyperactivity disorder (ADHD). By comparing the results of brain magnetic resonance imaging scans of 20 children with ADHD after 32 weeks of hippotherapy and the baseline of blood BDNF levels with the parameters of healthy children, it was proved that hippotherapy had a positive effect on the recovery of brain function in children with ADHD. Park et al. [10]discussed the effect of hippotherapy on gross motor function of children with CP. By analyzing the improvement of gross motor function of 34 children with CP after 8 weeks of hippotherapy, the presented results imply a positive effect of the equestrian therapy to improve motor function of children with CP. Above studies mainly used medical measurement methods to evaluate the effects of hippotherapy on gross motor function and behavioral disorders. Such an evaluation method is generally time-consuming and laborious, requiring higher cost output.

Current medical studies have shown that hippotherapy is effective for many diseases, but due to the inherent difficulties in collecting objective data and the lack of effective evaluation methods, the related research progress of hippotherapy is slow. With the development of micro-electro-mechanical system (MEMS), wireless communication and sensor network technology, wireless body sensor network (BSN) -a kind of wireless sensor network (WSN) [11], which is composed of multiple sensor nodes (each capable of data acquisition, processing and communication) placed on different parts of human body are gradually applied in the fields of medical rehabilitation [12], motion analysis [13] and so on. However, the evaluation of motor rehabilitation of children with CP mainly focuses on the monitoring of their motor coordination ability and joint movement, these are what BAN is good at. Therefore, it is feasible to apply BAN to the evaluation of the curative effect of hippotherapy.

Aiming at the current development of hippotherapy, this paper introduces a method of motor measurement and evaluation for children with CP based on body area sensor network. In our research, the motion data of children with CP during equestrian treatment were measured by arranging inertial sensor nodes on the motor dysfunction area of children with CP. One sensor fusion algorithm is adopted for sensor fusion whose accuracy is verified by optical system. In addition, via introducing the control group, the differences of motor coordination ability and gait parameters between children with CP and healthy children were discussed. The results show that our method can effectively measure the movement posture and gait parameters of children with CP during hippotherapy, which provides a basis for proving the effectiveness of hippotherapy.

2   System Platform and Experimental Description

In this section, the system hardware, participants and protocols of experiment will be introduced.

2.1   Experimental Scenario and Platform

In this research, the motion capture system was used (which is developed by our "LIS" Laboratory) to collect the raw sensor data in training. Our system consists several sensor nodes and one sink node, each sensor node equips with MEMS sensors and a radio frequency module. The motion information collected by the sensor, including acceleration, angular velocity and magnetic field intensity, will be written into the SD card in real time under working condition. The sink node contains a LoRa RF module, which works in 433MHz. The highest sample frequency can up 400 Hz. The MEMS sensors is one kind of industrial high precision inertial sensor-ADIS16448, which is equipped with a 3-axis gyroscope, a 3-axis accelerometer, and a 3-axis magnetometer, Table 1 shows their specifications. Figure 1 shows the hardware setup of the system.

2.2   Participants and Protocols

In our case study, four participants (1 healthy children, male; 3 children with CP, 1 male, 2 females) and one horse were recruited to participate in the experiment (see Table 2). The experimental site is Suzhou Industrial Park Boai School & Clinic, China. Suzhou Industrial Park Boai School & Clinic is a public welfare

Table 1. MARG data performances specifications

Unit	Gyroscope	Accelerometer	Magnetometer
Dimensions	3 axis	3 axis	3 axis
Dynamic range	±1000 deg/s	±18 g	±1900uT
Sensitivity (/LSB)	0.04 deg/s	0.833 mg	142.9uguass
Bandwidth (kHz)	330	330	25
Linearity (% of FS)	0.2	0.2	0.1

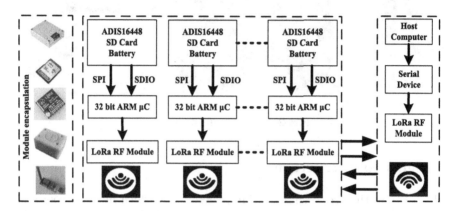

Fig. 1. The hardware of data acquisition system

school for disabled children donated by society, which has eight years experiences in hippotherapy. During the experiment, two therapists were also recruited to assist children and ensure safety.

Table 2. Participants' anthropometric details

Gender	Age (year)	Weight (kg)	Symptoms
Female	8	25.7	Hemiplegia with heel-toe, crouched gait
Female	10	29.6	Spastic diplegia of lower extremities
Male	12	30.2	Ataxia cerebral palsy, lower limb spasticity

During the experiment, ten inertial sensor nodes fitted on suitable nylon bandages were arranged on the surface of children' lumbar, chest, thigh, calf, upper arm and lower arm. Subsequently, the children ride on the horseback under the help of therapists, the groom leads the horse around a 30m×40m rectangular field and walks slowly. Therapists follow the horse on both sides to protect the children. After horse riding, all children will walk about 2 min in the designated corridor to collect gait data. Figure 2 shows the experimental scene.

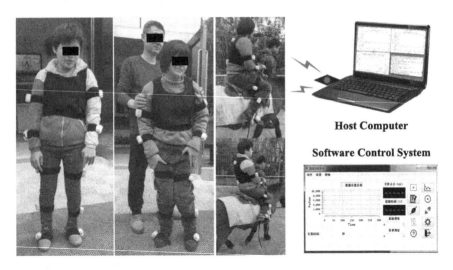

Fig. 2. The experiment scene

3   Algorithm Structure

In this section, the proposed algorithm is described, which includes coordinate definition, signal pre-processing, orientation estimation algorithm, the method of motion capture, respectively.

3.1   Coordinate Definition

In our research, three coordinate systems were defined as follows:

(1) Navigation coordinate system (NCS): In this research, NCS is defined as the North-East-Down coordinate system (see Fig. 3). In summary, the X axis points to the North, the Y axis is perpendicular to the equator and points to the East, and Z axis is perpendicular to the ground and points to the center of the earth, respectively.

(2) Sensor coordinate system (SCS): The sensor frame is defined as the axes of SCS in Fig. 3.

(3) Body coordinate system (BCS): In this paper, every segment has its own coordinate system and specific definition refers to Fig. 3.

3.2   Signal Pre-processing

In the processing of sensor data, white noise interference often exists in the raw sensor data. Therefore, signal pre-processing is essential to reduce the sensor error caused by white noise. In our research, the process of signal pre-processing can be summarized as follows:

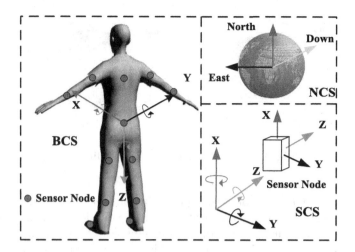

Fig. 3. The definition of coordinate system

Accelerometer: By analyzing the output of the accelerometer, it can be found that the outputs of the accelerometer contain more high-frequency components and the data oscillation is very serious. In order to filter the high-frequency part of the signal, a low-pass filter is used to filter the outputs of accelerometer.

Gyroscope: The error of the gyroscope is mainly on the zero drift, which can be simplified as the fluctuation of the output signal of gyroscope around the zero point in static state. In this paper, the weighted average filtering method is used to estimate the zero drift of gyroscope, so as to remove the influence of zero drift on the subsequent attitude calculation as much as possible.

Magnetometer: For magnetometer, it is mainly disturbed by the magnetic field of the surrounding environment, generally divided into soft iron interference and hard iron interference. In order to remove the local magnetic field interference, many studies have put forward relevant schemes [14] [15], among which an ellipsoid fitting method based on least squares [15] is effective. This method is also adopted by us to calibrate the magnetic field interference in this paper. Figure 4 shows the outputs of magnetometer before and after fitting. It can be found that before ellipsoid fitting, the outputs of magnetometer are approximately an ellipsoid and the center deviates from the origin, while the outputs of magnetometer are approximately a positive sphere after ellipsoid fitting.

3.3 Orientation Estimation Algorithm

In this research, our aim is to analysis the motor coordination function of children with CP. Motion coordination can be assessed by capturing children's movements. So orientation estimation algorithm should be used to measure the movements of children. In previous studies, there have been many related studies in such field, such as gradient descent algorithm [16], Kalman filter [17], complementary filter [18]. The main idea is to compute the estimation of orientation

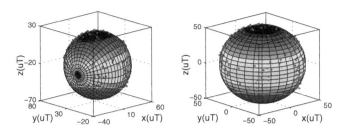

Fig. 4. The performance of ellipsoid fitting

through the optimal fusion of gyroscope, accelerometer, and magnetometer. In this paper, the gradient descent algorithm which is developed by Madgwick [16] is adopted for sensor fusion. In addition, on the basis of the original algorithm, the initial attitude calibration process is added to obtain more accurate results, and the process of algorithm is as follows.

(1) Initial Attitude Calibration

At first, considering the gimbal lock problem of euler angle and computational complexity of rotation matrix, quaternion representation is deployed in this research to describe the 3-D orientations of each limb. In general, a unit quaternion q can be expressed as

$$q = [q_0 \ q_1 \ q_2 \ q_3]^T \in H \tag{1}$$

where, $q_0 \in R$ and $[q_1 \ q_2 \ q_3]^T \in H$ are the scalar and the vector part of unit quaternion, respectively.

In order to express the movement of limbs in NCS, a series of attitude calibration should be conducted to make sure that the positions of sensors and limbs are fixed, which can guarantee the rotation quaternion between the sensor and corresponding body part is a fixed value. In our research, the calibration process is as follows: the subject is required to face the north and stand at up-right posture for a few seconds after he/she has worn the sensor nodes. In this way, the body frame BCS can be roughly overlapped with NCS. The initial alignment $q_{S,in}^N$ between SCS and NCS can be obtained by means of magnetometer and accelerometer as follows:

$$\phi_{in} = \arctan(a_s^y, a_s^z) \tag{2}$$

$$\theta_{in} = \arcsin(-a_s^x/g) \tag{3}$$

$$h_N^x = h_s^x \cos\theta_{in} + h_s^y \sin\theta_{in} \sin\phi_{in} + h_s^z \sin\theta_{in} \cos\phi_{in} \tag{4}$$

$$h_N^y = h_s^y \cos\phi_{in} - h_s^z \sin\phi_{in} \tag{5}$$

$$\varphi_{in} = -\arctan(h_N^y/h_N^x) \tag{6}$$

where, ϕ_{in}, θ_{in}, φ_{in} represent the roll, pitch and yaw, respectively; g indicates the acceleration of gravity, a_s^x, a_s^y, a_s^z and h_s^x, h_s^y, h_s^z represent three-axis acceleration and three-axis magnetic field after calibration, respectively. Then, the initial quaternion q_S^N can be calculated from Eq. (7) through the mutual transformation between quaternion and Euler angles.

$$q_S^N = \begin{bmatrix} c(\phi_{in}/2)c(\theta_{in}/2)c(\varphi_{in}/2) + s(\phi_{in}/2)s(\theta_{in}/2)s(\varphi_{in}/2) \\ s(\phi_{in}/2)c(\theta_{in}/2)c(\varphi_{in}/2) - c(\phi_{in}/2)s(\theta_{in}/2)s(\varphi_{in}/2) \\ c(\phi_{in}/2)s(\theta_{in}/2)c(\varphi_{in}/2) + s(\phi_{in}/2)c(\theta_{in}/2)s(\varphi_{in}/2) \\ c(\phi_{in}/2)c(\theta_{in}/2)s(\varphi_{in}/2) - s(\phi_{in}/2)s(\theta_{in}/2)c(\varphi_{in}/2) \end{bmatrix} \quad (7)$$

where c and s represent cos and sin functions, respectively. As the coordinate frame of each body segment is aligned with NCS during the initialization, resulting in $q_S^B = q_S^N$. Of course, it must be declared that the few seconds of initial sensor-to-segment calibration is suitable for the case where the surrounding magnetic field interference remains unchanged and that this static standing calibration happens at a certain location for a very short time.

(2) orientation update

In this paper, the gradient descent algorithm which is developed by Madgwick [16] is adopted for sensor fusion. The gradient descent algorithm is introduced in document. At here, we will make a briefly description. The core idea is to approximate the minimum deviation model by continuous recursive iteration. The objective function can be defined as Eq. (8).

$$f(q_S^N, d^N, s^S) = (q_S^N)^* \otimes d^N \otimes q_S^N - s^S \to 0 \quad (8)$$

where q_S^N donates an orientation of the sensor, d^N represents a predefined reference direction of the field in the earth frame, s^S is the measured direction of the field in the sensor frame. The fusion process can be represented as Eq. (9) where λ_t and $(1 - \lambda_t)$ are weights applied to each orientation calculation.

$$q_{S,t}^N = \lambda_t q_{S,\nabla,t}^N + (1 - \lambda_t) q_{S,\omega,t}^N \qquad 0 < \lambda_t < 1 \quad (9)$$

3.4   The Method of Motion Capture

According to the principle of human kinematics, a human dynamic model based on skeletal vector is constructed, as shown in Fig. 5. The feature of this model is that each skeleton is connected by joints and traversed from top to bottom with pelvis as root point, so that the human posture can be obtained by combining the vectors of each body segment.

The vectors of each skeletal segment are defined in Fig. 5. O_B represents zero point. The position of the pelvis can be represented by the skeletal vectors in Eq. (10).

$$d_{\eta,\gamma}^B = \varsigma_{\eta,\gamma} \delta_{\eta,\gamma} \in R^3 \quad (10)$$

where η and γ denote the label of segments and limbs respectively. $d_{\eta,\gamma}^B$ is the vector of a body segment represented in BCS. $\varsigma_{\eta,\gamma} \in R$ is the length of a body

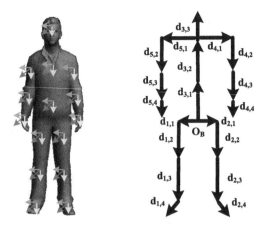

Fig. 5. The performance of ellipsoid fitting

segment. $\delta_{\eta,\gamma} \in R$ is the unit vector of a body segment in BCS. Through the initial attitude estimation, we can get q_S^B, After attitude updating, $q_S^N(t)$ can be measured. Thus the human body's posture in NCS can be expressed by Eq. (11).

$$q_B^N(t) = q_S^N(t) \otimes (q_S^B)^* \tag{11}$$

Then the posture of each limb vector under NCS can be expressed by Eq. (12).

$$d_{\eta,\gamma}^N(t) = q_{B,\eta,\gamma}^N(t) d_{\eta,\gamma}^B \tag{12}$$

where $d_{\eta,\gamma}^N(t)$ represents a vector of a body segment represented in NCS at time t. $q_{B,\eta,\gamma}^N(t)$ denotes the rotation quaternion of the corresponding skeletal segments converted from BCS to NCS at time t. At this moment, the position of each limb segment under NCS can be expressed by Eq. (13).

$$S_{\eta,\gamma}^N(t) = \sum_{t=0}^{n} d_{\eta,\gamma}^N(t) + O_N(t) \tag{13}$$

where $S_{\eta,\gamma}^N(t)$ is the position of joint between η, γ th and $\eta+1$, γ th body segments, $O_N(t) \in R$ is the position of the center of pelvis at time t in NCS.

4 Experimental Results and Algorithm Validation

In this section, the accuracy of our method and experiment will be conducted. Firstly, Vicon optical system will be used for evaluating the accuracy of our method. Secondly, the motor posture of children with CP during hippotherapy will be captured to assess their motor coordination ability.

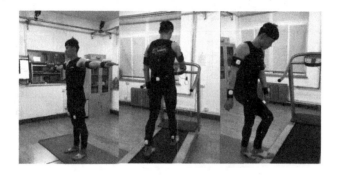

Fig. 6. The experimental scene of algorithm validation

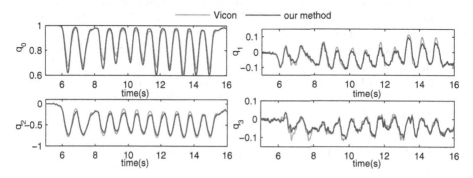

Fig. 7. The comparison of quaternion

4.1 Algorithm Validation

In this subsection, we use Vicon optical motion tracking system as a reference standard to verify the accuracy of the proposed algorithm. Vicon system is a well-known optical motion tracking system in the world, and its accuracy can reach 0.01 mm [19]. In this study, one participant participated in the measurement of the experiment. During the experiment, sensor nodes were arranged on the surface of the subject, and optical markers are arranged on the corresponding parts of the body. The experimental scene is shown in Fig. 6. The comparison of quaternion are shown in Fig. 7. It can be seen that the proposed method can track

Table 3. Estimation attitude comparison between our method and vicon

Angle	RMS(SD ± MEAN)(deg)	Correlation Coefficient
Yaw	1.2493(0.7313 + 0.5180)	0.9457
Pitch	0.2934(0.2183 + 0.0751)	0.9732
Roll	0.8249(0.4834 + 0.3415)	0.9581

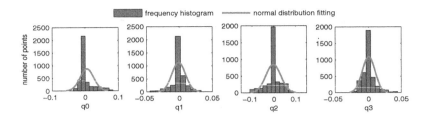

Fig. 8. Error statistics of quaternion

Vicon system accurately. Furthermore, the frequency histogram and normal distribution of quaternion are given in Fig. 8. It can be seen that the corresponding error mean and standard deviation of q0, q1, q2 and q3 are 0.0052, 0.0011, 0.0026, 0.0016 and 0.0116, 0.0105, 0.0141 and 0.0096, respectively. Table.3 lists the root-mean-square errors (RMSE) and correlation coefficients of the corresponding Euler angles. It can be seen that the corresponding RMSE are 1.2493, 0.2934 and 0.8249, the correlation coefficients are 0.9457, 0.9732 and 0.9581, respectively. The results show that our method is effective and estimation errors are well controlled.

4.2   Evaluation of Motion Coordination Ability

During the experiment, the inertial sensor nodes were arranged on the surface the pelvis, chest, upper arm, lower arm, thigh shank and feet of the children. With the help of the therapist, the children sat on the horseback and walked slowly. The children could adjust their posture by feeling the rhythm of the horse in the course of walking, so as to achieve the effect of improving muscle control. In this paper, we mainly measure the motor ability of children with cerebral palsy in the early stage of hippotherapy. In the experiment, in order describe the results clearly, a healthy child was introduced as a control group.

Figure 9 shows the raw sensor data of one child with CP in hippotherapy. Figure 10 shows the comparison of riding posture between CP and healthy children during hippotherapy. From Fig. 10, we can see that children with CP shows poor coordination with horses, posture distortion and can not control the balance of their limbs well at the early stage of treatment because of poor muscle tension and weak coordination ability. Figure 11 shows the contrast of joint angle between CP and healthy children. In Fig. 11, we mainly list the hip abduction/adduction and hip flexion/extension. We can see that in horse riding, children with cerebral palsy can not control their posture well because of their weak muscular tension, so their posture changes greatly during riding. Taking the hip flexion/extension for example, we can see the degree of flexion/extension of trunk corresponding to CP is usually large than healthy child. This indicates that children with CP have weak control over trunk balance, and muscle tone of waist is poor.

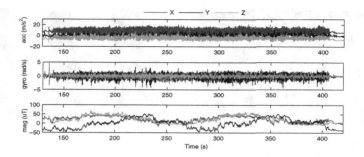

Fig. 9. The raw sensor data of one child with CP in hippotherapy.

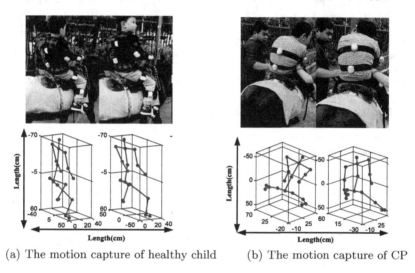

(a) The motion capture of healthy child   (b) The motion capture of CP

Fig. 10. The comparison of motion capture between healthy and CP

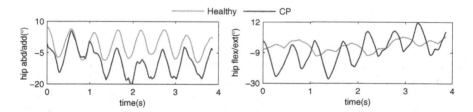

Fig. 11. Contrast of joint angle between healthy children and CP children.

In addition to the analysis of riding postures, we also analyzed the walking postures of CP and healthy children (see Fig. 12). Figure 12 shows that our method can effectively capture the child's movement posture. Through the comparison of CP and healthy children, it can be found that children with CP shows abnormally distorted when walking. In addition, we also counted the changes of

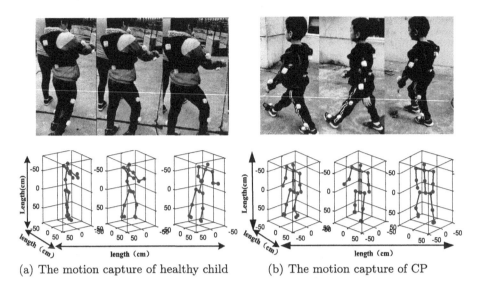

(a) The motion capture of healthy child   (b) The motion capture of CP

Fig. 12. The comparison of motion capture between healthy and CP

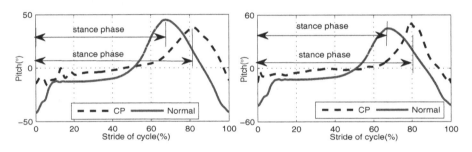

Fig. 13. Contrast of joint angle between healthy children and CP children.

the angle between foot plane and ground plane in the sagittal plane (equal to the pitch angle of foot) between CP and healthy children in walking. From Fig. 13, It can be found that the toe flexion is obvious and the dorsiflexion is very small in children with CP when walking normally. In addition, Fig. 13 shows that the proportions of stance phase of healthy children is about 65%, which is basically consistent with 60% of the actual measurements, while the children with CP maintained at about 80%, which indicates that the lower limbs of children with CP have motor deficits-crouch gait.

5   Conclusion

This paper introduces a method of motor measurement and evaluation for children with CP based on body area sensor network. The method uses wearable inertial sensors to measure the motor function of children with CP by sensor fusion algorithm, whose accuracy is verified by optical system. In addition, via introducing the control group, the differences of motor coordination ability and gait parameters between children with CP and healthy children were discussed. Generally speaking, our method can effectively measure the movement posture and gait parameters of children with CP during hippotherapy, which provides a basis for proving the effectiveness of hippotherapy.

Acknowledgment. we would like to express our sincere thanks to Dalian Qiyu Ipony Equestrian Club Co. Ltd and Suzhou Industrial Park Boai School & Clinic for their support of this study.

References

1. Leung, B., Chau, T.: Single-trial analysis of inter-beat interval perturbations accompanying single-switch scanning: case series of three children with severe spastic quadriplegic cerebral palsy. IEEE Trans. Neural Syst. Rehabil. Eng. **24**(2), 261–271 (2016)
2. Hegde, N., et al.: The pediatric SmartShoe: wearable sensor system for ambulatory monitoring of physical activity and gait. IEEE Trans. Neural Syst. Rehabil. Eng. **26**(2), 477–486 (2018)
3. Stanley, J., Peake, J., Buchheit, M.: The effect of hydrotherapy on cardiac parasympathetic recovery and exercise performance. J. Sci. Med. Sport **13**(supp–S1), 51–52 (2010)
4. Field, T., Largie, S., Diego, M., Manigat, N., Seoanes, J., Bornstein, J.: Cerebral palsy symptoms in children decreased following massage therapy. Early Child Dev. Care **175**(5), 445–456 (2005)
5. Naimo, P.S., et al.: Surgical intervention for anomalous origin of left coronary artery from the pulmonary artery in children: a long-term follow-up. Ann. Thorac. Surg. **101**(5), 1842–1848 (2016)
6. Wang, Z., et al.: Inertial sensor-based analysis of equestrian sports between beginner and professional riders under different horse gaits. IEEE Trans. Instrum. Meas. **67**(11), 2692–2704 (2018)
7. Debuse, D., Gibb, C., Chandler, C.: Effects of hippotherapy on people with cerebral palsy from the users perspective: a qualitative study. Physiotherapy Theory Pract. **25**(3), 174–192 (2009)
8. Lee, C.-W., Gil, K.S., Sik, Y.M.: Effects of hippotherapy on recovery of gait and balance ability in patients with stroke. J. Phys. Therapy Sci. **26**(2), 309–311 (2014)
9. Lee, N., Park, S., Kim, J.: Effects of hippotherapy on brain function, BDNF level, and physical fitness in children with ADHD. J. Exerc. Nutr. Biochem. **19**(2), 115–121 (2015)
10. Park, E.S., Rha, D.-W., Shin, J.S., Kim, S., Jung, S.: Effects of hippotherapy on gross motor function and functional performance of children with cerebral palsy. Yonsei Med. J. **55**(6), 1736–1742 (2014)
11. Wang, Z., Zhao, H., Qiu, S., Gao, Q.: Stance-phase detection for ZUPT-aided foot-mounted pedestrian navigation system. IEEE/ASME Trans. Mechatron. **20**(6), 3170–3181 (2015)
12. Qiu, S., Wang, Z., Zhao, H., Huosheng, H.: Using distributed wearable sensors to measure and evaluate human lower limb motions. IEEE Trans. Instrum. Meas. **65**(4), 939–950 (2016)

13. Yuan, Q., Chen, I.-M.: Human velocity and dynamic behavior tracking method for inertial capture system. Sens. Actuators **183**, 123–131 (2012)
14. Vicente, A.O., Garcia, G.R., Olivares, G., Górriz, J.M., Ramirez, J.: Automatic determination of validity of input data used in ellipsoid fitting MARG calibration algorithms. Sensors **13**(9), 797–817 (2013)
15. Kok, M., Schön, T.B.: Magnetometer calibration using inertial sensors. IEEE Sens. J. **16**(4), 5679–5689 (2016)
16. Madgwick, S.O.H., Harrison, A.J.L., Vaidyanathan, R.: Estimation of IMU and MARG orientation using a gradient descent algorithm. In: IEEE International Conference on Rehabilitation Robotics, pp. 1–7. IEEE, Switzerland (2011)
17. Zhang, Z., Meng, X., Wu, J.: Quaternion-based Kalman filter with vector selection for accurate orientation tracking. IEEE Trans. Instrum. Meas. **61**(10), 2817–2824 (2012)
18. Mahony, R., Hamel, T., Pflimlin, J.M.: Nonlinear complementary filters on the special orthogonal group. IEEE Trans. Autom. Control **53**(5), 1203–1218 (2008)
19. Oxford Metrics, Vicon Motion Systems (2019). https://www.vicon.com

Propagation

Channel Gain for a Wrist-to-Arm Scenario in the 55–65 GHz Frequency Band

Arno Thielens[1,2], Reza Aminzadeh[2(✉)], Luc Martens[2], Wout Joseph[2], and Jan Rabaey[1]

[1] Berkeley Wireless Research Center, Department of Electrical Engineering and Computer Sciences, University of California Berkeley, Berkeley, CA 94704, USA

[2] Department of Information Technology, Ghent University, IMEC, 9052 Ghent, Belgium
{arno.thielens,reza.aminzadeh}@ugent.be

Abstract. Wireless communication on the body is expected to become more important in the future. This communication will in certain scenarios benefit from higher frequencies of operation and their associated smaller antennas and potentially higher bandwidths. One of these scenarios is communication between a wristband and wearable sensors on the arm. In order to investigate the feasibility of such a scenario, propagation at 55–65 GHz along the arm is measured for two configurations. First, for increasing separation distances along the arm, and second for a transmitter is rotationally placed around the wrist. Two channel gain models are fitted to the data and used to obtain a channel gain exponent in the first configuration and loss per angle of rotation in the second configuration. These models are relevant inputs for the design of future wearable wireless systems.

Keywords: Body Area Networks · 5G communication · mm-wave propagation

1 Introduction

There is a growing interest in Body Area Networks (BANs). These collections of wireless, body-worn sensors and actuators are envisioned to enable a large amount of wearable applications [1, 2]. A standard for wireless communication in BANs (IEEE 802.15.6) [3] has been developed and several applications already exist [1, 2]. There are three types of communication within a BAN: on-body communication between two body-worn nodes, off-body communication between a body-worn node, and body surface to intra-body communication between a body-worn node and an implanted node [3]. The current generation of BANs mainly operate below 6 GHz. However, there is a trend in wireless research, for example in 5th generation networks, to consider higher frequency bands. One of these potential frequency bands is the V-band (40–70 GHz), where a license-free frequency band is allocated around 60 GHz (57–64 GHz in the US). The advantages of using this relatively high frequency band is the

L. Mucchi et al. (Eds.): BODYNETS 2019, LNICST 297, pp. 349–359, 2019.
https://doi.org/10.1007/978-3-030-34833-5_26

use of smaller antenna (arrays) and higher bandwidths. Two aspects that are very appealing for BANs as well.

An application that could benefit greatly from 60 GHz communication is the wristband to arm scenario illustrated in Fig. 1. It is conceivable that a wristband (of for example a smart watch) contains multiple interconnected antennas that work at 60 GHz and cover an arm with several scattered wireless sensors, for example: Electromyography (EMG), skin impedance, blood oxygenation, and blood oximetry sensors that are not necessarily all on the same location. Using the right protocol and antenna combiners, such a wristband array could be used for on-body beam steering [4] or Multiple Input Multiple Output (MiMo) communication [5]. This will provide premium channel gains and signal-to-noise and signal-to-interference ratios. In order to enable such a network, the propagation along the arm needs to be studied first. In particular, the channel loss or equivalently gain [6, 7] that can exist between such nodes.

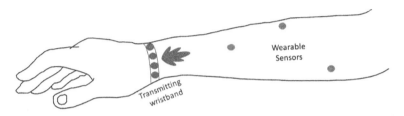

Fig. 1. Illustration of the concept of a wristband with multiple 60 GHz transmitters communicating with several wearable sensors on the arm.

There have been previous studies of on-body antennas at 60 GHz [8–10] and on-body channel loss measurements at 60 GHz [8, 11–13]. However, the number of studies is limited and are either based on measurements and simulation using phantoms [8, 11, 13] or only consider certain fixed links (fixed transmitter (TX) and receiver (RX)) on the human body such as "shoulder to ankle", "wrist to head" [8, 12] and do not provide insight into the relationship between channel loss and propagation distance. We did not find previous publications that study propagation along the arm at 60 GHz. Therefore, the goals of this study were the following: (1) execute channel gain measurements at 60 GHz as function of distance along the arm of real humans, (2) execute channel gain measurements for rotated TX antennas on the wrist that emulate a wristband with multiple antennas, and (3) develop a channel gain model for propagation in that scenario.

2 Materials and Methods

2.1 Theory

Propagation of vertically (V) and horizontally (H) polarized electromagnetic fields on a flat conductive surface has been described in literature [14, 15] and more specific at 60 GHz in [11]. For a V-polarized wave, the electric field E_r at the location of a receiver at a height of h_r and distance d from a transmitter at height h_T, can be expressed (near the surface) as [11, 14, 15]:

$$E_r = E_{QS} + E_{geom} + E_{surf}$$ (1)

with E_r the electric field at the receiver, E_{QS} is the quasi-static field, E_{geom} is the geometrical-optics field, and E_{surf} is the Norton Surface wave. The relative amplitudes of the last two terms depend on d, h_r, h_T, the dielectric parameters of the conductive surface, and the transmitter and receiver parameters. Expressions for both terms can be found in [11, 14, 15]. The validity of this approximation is discussed in [11] and requires that h_T and h_R are maximally a couple of millimeters. The first term in Eq. 1 governs the near-field transmission (quasi-static coupling) and has a $1/d^3$ dependency. At 60 GHz, this component is small at propagation distances of several centimeters [11]. The second and third terms will be the dominant in the channel measurements executed in this study (see Sect. 2.2). Both terms have a $1/d^2$ dependency [11], which has led to the proposal of the following channel gain/loss model in [11]:

$$G(d) = G(d_0) - 10.n.log_{10}\left(\frac{d}{d_0}\right) + X_\sigma$$ (2)

with G the channel gain in decibels, d_0 an arbitrary reference distance, n the channel gain exponent, and X_σ the lognormal variance on the pathloss. As [11] proposes a $1/d^2$ dependency of the surface waves, they predicted and found an $n = 4$ for the channel loss, which is a power that scales with E_r^2 [11].

Another analysis can be done for H-polarized waves, leading to a similar channel gain model [11]. Therefore, this model will be used in Sect. 2.3 to process the measurement data.

The dependencies of channel gain over distance assume perfect alignment in terms of polarization. However, in the case of a wristband containing several transmitting antennas, there will be a polarization mismatch between TX and RX. Moreover, the field will propagate along a curved surface instead of an approximately straight path. The polarization mismatch between two linearly-polarized antennas can be described using [16]:

$$g(\psi) = g(0°).cos^2(\psi)$$ (3)

with g the linear channel gain and ψ the angle between the polarizations of the receiver and the transmitter. This mismatch will decrease channel gain as the TX-RX pair is rotated over angles between 0° and 90° relative to one another and increase again for further rotations beyond 90° up to 180°. Channel gain along a curved surface is commonly described using an exponential dependency [17]:

$$G(d) = G(0) + 10.log_{10}\left(e^{-\alpha d}\right) + X_\sigma$$ (4)

with G the channel gain in decibels, α the loss per unit distance, and X_σ a lognormally distributed parameter with zero mean and variance (σ^2), which is the measured variance on the pathloss. Of course, d is also a function of the angle ψ when two antennas are rotated with respect to one another along the arm. Equations 3 and 4 both cause a decrease in channel gain between $0°$ and $90°$ rotation of linearly polarized TX and RX relative to one another. However, while Eq. 4 predicts a further increase in channel gain between $90°$ and $180°$, Eq. 3 predicts an increase due to a better polarization match. Therefore, an interesting option is the use of a two-slope channel loss model like the one proposed in [18]:

$$G(\theta) = G(0°) - \alpha_1.|\theta| \text{ for } \theta \epsilon[-\theta_c, +\theta_c]$$
$$G(\theta) = G(\theta_c) - \alpha_2.|\theta| - \theta_c \text{ for } \theta \epsilon[-\pi, -\theta_c] \text{ and } \theta \epsilon[\theta_c, \pi] \qquad (5)$$

with θ the angle of rotation around the arm, θ_c the transition angle, and α_1 and α_2 the two losses over distance with $\alpha_1 > \alpha_2$.

2.2 Measurements

The goal of our measurements was to emulate a wristband for a wearable sensor communication application on the arm. To this aim, channel gain was measured along the arm for two scenarios: (1) transmission along the arm and (2) communication between a rotated transmitter and a fixed receiver, in a frequency band from 55 to 65 GHz. The wireless on-body propagation was studied for the scenarios illustrated in Fig. 2.

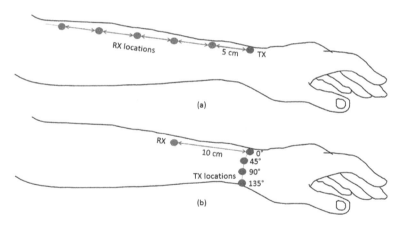

Fig. 2. On-body channel gain measurement scenarios for (a) propagation along the arm and (b) propagation around the arm at fixed separation distance.

This channel gain was measured on the left arm of three male subjects with heights and body masses of 191 cm and 83 kg, 169 cm and 75 kg, and 172 cm and 58 kg, respectively.

The procedure for measuring channel gain was as follows (first scenario). Linearly-polarized horn antennas (QMS-00475, Steatite Antennas, UK) resonating in a frequency band around 60 GHz were placed on the left arm of the subjects at a minimum separation distance of 5 cm on the arm of the subject. The TX was always placed on the wrist (h_T = 5 mm), while the RX (h_r = 5 mm) was moved away from the TX in steps of 5 cm up to a separation distance of 45 cm, see Fig. 2(a). Distances are measured in between horn apertures. The horn antennas were placed in two configurations: H-polarization, i.e. polarization parallel to the skin and V-polarization, i.e. polarization orthogonal to the skin. Figure 3 shows an illustration of the measurement setup on subject 1.

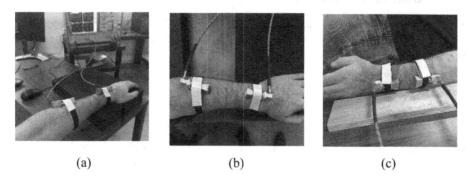

(a)   (b)   (c)

Fig. 3. Measurement setup on the body of the channel gain measurements (a) and (b) H-configuration, (c) V-configuration.

The horn antennas were connected to a Vector Network Analyzer (ZVA 67, Rohde & Schwarz, Munich, Germany), which swept over a frequency band from 55–65 GHz in 201 frequency steps. 30 sweeps of all two-port S parameters were registered for every measurement configuration and averaged for processing.

An additional on-body configuration (second scenario) was studied for subject 1 where the TX and RX were aligned and placed at 10 cm separation distance, see Fig. 2 (b). In this case the TX was again located on the wrist and rotated along the wrist over 360° in approximate steps of 45°. The RX was static during this rotation. The goal of this measurement is to emulate a wristband containing multiple TX antennas. Both antenna polarizations were again considered in this setup.

2.3   Data Analysis

The S_{21} and S_{12} parameter were pooled for every measurement configuration and separation distance, leading to 60 samples per step in distance. These were fed into a log-linear fit using the channel gain model shown in Eq. 2. d_0 was chosen to be 10 cm in this fit. The fit resulted in values for $G(d_0)$ and the channel gain exponent n. The average deviation σ was calculated by averaging the difference (in decibels) between the fitted model and the measurement data.

The S_{21} and S_{12} parameters obtained during the rotational measurements were pooled again for every measurement configuration and angle of rotation. Measurements were also pooled for measurements with equal amplitude in rotation angle and opposite sign (for example 45° and −45° were pooled) leading to 120 samples per angle. Based on Eq. 3 we enforced a transition angle of 90° and fitted two slopes to the measurements at angles $|\theta| < 90°$ and $|\theta| > 90°$ in order to obtain α_1 and α_2. The average deviation σ was calculated using the same procedure.

3 Results and Discussion

3.1 Measurements Along the Arm

Figure 4 shows the results of the channel gain measurements along the arm at 55 GHz, 60 GHz, and 65 GHz, alongside the channel gain model described by Eq. 2, fitted to the data.

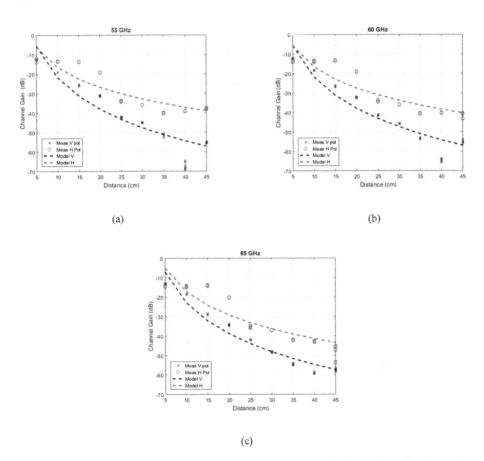

Fig. 4. Channel gain measurements along the arm of subject 1 in the configuration shown in Fig. 1 at (a) 55 GHz, (b) 60 GHz, and (c) 65 GHz.

The parameters of the channel gain model (Eq. 2) are shown in Table 1. The channel gain exponents listed in Table 1 are between 3.4 and 5.7, while channel gains at 10 cm were found in a −25 to −16 dB range. The parameters for the different subjects were found to be comparable. We found lower channel gain exponents for the H-polarized antennas in comparison to V-polarized antennas for subjects 1 and 3, while for subject 2, the channel loss exponent was slightly higher for H-polarization. This might be due to the higher body mass index (BMI) of subject 2 w.r.t. BMI of subjects 1 and 3. The channel gain at 10 cm decreased with frequency. This was expected as larger relative distances in comparison to the wavelength had to be covered at higher frequencies (smaller wavelengths), which implies a lower channel gain [11]. Our results demonstrate a good agreement with literature. For instance [11] reported channel gain exponents from 3.5 up to 4 for a 60 GHz dipole above a human skin phantom. The theory presented in [11] does predict a path loss exponent of exactly $n = 4$. A path loss exponent of $n = 4$ is consistent with surface waves [11]. Most of the values we found were higher than 4, which indicates that probably there were some near field data (exponent > 4) included in the measurements. In [19], a pathloss exponent of 3.6 was reported for two rectangular waveguides at 60 GHz on a skin phantom. In addition, [19] showed that different textiles have negligible effect on the channel gain at 60 GHz, which suggests that our measurements are usable for situations in which the arm is covered by clothing. The variation on the path loss (σ) is around 5 dB. For the horizontally polarized antennas on each of the three subjects the σ slightly increases with increasing the frequency. Similar behavior is observed for vertically polarized horns (except subject 1).

In comparison to literature at lower frequencies, the channel gain exponents found in this study were generally higher. Channel gain along the arm was studied from

Table 1. Parameters of the channel gain model presented in Eq. 2.

Subject & Frequency	G(10 cm) (dB)		n		$\sigma(dB)$	
	H	V	H	V	H	V
Subject 1						
55 GHz	−16	−22	3.4	5.4	5.3	5.9
60 GHz	−17	−22	3.6	5.4	5.5	5.1
65 GHz	−17	−23	4.0	5.3	6.1	3.7
Subject 2						
55 GHz	−17	−22	4.7	4.4	3.6	3.2
60 GHz	−18	−23	4.8	4.6	3.7	3.7
65 GHz	−18	−23	4.7	4.5	4	3.8
Subject 3						
55 GHz	−19	−24	5.1	5.3	4.3	4.3
60 GHz	−19	−25	5.1	5.5	4.4	4.5
65 GHz	−19	−25	5	5.7	4.6	5.4

0.45–2.4 GHz in [7] for separation distances from 10–50 cm using the same model as presented in Eq. 2, resulting in channel gain exponents between 0.6 and 3.2. The values in [7] were obtained for indoor environments where reflections were present. This generally leads to lower path loss exponents [3]. In the contrary, in this study a very low amount of reflections was expected due to the higher frequencies, which would result in higher channel gain exponents. The IEEE channel gain model [3] valid at 0.4–11 GHz found channel gain exponents from 0.5–2 in indoor environments and 1.7–4.5 in anechoic conditions. The highest channel gain exponents in [3] were found between 3–11 GHz. [20] measured channel gain at 2.45 GHz using dipoles in the H-polarization on the arm from 5–30 cm and found a channel gain exponent of 3.4.

3.2   Measurements Around the Arm

Figure 5 shows the channel gain as a function of the rotation around the wrist of the TX at 10 cm from the RX antenna.

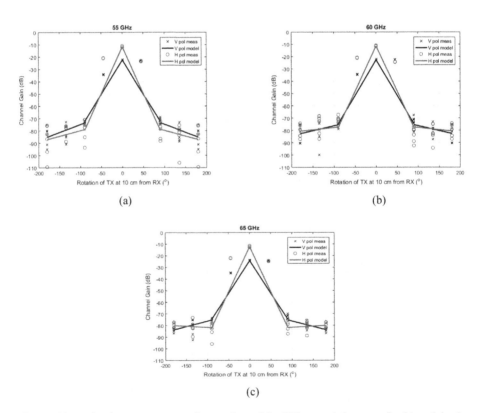

Fig. 5. Channel gain measurements for rotation of the TX around the arm of subject 1 in the configuration shown in Fig. 1 at (a) 55 GHz, (b) 60 GHz, and (c) 65 GHz.

The parameters of the channel gain model shown in Eq. 5 are shown in Table 2. The loss per angle listed in Table 2 ranges from -0.02 to 0.77 dB/°. The loss per degree was significantly higher for the angles $|\theta| < 90°$ (α_1) in comparison to $|\theta| > 90°$ (α_2) as expected in Sect. 2.1. This justified our choice of $\theta_c = 90°$ and was also in line with the results found in [18] at lower frequencies for propagation around the human body. The V-polarization had lower losses α_1 for rotation angles <90° in comparison to H-polarization. It seems that since H-polarization is parallel to the arm, rotating the antennas results in a higher diffraction loss around the arm. On the contrary, the losses per angle α_2 are higher for V-polarization in comparison to H-polarization. Potentially, a better fit could be obtained by using a three-slope model instead of a two-slope model. Most of the loss (on a logarithmic scale) occurred between 45° and 90°, which corresponded well with Eq. 3. Measurements with more angular resolution should be executed to determine this.

Table 2. Parameters of the channel gain model in Eq. 5 fitted to measurements on subject 1.

Frequency	α_1 (dB/°)		α_2 (dB/°)		σ (dB)	
	H	V	H	V	H	V
55 GHz	0.76	0.56	0.091	0.13	7.5	4.6
60 GHz	0.73	0.58	0.037	0.080	5.2	2.8
65 GHz	0.77	0.56	−0.020	0.093	2.6	1.6

The losses per angle α_1 for $|\theta| < 90°$ were found to be relatively large and would make communication with a single antenna at 60 GHz around the arm ($|\theta| > 90°$) rather difficult, since we measured 50–70 dB loss over 90° rotation. However, this opens up opportunities for good signal-to-interference ratios for channels that are 90° rotated towards one another on the arm (assuming similar path gains as both TX and RX would rotate around the arm). An important note here is that the used antennas have a high gain (19 dBi at 60 GHz) and narrow radiation pattern (3 dB beam width of 14° to 24°) in comparison to what can be expected from smaller on-body antennas.

4   Conclusion

Propagation of electromagnetic waves at frequencies from 55 to 65 GHz was studied in a wrist-to-arm scenario. To this aim antennas tuned to that frequency band were placed on the left arm of three subjects in two measurement scenarios that are representative for communication from a wristband to an arm-worn sensor: (1) transmission along the arm and (2) communication between a rotated transmitter and a fixed receiver. A log-linear model, normalized to the channel gain at 10 cm antenna separation, was fitted to the measured scattering parameters obtained in the first scenario, resulting in an estimation of channel gain exponents. A dual-slope model was fitted to the data obtained in the second scenario (rotation scenario) in order to obtain two loss factors that describe the loss in channel gain per rotational angle around the wrist. In the along the arm scenario, channel gain exponents between 3.4 and 5.7 were obtained, in comparison to a theoretically expected value of 4. The channel gains at 10 cm ranged from −25 to −16 dB. The measured losses per angle in the second scenario ranged from −0.02 to 0.77 dB/° with significantly lower losses for rotational angles beyond 90°. The loss per angle for rotation from 0° to 90° was found to be higher than 0.56 dB/°, while this quantity is smaller than 0.13 dB/° for additional rotations beyond 90° up to 270°. This suggests the potential for simultaneous operation of multiple wireless channels in the studied frequency band on the same arm with favorable signal-to-interference ratios.

Acknowledgment. A. Thielens is a post-doctoral Fellow of Flanders Innovation and Entrepreneurship under grant No. 150752. A.T. has received funding from the European Union's Horizon 2020 research and innovation programme under the Marie Skłodowska-Curie grant agreement No 665501 with the research Foundation Flanders (FWO). A.T. is an FWO [PEGASUS]² Marie Skłodowska-Curie Fellow.

References

1. Chen, M., Gonzalez, S., Vasilakos, A., Cao, H., Leung, V.C.: Body area networks: a survey. Mobile Netw. Appl. **16**, 171–193 (2011)
2. Ghamari, M., Janko, B., Sherratt, R.S., Harwin, W., Piechockic, R., Soltanpur, C.: A survey on wireless body area networks for ehealthcare systems in residential environments. Sensors **16**, 831 (2016)
3. IEEE, P802.15 Working Group for Wireless Personal Area Networks (WPANs). Channel Model for Body Area Network (BAN). IEEE P802.15-08-0780-09-0006, April 2009
4. Anderson, M.G., Thielens, A., Wielandt, S., Niknejad, A., Rabaey, J.M.: Ultra-low power on-antenna beamforming for antenna arrays using tunable passives. IEEE MTT Lett. **29**(2), 158–160 (2019)
5. Marinova, M., et al.: Diversity performance of off-body MB-OFDM UWB-MIMO. IEEE Trans. Antennas Propag. **63**, 3187–3197 (2015)
6. ITU standard
7. Thielens, A., et al.: A comparative study of on-body radio-frequency links in the 420 MHz–2.4 GHz range. Sensors **18**(12), E4165 (2018)
8. Pellegrini, A., et al.: Antennas and propagation for body-centric wireless communications at millimeter-wave frequencies: a review. IEEE Antennas Propag. Mag. **55**(4), 262–287 (2013)
9. Chahat, N., Zhadobov, M., Le Coq, L., Sauleau, R.: Wearable endfire textile antenna for on-body communications at 60 GHz. IEEE Antennas Wirel. Propag. Lett. **11**, 799–802 (2012)
10. Chahat, N., Zhadobov, M., Sauleau, R.: 60-GHz textile antenna array for body-centric communications. IEEE Trans. Antennas Propag. **AP-61**, 1816–1824 (2013)
11. Chahat, N., Valerio, G., Zhadobov, M., Sauleau, R.: On-body propagation at 60 GHz. IEEE Trans. Antennas Propag. **AP-61**, 1876–1888 (2013)
12. Hall, P.S., et al.: Advances in antennas and propagation for body centric wireless communications. In: Proceedings of the Fourth European Conference on Antennas and Propagation, Barcelona, Spain, 12–16 April 2010 (2010)
13. Petrillo, L., Mavridis, T., Sarrazin, J., Dricot, J.-M., Benlarbi-Delai, A., et al.: BAN working frequency: a trade-off between antenna efficiency and propagation losses. In: Conference EuCAP 2014, La Haye, Netherlands, April 2014 (2014)

14. Norton, K.A.: The propagation of radio waves over the surface of the earth and in the upper atmosphere—part I ground-wave propagation from short antennas. Proc. IRE **24**(10), 1367–1387 (1936)
15. Bae, J., Cho, H., Song, K., Lee, H., Yoo, H.-J.: The signal transmission mechanism on the surface of human body for body channel communication. IEEE Trans. MTT **60**(3), 582–593 (2012)
16. Balanis, C.A.: Antenna Theory. Wiley, Hoboken (1984)
17. Fort, A., Keshmiri, F., Crusats, G.R., Craeye, C., Oestges, C.: A body area propagation model derived from fundamental principles: analytical analysis and comparison with measurements. IEEE Trans. A&P **58**(2), 503–513 (2010)
18. Ryckaert, J., De Doncker, P., Meys, R., De Le Hoye, A., Donnay, S.: Channel model for wireless communication around human body. Electron. Lett. **40**(9), 543–544 (2004)
19. Guraliuc, A.R., Zhadobov, M., Valerio, G., Chahat, N., Sauleau, R.: Effect of textile on the propagation along the body at 60 GHz. IEEE Trans. Antennas Propag. **62**(3), 1489–1494 (2014)
20. Reussens, E., et al.: Characterization of on-body communication channel and energy efficient topology design for wireless body area networks. IEEE Trans. Inf. Technol. Biomed. **13**(6), 933–945 (2009)

WBAN Radio Channel Characteristics Between the Endoscope Capsule and on-Body Antenna

Mariella Särestöniemi[1(⊠)], Carlos Pomalaza Raez[2], Markus Berg[1], Chaïmaâ Kissi[3], Matti Hämäläinen[1], and Jari Iinatti[1]

[1] Centre for Wireless Communications, University of Oulu, Oulu, Finland
mariella.sarestoniemi@oulu.fi
[2] Department of Electrical and Computer Engineering, Purdue University, West Lafayette, USA
[3] Electronics and Telecommunication Systems Research Group, National School of Applied Sciences (ENSA), Ibn Tofail University, Kenitra, Morocco

Abstract. This paper presents a study on the radio channel characteristics between an endoscope capsule and an on-body antenna in different parts of the small intestine with different on-body antenna location options. The study is conducted using finite integration technique based electromagnetic simulation software CST and one of its anatomical voxels. An endoscope capsule model with a dipole antenna is set inside different areas of the small intestine of the voxel model. A recently published highly-directive on-body antenna designed for on-in-body communications is used in the evaluations. Different rotation angles of the capsule are also considered both with a layer model and a voxel model. It is found that radio channel characteristics vary remarkably depending on the antenna location in the small intestine and location of the on-body antenna. Thus, the on-body antennas should be located carefully to ensure coverage over the whole intestine area. However, the path loss does not only depend on the distance between a capsule and the on-body antenna but also on the tissues between the capsule and on-body antennas. Furthermore, orientation of the capsule has also strong impact when linearly polarized antennas are used.

Keywords: Capsule endoscopy · Directive antenna · Gastrointestinal monitoring · Implant communications · Ultra wideband · Wireless Body Area Networks

1 Introduction

Capsule endoscopy has become a popular method to investigate the gastrointestinal (GI) tract area due to its several advantages: it is reliable, painless, and comfortable way to examine especially the small intestine (SI) area, which is not easily reached with the conventional endoscopy techniques. In the capsule endoscopy, the patient just swallows a small pill, which contains a camera and transmitter, and wears a monitoring device on the waist where the data from the capsule is transmitted [1, 2].

© ICST Institute for Computer Sciences, Social Informatics and Telecommunications Engineering 2019
Published by Springer Nature Switzerland AG 2019. All Rights Reserved
L. Mucchi et al. (Eds.): BODYNETS 2019, LNICST 297, pp. 360–373, 2019.
https://doi.org/10.1007/978-3-030-34833-5_27

Different techniques are used to transmit the data from the capsule to the on-body device. Ultra wideband (UWB) has recently become an attractive alternative for the communication link since it enables reliable and high-data rate data transfer with low power consumption and simple electronics. Besides, large bandwidth enables high resolution for the images [3, 5]. The frequency bandwidth determined by the IEEE 802.15.6 standard for Wireless Body Area Networks (WBAN) [6] is 3.1–10.6 GHz. The propagation losses in the tissues increase as the frequency increases. Thus, the lower part of the UWB band is usually considered for the capsule endoscopy application [3–5].

Smooth design of transceivers require deep knowledge of the channel characteristics and propagation within the tissues. Thus, there are several UWB channel models and propagation studies presented in the literature for wearable and implant communication systems in the human abdomen area [7–17]. Furthermore, the research in antenna design, both for capsule antennas as well as for on-body receiver antennas, has been active recently [18–25]. Channel characteristics between the capsule antenna and on-body antenna is studied e.g. in [3, 5, 7, 24]. In-body power distribution in the abdominal area was studied in detail in [7]. It was shown that the power inside the abdomen area is distributed depending on the tissues and antenna locations. Even challenging locations in the small intestine area can be reached with appropriate on-body antenna locations.

This paper is continuation of [7] by presenting UWB-WBAN channel characteristics between the endoscope capsule and recently published high-directive on-body antennas in different parts of the SI. Two different on-body antenna location options, both suitable for capsule endoscopy, are considered. Frequency and time domains are considered. Furthermore, the impact of the capsule's rotation angle is studied on the channel characteristics both with a layer model and the voxel model.

The paper is organized as follows: Sect. 2 describes the study case, i.e., voxel model, antennas, and antenna locations. Section 4 presents the results for channel characteristics between the endoscope capsule and on-body antenna as well as the impact of the rotation angles. Conclusions are given in Sect. 5.

2 Study Case

Since this paper is continuation of the research presented in [7], the study case can be studied more in detail in [7]. However, this section briefly repeats the most essential information for ease reading.

2.1 Voxel Model

Simulations were conducted using the electromagnetic simulation software CST MicroWave Studio [26], which is based on finite integration technique (FIT). CST provides several voxel models, among which we selected an anatomical voxel model Laura, presented in Fig. 1a. Laura corresponds to lean female body with resolution of 1.87 cm × 1.87 cm × 1.87 cm. Cross-section of the voxel model's abdomen area on the navel line is shown in Fig. 1b.

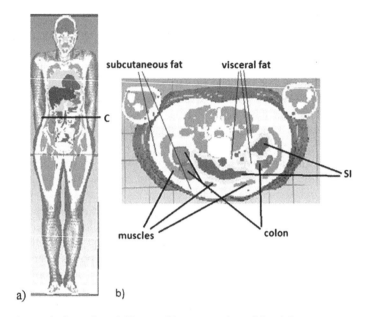

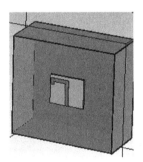

Fig. 1. (a) Anatomical voxel model Laura, (b) cross section of the abdomen area presenting the subcutaneous and visceral fat.

2.2   On-Body Antenna and Antenna Locations

In this study case, we use a cavity-backed low-band UWB antenna designed for on-in-body communications. The antenna is presented in Fig. 2 [18]. This antenna is designed to work in the frequency band 3.75–4.25 GHz. Two different antenna location options were considered, both of them are suitable for monitoring purposes [7]. The antenna location options are presented in the Fig. 3a–b.

Fig. 2. A cavity-backed low-band UWB on-body antenna designed for in-body communications.

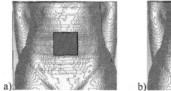
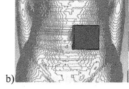

Fig. 3. Location of the on-body antenna (a) on the navel, (b) on the side.

2.3 Capsule Model

In this study, we use a simplified capsule model, in which a simple dipole antenna is embedded in the plastic capsule shell, as presented in Fig. 4a–b, respectively. The capsule itself has realistic dimensions: 11 mm × 25 mm, corresponding to the size of the commercial capsules nowadays. The dipole antenna is omnidirectional and it is designed to work at the frequency 4 GHz. The reflection coefficient S11 and the radiation pattern of the dipole antenna are presented in Fig. 5a–b, respectively.

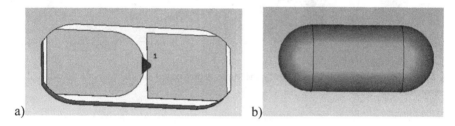

Fig. 4. (a) dipole antenna inside the capsule, (b) capsule shell

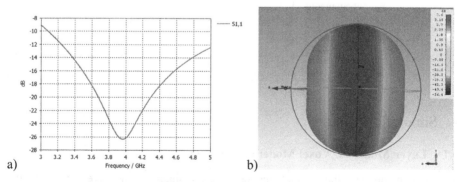

Fig. 5. (a) S11 and (b) radiation pattern of the antenna.

3 Layer Model

The layer model used in this study is presented in Fig. 6a. Tissue thicknesses in the layer model correspond to the thicknesses of the voxel model in the cross-section C in Fig. 1 with antenna location option 2 shown in Fig. 6b. The location of the capsule in the small intestine is included in the voxel model as well. The thicknesses of the different layers are summarized in Table 1. One should note that the thicknesses of different layer models may vary depending which part of the abdomen is considered. Table 1 also summarizes the dielectric properties of these tissues to describe different propagation properties [27].

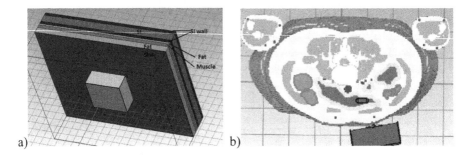

Fig. 6. (a) Layer model designed using the dimensions based on (b) antenna location 2 and cross-section C.

Table 1. Layer model dimension and dielectric properties of tissues at 4 GHz.

	Thickness [mm]	Permittivity	Conductivity
Skin	1.4	36.6	2.34
Fat subcutaneous	15	5.13	0.183
Muscle	9	50.8	3.01
Fat (visceral)	4	5.13	0.183
SI wall	8	50.82	3.105
SI content	20	51.7	4.62

4 Simulation Results

4.1 Layer Model vs. Voxel Model Comparison

This section compares the channel characteristics obtained with the layer model and the voxel model. The frequency domain results - path loss - and time domain results - impulse responses (IR) - obtained by performing inverse fast Fourier transform (IFFT) for the S21, for the layer model and voxel model are presented in Fig. 7a–b, respectively. As one can note, there is clear difference between the results obtained using the layer model and the voxel model both in frequency and time domains. In the frequency range of interest, i.e. at 3.75–4.25 GHz, the channel parameters S21, which corresponds to path loss, is even 10 dB lower with the layer model than with the voxel model. In the time domain, the levels of the first three peaks are 10 dB lower with the layer model.

The reason for this tendency is conjectured to be due to two reasons: (1) the pixels of the voxel model has more space between the antenna and the skin, which improves the antenna performance [18] and hence may improve the channel characteristics as explained in [14]. (2) The layer model mainly takes account the simple direct propagation through the tissues whereas the voxel model includes the impact of more complex indirect propagation paths, e.g. through the fat layer, as explained in [7, 8].

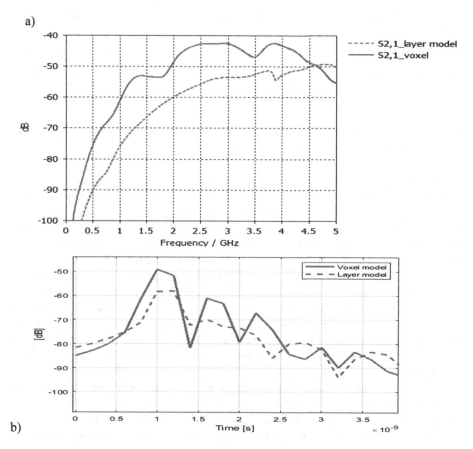

a)

b)

Fig. 7. (a) Frequency and (b) time domain comparison between the voxel model and layer model results.

4.2   On-Body Antenna Location 1

In this section, we present channel characteristics between the capsule and the low-band UWB cavity-backed on-body antenna at the cross-section A (see Fig. 1) with different antenna location options. The channel characteristics are evaluated at three different capsule locations, which are presented in Fig. 8. In the option "a", the capsule is in the middle of the SI at the cross-section B, i.e., the distance between the on-body antenna and the capsule is the smallest. In the capsule location option "b", the antenna is on the front-left part of the SI, and in the capsule location option "c", the antenna is on the right back part of the SI. These capsule location options are chosen to cover the most interesting parts of the SI in terms of in-body power distribution studies presented in [7].

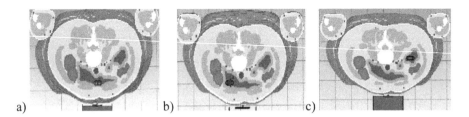

Fig. 8. Locations of the capsule (a) in the middle of the SI's front part, (b) in the left side of the SI's front part, (c) in the right side of the SI's back part.

The frequency and time domain channel characteristics are presented in Fig. 9a–b, respectively. Evidently, the path loss is lowest as the capsule is located in the middle of the SI (case a), since the distance between the capsule and the on-body antenna is smallest and since the part of the signal may travel without passing the muscle layer, as explained in [7] and [8]. Instead, the path loss difference between the cases b and c is surprisingly small in the frequency range of interest, although "c" is clearly further from the on-body antenna than in the case "b". Actually at 3.8 GHz, the path loss in location "b" is even higher than at point "c". Since there are no remarkable differences in the antennas' radiation patterns toward point "b" and "c", as presented in [18], the reason for this phenomenon can be found from the propagation paths. For the point "c", there is a propagation path option through the fat layer, in which the losses are minor, as explained in [7, 8, 12, 13]. Instead, for the point "b", most of the signal needs to travel through the small intestine tissue, in which the losses are high.

In the time domain, as the IFFT is performed for the whole bandwidth, the differences are clearer. Besides, the shapes of the IRs differ from each other remarkably. The further away the capsule is from the on-body antenna, the richer is the IR with larger number of significant propagation paths, which appear as the signal propagates inside the body avoiding the most challenging tissues.

The path loss in the case of point "c" is excessive to provide enough strong communications link between the capsule and the on-body antenna. Thus, we need to evaluate the channel characteristics when the on-body antenna is located on the side of the abdomen as well. The next subsection channel characteristics with the antenna location option 2.

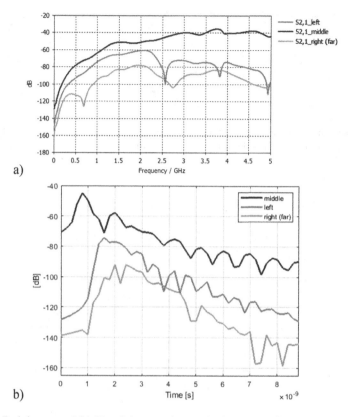

a)

b)

Fig. 9. (a) Path losses and (b) IRs of the capsule – on-body antenna link at the antenna location option 1.

4.3   On-Body Antenna Location 2

Next, we evaluate the channel characteristics with the antenna location option 2. Capsule locations are presented in Fig. 10a–c as (a) left (the furthest possible location), (b) middle (the second furthest location) and (c) in the right side of the SI's back part. The frequency and time domain channel characteristics are presented in Fig. 11a–b. The channel is naturally at strongest in the capsule location "b", since the distance between the capsule and the on-body antenna is the smallest of these presented cases. The channel at capsule location "a" is stronger than in the location "c", although the distance between the capsule and the on-body antenna is larger in the case of "a" The path loss is even 10 dB higher at the location "c" than in the location "a" at 3.75 GHz. Instead, at 4–4.25 GHz, the path loss is same. In the time domain, the difference is the strongest for first two peaks.

The channel in the point "a" is stronger than in the point "c" due to the more favorable propagation paths towards the on-body antenna. For instance in the case of point "a", according to the voxel model's cross-section, the signal can propagate through the fat layer without passing the muscle layer, which is known to be the among

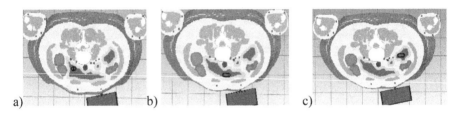

Fig. 10. Locations of the capsule (a) in the middle of the SI's front part, (b) in the left side of the SI's front part, (c) in the right side of the SI's back part.

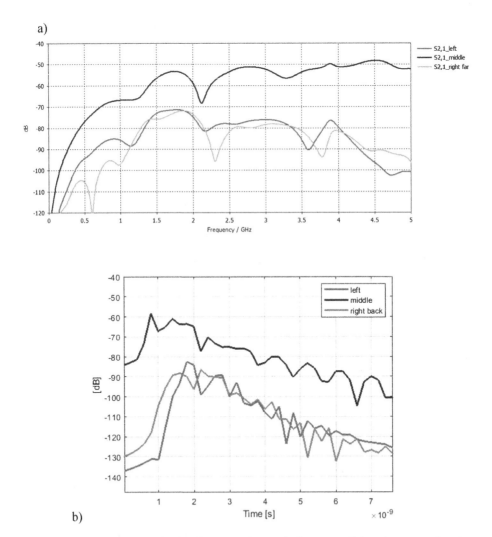

Fig. 11. (a) Path losses and (b) IRs of the capsule – on-body antenna link at the antenna location option 2.

the worst tissues for the propagation. Instead, in the point "c", the signal has to pass the muscle layer before reaching the on-body antenna, which reduced the power more. These inbody power distribution and propagation path issues are explained more in detail in [7].

The path loss with the antenna location option 2 in the point "c" is still high, though slightly lower than with the antenna location option 1. To ensure good communication link between the capsule and the on-body antenna in the location "c", one receiving on-body antenna should be placed further from the navel area towards sides of the body. Besides, it is essential to have more than one on-body antenna in the capsule endoscopy operations.

4.4   Impact of the Rotation on the Channel Characteristics

Layer Model Results

In this subsection we present the impact of the capsule's rotation angle on the channel characteristics. Since the antennas are linearly polarized, the rotation angle is assumed to have a clear impact on the power loss.

First, the impact is evaluated with the layer model for simplicity. We evaluated the rotation angles 0°, 45° and 90°, as shown in Fig. 12a–c. As one can note, rotation of the capsule impacts clearly on the channel characteristics both in frequency and time domains. Naturally, the difference is largest between the rotation angles 0° and 90°. The path loss difference is maximum 13 dB within the frequency range of the interest. The smallest path loss difference is 4 dB at 4 GHz. In time domain, the largest difference can be seen in the level and the shape of the IR's main peaks. The level difference is up to 8 dB in the main peaks (Fig. 13).

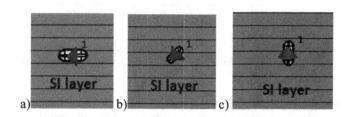

Fig. 12. Rotation angles of the capsule (a) 0°, (b) 45°, and (c) 90° with layer model

Voxel Model Results

The impact of the rotation is evaluated for the case with the on-body antenna and capsule location presented in Fig. 6b. The thickness of the tissues just below the antenna in this scenario is the same as with the layer model. We evaluated the rotation angles 0°, 45° and 90°, which are presented in vertical cross-sections in Fig. 14a–c.

Figure 15a–b present the channel characteristics with different rotation angles of the capsule in frequency and time domains, respectively. As one can note from Fig. 15a, there is only minor differences in the path losses between the rotation angle cases 0° and 45° in the frequency range 2–5 GHz. Instead, with the rotation angle 90° the path loss is

a)

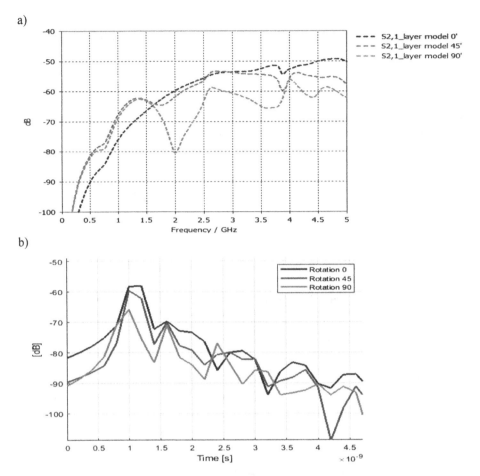

b)

Fig. 13. Channel characteristics between the capsule – on-body antenna link with different rotation angles of the capsule in (a) frequency domain and (b) time domain, layer model results.

10–17 dB lower than with rotation angles 0 and 45 in the frequency band of the interest. Similar tendency can be found in the main peaks of the IRs presented in Fig. 15b: the level of the main peak is approximately same for the cases with the rotation angle 0 and 45, whereas the main peak obtained with the rotation angle 90° is 6 dB lower. Interestingly, the level of the second peak is the highest for the case with the rotation angle 90°. In general, the rotation angle changes clearly the shape of the IR after the main peak: the timing, width, and level of the side peaks very remarkably. Hence, the rotation of the capsule affects on the propagation path which the signal choses.

When comparing the impact of the rotation obtained with layer model and voxel model, one can note similarities only in the path loss behaviour. Naturally, the level difference is same as explained in Subsect. 3.1. In time domain, there are clear differences between the side peaks obtained using the layer model and voxel model. It is obvious that the rotation affects on the propagation paths, which can not be investigated accurately with the simple layer models. The impact of the rotation on the channel characteristics will be studied more in detail with the voxel models in the extension of this paper.

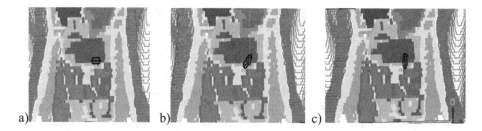

Fig. 14. Rotation angles of the capsule (a) 0°, (b) 45° and (c) 90°.

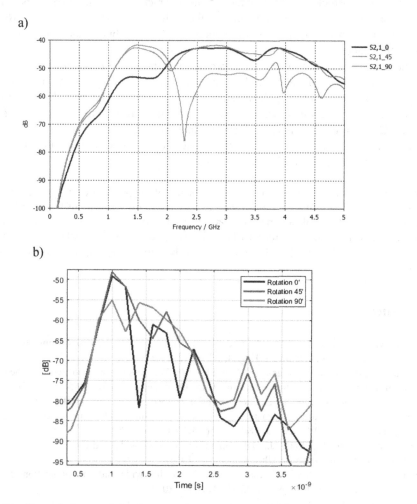

Fig. 15. Channel characteristics between the capsule – on-body antenna link with different rotation angles of the capsule in (a) frequency domain and (b) time domain.

5 Conclusions

This paper presents a study on the radio channel characteristics between the capsule endoscope and the high-directive on-body antenna in different parts of the small intestine with different on-body antenna locations. The study was conducted using finite integration technique based electromagnetic simulation software CST and its anatomical voxel model. A capsule endoscope with a dipole antenna was set inside different areas of the small intestine of the voxel model. The impact of the different rotation angles of the capsule on the channel characteristics was also evaluated both with a layer model and a voxel model. It is found that the radio channel characteristics varied remarkably depending on the capsule location in the small intestine and location of the on-body antennas. Thus, the locations of on-body antennas should be carefully selected to ensure coverage over the whole intestine area. Furthermore, orientation of the capsule had also clear impact on the channel characteristics when linearly polarized antennas are used. The largest difference in the path losses of different cases is 16 dB. In the main peaks of the IR's the difference is only 6 dB but in the side peaks, the difference is larger.

The results presented in this study provide insight on the channel characteristics, which could be obtained when a highly directive on-body UWB antenna is used. In this study, we used a simple dipole antenna on the capsule. The path loss could be diminished even more with circular-polarized antennas, either on the body or inside the capsule. Our future target is to evaluate channel characteristics with different highly-directive antennas and also with more realistic capsule structure. Furthermore, the impact of the rotation is studied more in detail.

Acknowledgements. This research has been financially supported by the project WBAN Communications in the Congested Environments and in part by Academy of Finland 6Genesis Flagship (grant 318927). Ilkka Virtanen, Timo Mäkinen, and Jari Sillanpää from University of Oulu deserve acknowledgement for their help to enable the exhaustive simulations. Dr. Marko Sonkki from CWC, University of Oulu, is acknowledged for his participation on the on-body antenna design.

References

1. Ciuti, G., Menciassi, A., Dario, P.: Capsule endoscopy: from current achievements to open challenges. IEEE Rev. Biomed. Eng. **4**, 59–72 (2011)
2. Neumann, H., Fry, L.C., Nägela, A., Neurath, M.F.: Wireless capsule endoscopy of the small intestine: a review with future directions. Curr. Opin. Gastroenterol. **30**(5), 463–471 (2014)
3. Ara, P., Yu, K., Cheng, S., Dutkiewicz, E., Heimlich, M.C.: Human abdomen path-loss modeling and location estimation of wireless capsule endoscope using round-trip propagation loss. IEEE Sens. J. **18**(8), 3266–3277 (2018)
4. Chavez-Santiago, R., Wang, J., Balasinham, I.: The ultra wideband capsule endoscope. In: International Conference on Ultra Wideband (2013)
5. Stoa, S., Chavez-Santiago, R., Balasinham, I.: An ultra wideband communication channel model for capsule endoscopy. In: ISABEL 2014 (2014)

6. IEEE Standard for Local and metropolitan area networks _Part 15.6: Wireless Body Area Networks. IEEE Std 802.15.6-2012, pp. 1–271 (2012)

7. Särestöniemi, M., Pomalaza-Raez, C., Berg, M., Kissi, C., Hämäläinen, M., Iinatti, J.: In-body power distribution for abdominal monitoring and implant communications systems, ISWCS, September 2019

8. Särestöniemi, M., Pomalaza-Raez, C., Berg, M., Kissi, C., Hämäläinen, M., Iinatti, J.: Fat in the abdomen as a propagation medium in WBAN applications, Bodynets 2019 (2019)

9. Khaleghi, A., Chávez-Santiago, R., Liang, X., Balasingham, I., Leung, V.C.M., Ramstad, T. A.: On ultra wideband channel modeling for in-body communications. In: Proc. IEEE International Symposium on Wireless Pervasive Computing (ISWPC), 5–7 May 2010

10. Teshome, A., Kibret, B., Lai, D.T.H.: A review of implant communication technology in WBAN, progresses and challenges. IEEE Rev. Biomed. Eng. **12**, 88–99 (2018)

11. Leelatien, P., Ito, K., Saito, K., Sharma, M., Alomainy, A.: Channel characteristics and wireless telemetry performance of transplanted organ monitoring system using ultrawideband communication. IEEE J. Electromagnet. RF Microwaves Med. Biol. **2**, 94–101 (2018)

12. Asan, N.B., et al.: Intra-body microwave communication through adipose tissue. Healthc. Technol. Lett. **4**, 115–121 (2017)

13. Asan, N.B., et al.: Characterization of fat channel for intra-body communication at R-band frequencies. MDPI Sens. **18**(9) (2018)

14. Särestöniemi, M., et al.: Measurement and simulation based study on the UWB channel characteristics on the abdomen area. In: ISMICT 2019 (2019)

15. Särestöniemi, M., Kissi, C., Pomalaza-Raez, C., Hämäläinen, M., Iinatti, J.: Impact of the antenna-body distance on the UWB on-body channel characteristics. In: ISMICT 2019 (2019)

16. Särestöniemi, M., Kissi, C., Pomalaza Raez, C., Hämäläinen, M., Iinatti, J.: Propagation and UWB channel characteristics on human abdomen area. In: EUCAP 2019 (2019)

17. Li, J., Nie, Z., Liu, Y., Wang, L., Hao, Y.: Characterization of in-body radio channels for wireless implants. IEEE Sens. J. **17**(5), 1528–1537 (2017)

18. Kissi, C., Särestöniemi, M., Raez, C.P., Sonkki, M., Srifi, M.N.: Low-UWB directive antenna for wireless capsule endoscopy localization. In: BodyNets 2018 (2018)

19. Kissi, C., et al.: Low-UWB receiving antenna for WCE localization. In: ISMICT 2019 Conference (2019)

20. Kissi, C., et al.: Low-UWB antennas in vicinity to human body. In: ISMICT 2019 Conference (2019)

21. Kissi, C., et al.: High-directivity antenna for low-UWB body area networks applications. In: International Symposium on Advanced Electrical and Communication Technologies (ISAECT), pp. 1–6 (2018)

22. Bao, Z.: Comparative study of dual-polarized and circularly-polarized antennas at 2.45 GHz for ingestible capsules. Trans. Antennas Propag. **67**(3), 1488–1500

23. Lei, W., Guo, Y.-X.: Design of dual-polarized wideband conformal loop antenna for capsule endoscopy systems (2017)

24. Yazdandoost, K.Y.: Antenna for wireless capsule endoscopy at ultra wideband frequency. In: International Symposium on Personal, Indoor, and Mobile Radio Communications (PIMRC) (2017)

25. Lee, S.H., et al.: A wideband spiral antenna for ingestible capsule endoscope systems: experimental results in a human phantom and a pig. IEEE Trans. Biomed. Eng. **58**, 1734–1741 (2011)

26. CST Microwave Studio. http://www.cst.com

27. https://www.itis.ethz.ch/virtual-population/tissue-properties/database

Analysis of Channel Characteristic for Body Channel Communication Transceiver Design

Jaeeun Jang$^{(\boxtimes)}$ and Hoi-Jun Yoo

KAIST, Yuseong-Gu, Daejeon 34141, Republic of Korea
jaeeun.jang@kaist.ac.kr

Abstract. In this paper, body channel communication and its channel characteristic are investigated through measurement. Previously, the body channel communication has limitation in channel bandwidth due to its fluctuation. To verify orientation, 4 independent systemic factors are under test; (1) the size of the signal electrode attaching on the skin, (2) the size of the ground plane (GND) electrode that is not attaching on the skin, (3) the channel distance between TX and RX through human body, and (4) the length of cable connecting between the transceiver hardware and signal electrode. The size of the electrode and channel communication does not have a high correlation, However, the cable length between electrode and device shows a large variation. The newly proposed results are useful for hardware design and allow larger utilizable channel bandwidth that is promising for future BCC hardware design.

Keywords: Analysis · Body area network · Body channel communication · BCC · Channel · High data rate · Measurement · Wide-band

1 Introduction

Wireless body area network (WBAN) is considered to be an increasingly important technology in our lives. WBAN is one of the most closely engaged communication solutions in the near-human body. It is dedicated to targeting several of miniaturized sensor nodes, portable, multi-media devices, diagnostics, and patients monitoring applications. Especially, IEEE 802.15.6 standard was proposed in early 2010s to support wireless connectivity among devices in, on, and around the human body. The IEEE 802.15.6 WBAN standard consists of three PHYs: ultra-wide-band (UWB) PHY, narrow-band (NB) PHY, and body channel communication (BCC), that is labeled as human body communication (HBC) [1]. The BCC that uses the human body as a communication medium is considered as an energy-efficient PHY since it adopts high conductivity human body as a communication medium, and its low-frequency band enables low power communication. Compare to UWB and NB, BCC signal attenuation near the human body is significantly lower since signal energy absorption in human body tissue decreases [2]. So to say, BCC is one of the most remarkable PHY for hardware design in terms of energy efficiency.

The BCC hardware design research has continued to satisfy key specification such as low-cost, low-power, quality of service (QoS) scalability and so on. The main target applications of BCC can be classified as Fig. 1. First, applications can be grouped as

© ICST Institute for Computer Sciences, Social Informatics and Telecommunications Engineering 2019
Published by Springer Nature Switzerland AG 2019. All Rights Reserved
L. Mucchi et al. (Eds.): BODYNETS 2019, LNICST 297, pp. 374–383, 2019.
https://doi.org/10.1007/978-3-030-34833-5_28

physiological signal monitoring that includes wearable healthcare, patent status monitoring through sensor network coexistence. In the case of physiological, moderate data rate (<1 Mbps), ultra-low-power operation, and high network scalability are highly desired. The 802.15.6 HBC standard is a good fit for these applications since it emphasizes expandability to build sensor network and moderate, and variable data rate up to 1.3125 Mb/s. Second, multimedia applications typically operated under one-to-one connection, and require dedicated hardware design to support high data rate (>10 Mbps) with high energy efficiency. For these applications, the superior concern is low-power consumption, high data-rate for energy efficiency [3]. From the conceptual proposal of capacitive coupling approach [4], BCC researches firstly focused on sensor network applications [5–7], and move on to the high speed, multimedia applications [8, 9].

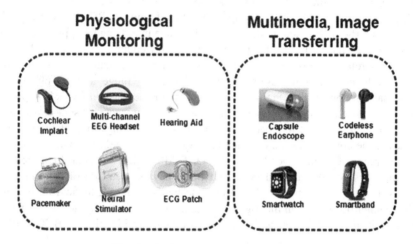

Fig. 1. Typical applications of WBAN

For such a hardware design, understand body channel environment is one of the key requirements because; (1) the electrode contact is utilized in BCC instead of antenna interface in RF communication [10]; (2) BCC frequency band located in a boundary of near-field and far-field communication. (3) Communication channel should be characterized before hardware design to set the design parameters and check available channel bandwidth. Especially, verifying both of channel gain or attenuation, and bandwidth should be accompanied. In previous work [11], the body channel bandwidth is verified from 30 MHz to 120 MHz and its bandwidth is verified up to 200 MHz in [9]. However, the detailed measurement process and investigation were not precisely investigated in [9]. For the BCC transceiver design, the electrode, electrode to transceiver interface, and body channel should be considered together since each of the components can affect communication performance.

In this paper, more details of body channel communication verification would be covered. From the review of the measurement setup, measurement to verify the effect of electrodes and cable will be introduced. After that, the paper concludes with a summary.

2 Body Channel Measurement

2.1 Previous Body Channel Measurements

The earliest human communication model is modeled as a closed loop between the transmitter (TX), receiver (RX) electrodes, and it is realized as capacitive coupling to the human body and earth ground [4]. In particular, the human body itself is modeled on a single node under the assumption of the perfect conductor. This model has the advantage that it is very simple to get intuition and valid for very low frequencies (<few MHz range). However, the model has limitation in that it is very inadequate according to the increase of the distance because the finite impedance of the human body itself is not considered. In order to compensate such a limitation, [11] proposed a distributed RC modeling by assuming the torso of the human body as a T-shape and dividing the human body into multiple distributed unit of RC (resistor-capacitor) networks. The RC distributed model has an advantage that it can be applied to a higher frequency (100 MHz or more). However, in the high frequency band, it has limitation in the low correlation between model and practical measured data. As shown in Fig. 2, there was a fluctuation in the case of the higher frequency range, and this phenomenon was the main reason for limiting the communication bandwidth in BCC. The previous study [12] showed that the frequency and the communication distance becomes a deterministic parameter of the mechanism of the signal propagation. As the frequency increases or the communication distance increases, the near field dominates at the low-frequency range. On the other hands, the far-field dominates in the high frequency region and it is possible to find switching frequency point inside of communication band. As a result, it can be concluded that the hard-to-control far-field term induces certain channel fluctuation in the higher frequency range. So to say, to release far-field occupation in the signal propagation becomes a key consideration in BCC hardware design.

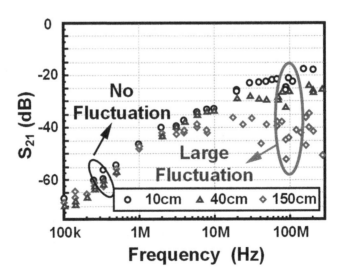

Fig. 2. Channel measurement results reported in [11]

The system design factors that can determine the characteristics of BCC channel are analyzed as follows; (1) the size of signal electrode attaching on the skin, (2) the size of the ground plane (GND) electrode that is not attaching on the skin, (3) the channel distance between TX and RX through human body, and (4) the length of cable connecting between the transceiver hardware and signal electrode. Figure 3 shows a generalized diagram of channel model, measurement setup and each of the factors (highlighted in red color). As shown in the figure, the electrode is responsible for the interface between TX, RX, and the human body. The transmitted signal is attenuated through the body channel and measured by a spectrum analyzer or a power detector capable of measuring received signal strength. In the case of measurement using a spectrum analyzer, it is difficult to implement the actual communication environment strictly. Considering impedance matching in the BCC is less feasible due to the variation in contact impedance, and it is difficult to consider the input impedance of the receiver [13]. In addition, the GND plane of spectrum analyzer may affect channel gain. However, it shows low influence in the overall bandwidth of the channel curve, so for the tendency analysis, the spectrum analyzer can be an appropriate solution.

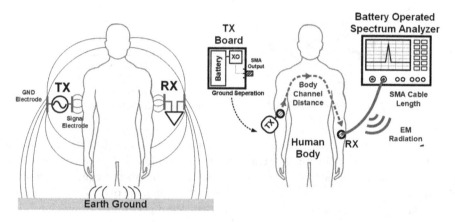

Fig. 3. Conceptual capacitive body channel model diagram, and channel measurement setup

The power detector or received signal strength indicator (RSSI) is used to overcome the disadvantages. In this case, the measurement setup becomes more complicated since frequency fundamental tone should be carefully measured. This paper mainly focuses on the measurement of the parameter's effect on channel tendency, so spectrum analyzer is adopted. Based on human body test, the commercial Keysight N9935A is utilized to isolate the GND plane coupling cost-efficiently. The TX is implemented as a customized PCB design, and signal frequency can be set by switching the crystal oscillators. Since the output spectrum power of each frequency may differ, so channel gain is obtained based on frequency-dependent calibration. Based on the measurement setup, 4 factors are measured and investigated.

2.2   Channel Effect Measurement with Variable: Signal Electrode Size

Figure 4(a) shows customized test electrodes for the verifying effect of electrode size. The electrode material is based on an attachable copper plate and electrode body is selected square-shaped Polypropylene (PP) plastic to reduce the unwanted effect. Each of electrode plate is connected to SMA connector through soldering. The length of the electrode side is varied from 2 cm to 5 cm. The electrode is connected to the TX board and spectrum analyzer without interconnecting cable.

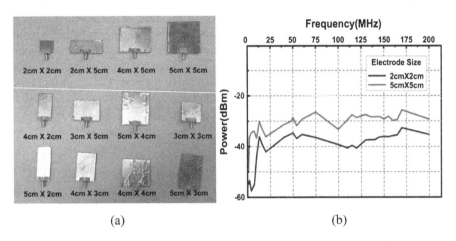

(a)   (b)

Fig. 4. (a) Tested electrodes setup (b) measured channel gain results

Figure 4(b) shows channel gain measurement results. Up to 200 MHz frequency is tested and the 2 cm × 2 cm and 5 cm × 5 cm case is plotted. The singularity of the plot is due to a limited number of frequency selection. With more frequency sampling, the smoother curve can be obtained. As shown in the figure, the overall curve tendency is maintained according to electrode size variation. The signal strength variation is less than 10 dB and it is because of different skin to the contact area. The overall bandwidth is maintained relative flatness up to high frequency range.

2.3   Channel Effect Measurement with Variable: GND Electrode Size

In the BCC, TX and RX GND planes are isolated and closed loop is modeled by capacitive coupling manner. Under the assumption of virtual earth GND, the ground node can be coupled directly or indirectly through the earth GND coupling. This indicates that not only larger forward path coupling (between TX signal electrode and RX signal electrode) but also larger return path coupling (between TX GND plane and RX GND plane) may increase channel gain. Figure 5 shows three classifications of electrode configuration in capacitive coupling BCC. Figure 5(a) shows the first configuration that both the signal electrode and GND electrodes attached to the body directly. In this case, the body is assumed as an impedance network and TRX signaling is modeled as a current driving method. However, since the low impedance GND electrode is attached very near to the human body, so that signal attenuation is relatively higher. Figure 5(b) shows approach without attaching GND electrode to the body. The GND coupling can be modeled as capacitive coupling through body and air. It has a benefit on low-power design since body channel decrease channel attenuation. On the other hand, channel status may suffer environmental variation since GND is opened. Figure 5(c) is the case of GND is embedded in PCB board. This approach mitigates the drawback of open GND, but careful design effort is required. In this measurement, open GND approach is utilized since it has more flexibility to adjust GND plane size.

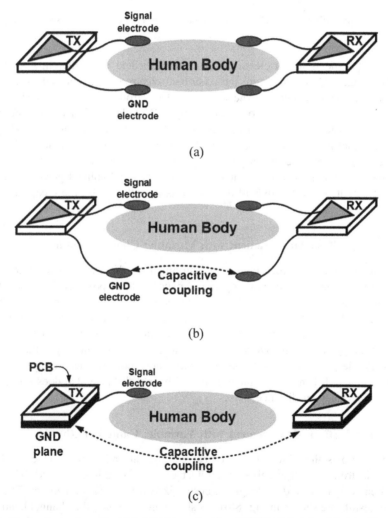

Fig. 5. Electrode configuration (a) Attaching signal and GND electrode. (b) Attaching signal electrode and floating GND electrode. (c) Signal electrode attaching and integrated GND plane in PCB

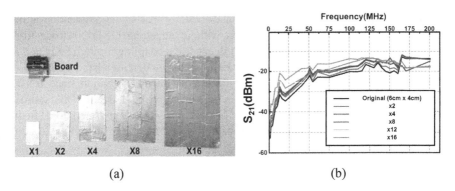

Fig. 6. (a) Tested different size of electrodes and custom TX board (b) measured channel gain results

Figure 6(a) shows tested electrodes that are fabricated in a different size. With a basic customized TX board setup, the additional electrode is connected to the board GND plane through soldering. The basic GND electrode size is designed as 6 cm 4 cm and its size are varied up to 16 times larger GND plane size, as a maximum case consideration. Figure 6(b) plotted measured results. With the increase of GND plane size, the channel gain increase slightly, and overall channel gain variation is less than 10 dB. It induces that the return path coupling increase channel gain but its contribution does not affect linearly so that does not occupy the dominant portion. Also, the remarkable point is that the overall bandwidth is not affected by the GND plane size directly.

2.4   Channel Effect Measurement with Variable: Channel Distance

Figure 7(a) describes the measurement environment in the variation of channel distance. To reduce the effect of another parameter such as body position, from torso to leg part is chosen and the test body is fixed for measurement. The communication distance is varied from 20 cm to 160 cm distance, and the wet electrode is selected to improve reliable contact. The measured results are shown in Fig. 7(b). With the increase of communication distance, the overall signal attenuation increase linearly in the dB scale. The remarkable point is that still, the bandwidth does not vary according to communication distance. It can be concluded that the channel distance also does not a major factor to affect channel distance.

2.5   Channel Effect Measurement with Variable: Cable Length

Figure 8(a) shows the different size of cables. By varying connection cable length between electrode and transceiver, the effect of cable length is verified. The SMA shielded cable is used and its length is customized from 5 cm to 100 cm. The measurement results are shown in Fig. 8(b). As shown in the figure, the channel bandwidth is maintained up to 200 MHz within the case of 5 cm. However, with an increase of cable length, the channel fluctuation is accelerated, and in the case of 100 cm, the

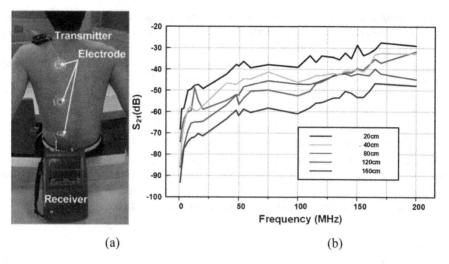

(a)   (b)

Fig. 7. (a) Measurement setup for distance variation effect (b) measured channel gain results

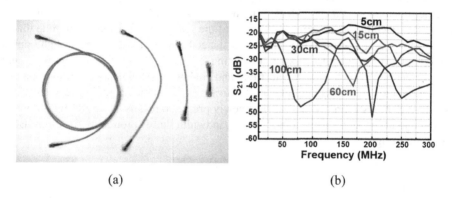

(a)   (b)

Fig. 8. (a) Tested cables with different length (b) measured channel gain results

overall fluctuation is more than 30 dB range which is undesirable. There are two reasons for this phenomena. First, even though the cable is shielded by the metallic cover, non-linear signal radiation occurs through the long cable. Since such a cable is inherently twisted or bent, the radiation pattern induces non-uniform bandwidth pattern in the channel. Secondly, without impedance matching, certain standing wave pattern can be assumed through a long cable. Such a pattern can generate channel fluctuation and overall channel communication bandwidth is strictly limited. This result shows that the long cable between devices and electrode affect channel condition and on the other hands, it means that available bandwidth can be extended up to 200 MHz range in the case of short cable usage. Moreover, typical wearable and portable applications do not integrate such a long cable, the verified results can be generalized to overall BCC transceiver hardware design.

Increasing available channel bandwidth can be considered as a superior advantage in hardware design. Larger bandwidth directly connected to potential with increasing transceiver data rate and reduces the filtering overhead in the hardware design. However, there are other considerations in the BCC. Due to the presence of the body antenna effect, an external FM radio band from 80 MHz to 110 MHz acts as an interference in the communication. The contact status may affect the channel condition. In the case of stable contact, the signal path can be modeled as a resistive path. But in the case of separation, the signal path operates like a serial capacitive coupled path. So the additional signal attenuation may vary channel status. In spite of several design challenges, BCC can be advantageous as an efficient and low power communication solution. Note that such efforts are generally applied to the RF hardware design also. The influence of the cable and channel characteristics covered in this paper can give intuition and help for understanding the nature of BCC hardware design.

3   Conclusion

In this paper, multiple parameters that can affect channel characteristics is discussed. The previous research has limitation in channel bandwidth up to 100 MHz range due to channel fluctuation. 4 independent systemic factors are under test; (1) the size of signal electrode attaching on the skin, (2) the size of the ground plane (GND) electrode that is not attaching on the skin, (3) the channel distance between TX and RX through human body, and (4) the length of cable connecting between the transceiver hardware and signal electrode. The size of the electrode and channel communication does not have a high correlation with channel fluctuation. However, the cable length between electrode and device shows a large variation. The newly proposed results are useful for hardware design and allow larger utilizable channel bandwidth that is promising for future BCC hardware design.

References

1. IEEE Computer Society: IEEE standard for local and metropolitan area networks: part 15.6 wireless body area networks. IEEE Standards Association. IEEE Computer Society. Accessed 29 Feb 2012
2. Bae, J., Song, K., Lee, H., Cho, H., Yoo, H.: A 0.24–nJ/b wireless body-area-network transceiver with scalable double-FSK modulation. IEEE J. Solid-State Circ. **47**(1), 310–322 (2012)
3. Jang, J., Bae, J., Yoo, H.: Understanding body channel communication. In: Custom Integrated Circuit Conference (2019)
4. Zimmerman, T.: Personal area networks (PAN): near-field intra-body communication. IBM Syst. J. **35**(34), 609–617 (1996)
5. Song, S.J., Cho, N., Kim, S., Yoo, J., Yoo, H.J.: A 2 Mb/s wideband pulse transceiver with direct-coupled interface for human body communications. In: 2006 IEEE International Solid State Circuits Conference - Digest of Technical Papers, San Francisco, CA, pp. 2278–2287 (2006)

6. Song, S., Cho, N., Kim, S., Yoo, J., Choi, S., Yoo, H.: A 0.9 V 2.6 mW body-coupled scalable PHY transceiver for body sensor applications. In: 2007 IEEE International Solid-State Circuits Conference. Digest of Technical Papers, San Francisco, CA, pp. 366–609 (2007)
7. Cho, N., Lee, J., Yan, L., Bae, J., Kim, S., Yoo, H.: A 60 kb/s-to-10 Mb/s 0.37nJ/b adaptive-frequency-hopping transceiver for body-area network. In: 2008 IEEE International Solid-State Circuits Conference - Digest of Technical Papers, San Francisco, CA, pp. 132–602 (2008)
8. Lee, J., et al.: 30.7 A 60 Mb/s wideband BCC transceiver with 150pJ/b RX and 31pJ/b TX for emerging wearable applications. In: 2014 IEEE International Solid-State Circuits Conference Digest of Technical Papers (ISSCC), San Francisco, CA, pp. 498–499 (2014)
9. Cho, H., Kim, H., Kim, M., Jang, J., Bae, J., Yoo, H.: 21.1 A 79pJ/b 80 Mb/s full-duplex transceiver and a 42.5 μW 100 kb/s super-regenerative transceiver for body channel communication. In: 2015 IEEE International Solid-State Circuits Conference - (ISSCC) Digest of Technical Papers, San Francisco, CA, pp. 1–3 (2015)
10. Song, S., Cho, N., Yoo, H.: A 0.2-mW 2-Mb/s digital transceiver based on wideband signaling for human body communications. IEEE J. Solid-State Circ. 42(9), 2021–2033 (2007)
11. Cho, N., Yoo, J., Song, S., Lee, J., Jeon, S., Yoo, H.: The human body characteristics as a signal transmission medium for intrabody communication. In: IEEE Transactions on Microwave Theory and Techniques, vol. 55, no. 5, pp. 1080–1086, May 2007
12. Bae, J., Cho, H., Song, K., Lee, H., Yoo, H.: The signal transmission mechanism on the surface of human body for body channel communication. In: IEEE Transactions on Microwave Theory and Techniques, vol. 60, no. 3, pp. 582–593, March 2012
13. Bae, J., Yoo, H.: The effects of electrode impedance on receiver sensitivity in body channel communication. Microelectron. J. 53, 73–80 (2016)

MAC Protocol with Interference Mitigation Using Negotiation Among Coordinators in Multiple Wireless Body Area Networks

Shunya Ogawa[1]([✉]), Takahiro Goto[1], Takumi Kobayashi[1], Chika Sugimoto[1], and Ryuji Kohno[1,2]

[1] Graduate School of Engineering Science, Yokohama National University, 79-5 Tokiwadai, Hodogaya-ku, Yokohama, Kanagawa 240-8501, Japan
{ogawa-shunya-md,goto-takahiro-wx,kobayashi-takumi-ch,chikas, kohno}@ynu.jp
[2] Centre for Wireless Communications, Faculty of IT and EE, University of Oulu, Linnanmaa, P.O. Box 4500, 90570 Oulu, Finland
ryuji.kohno@oulu.fi

Abstract. In this paper Cwe propose a new MAC protocol in presence of multiple wireless Body Area Network (BANs) which can for reduce inter-WBAN interference and improve overall performance of all BANs. A BAN system consists of a coordinator and some sensor nodes. When coverages of multiple BANs are overlapped, some packets transmitted from sensor nodes of different BANs cause interference. Although an international standard for wireless medical BAN, i.e. IEEE802.15.6 can reduce intra-WBAN interference within a single BAN, inter-WBAN interference caused by coexistence of multiple BANs can not reduce effectively. Therefore, this paper proposes such a new MAC protocols method that coordinators of overlapped BANs can negotiate among coordinators of BANs. In addition, to enable priority control which is a feature of the standard, we propose a method that changes parameters of the proposed method according to priority of packets. Throughput and delay time of the proposed scheme are illustrated by simulation, in which it is convinced that the proposed scheme can improve overall performance such as throughput and delay considering efficiency of priority control.

Keywords: Multiple WBAN · IEEE802.15.6 · MAC · Interference mitigation · Negotiation among coordinators

1 Introduction

Wireless Body Area Network (WBAN) is a technology for health care. WBAN is constructed with wearable or implant sensors and coordinators placed around the human body. It can monitor personal health conditions by using psysiological and biological information from sensors. WBAN is not only applied for

© ICST Institute for Computer Sciences, Social Informatics and Telecommunications Engineering 2019
Published by Springer Nature Switzerland AG 2019. All Rights Reserved
L. Mucchi et al. (Eds.): BODYNETS 2019, LNICST 297, pp. 384–393, 2019.
https://doi.org/10.1007/978-3-030-34833-5_29

medical applications, but also applied for non-medical application, research has progressed in recent years [3]. In WBAN, it is important to satisfy flexible quality of service (QoS) and latency, because allowable delay time is different between medical and non-medical information.and many paper discuss this problem [7,8].

IEEE802.15.6 was published as a international standard for WBAN and it standardize PHY layer and MAC layer [1]. As shown in Table 1, standard defines user priority (UP) and it can control QoS. There are two protocols in MAC layer such as contention base protocol and contention free protocol [2], and there are three access modes in standard, one of them is called superframe and it consists of beacon, contention access period such a CSMA/CA and contention free period.

In intra-WBAN, the coordinator schedules many sensor nodes so that they can send packets at the same time without interfering with each other, and can co-exist in a single BAN. Since WBAN move with people, when many people with WBAN enter into the communication range of each other, interference will occur between WBANs. Therefore, the interference of coexistent WBAN is a problem, and to solve this interference problem an appropriate MAC protocol is required [5], and many paper discuss this problem [4,6]. The standard IEEE802.15.6 only provides a basic outline and interference within a single BAN. Although intra-WBAN interference can be avoided by using an access technology such as TDMA, inter-WBAN interference caused by coexistence of many BANs can not be avoided. This is because coordination between coordinators of different WBANs is not done, and collisions occur if the transmission periods of packets is overlapped.

In order to solve this problem, in this paper, negotiation was performed among the coordinators, which was not recognized in the standard. Thereby enable to schedule among different BANs, and reduce interference. In addition to interference mitigation, we also consider different QoS requirements.

Table 1. IEEE802.15.6 Priority Mapping

User priorit	Traffic designation
0	Background (BK)
1	Best effort (BE)
2	Excellent effort (EE)
3	Video (VI)
4	Voice (VO)
5	Medicald data or network control
6	High-priority medical data or network control
7	Emergency or medical implant event report

2   Overview of IEEE802.15.6 MAC Protocol

This chapter describes the features of the conventional IEEE802.15.6 MAC protocol [1]. Specifically, it shows two access control methods and access modes.

2.1   CSMA/CA

CSMA/CA is a contention based protocol. If the node has a packet, it checks whether the channel is idle. If it is idle it decrements the backoff counter that set based on contention window (CW) by 1. When the backoff counter becomes 0. The backoff counter takes different values depending on UP. Specifically, high UP makes it easy to take a low value, and it enables priority control.

2.2   Polling

Polling is a contention free protocol, in which the coordinator assigns slots for packets to specific noeds. Therefore, in polling, packet collisions do not occur, so reliable communication can be performed.

2.3   Access Mode

There are three access mode in standard and one is beacon mode with superframes. Figure 1 shows the structure of Superframe. B shown in Fig. 1 is a beacon, which is transmitted from the coordinator to all sensor nodes in the communication range, and has the role of informing the start of Superframe and the configuration of Superframe. Also, the structure of Superframe can be roughly divided into two: CAP (Contension Access Period) and CFP (Contention Free Period). EAP (Exclusive Access Phase), RAP (Random Access Phase), and CAP (Contention Access Phase) shown in Fig. 1 are CAP, and MAP (Managed Access Phase) is CFP. EAP is a section that handles only User Priority 7 packets, which are emergency and implant information. RAP is an interval that handles all packets. CAP is an interval when B2 is in Superframe, and CAP is an interval that handles all packets. MAP is a section in which the coordinator gives each sensor node the right to transmit packets and can communicate without collisions. In addition, the coordinator is designed to be able to change the length, ratio between CAP and CFP and the length of Superframe itself.

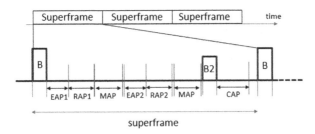

Fig. 1. Beacon mode with superframe in IEEE802.15.6

3   MAC Protocol with Interference Mitigation Using Negotiation Among Coordinators

IEEE802.15.6 has the problem that it can not avoid inter-WBAN interference. This is because coordination between coordinators of different WBANs is not done, and collisions occur if the transmission periods of packets is overlapped. In order to solve this problem, in this paper, negotiation was performed among the coordinators, which was not recognized in the standard, Thereby enable to schedule among different BANs, and reduce interference.

3.1   Negotiatiom Among Coordinators

Information obtained by negotiation between coordinators is sharing of overlap situation of each BAN. When an overlapping sensor node and the sensor node under its control transmits a packet simultaneously, contention will occur and packets will be destroyed. Therefore, if there are overlap nodes, they do not send packets simultaneously.

We assume that overlap situations are shared among coordinators. So, we show the procedure of how to identify overlap situations.

1. Since BAN uses UWB communication, they can share the distance (between coordinators, between coordinators and sensor nodes, etc.).
   By sharing the distance between a sensor node and the coordinator, it is possible to identify whether the node is within its communication range or not. However, just by distance, they does not know that sensor nodes belongs to which WBAN system.
2. Use the address of the sensor node given for each BAN.
   The MAC layer has the role of defining the MAC address for identifying the wireless device in the preamble part of the frame, so the address differs for each sensor node. By sharing this address among the coordinators, it is possible to identify whether a sensor node belong to own BAN or another BAN.

For example, in the case of Fig. 2, by identifying the distance and address between nodes, it is possible to identify which node causes interference.

3.2   Interference Mitigation MAC Protocol

The basic concept of this proposed method is sharing the overlap situation to identify the nodes that cause interference. Therefore, by sharing the overlap situation, coordinator with each BAN configure superframe in order not to send packets at the same time.

Interference Mitigation MAC Protocol in CFP
In CFP, inter-WBAN interference occurs when transmission rights are assigned to a overlapped of each BANs sensor node. In order to solve this problem, the

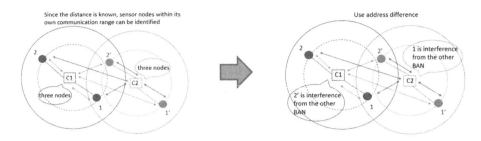

Fig. 2. How to identify overlap situations

structure of MAP of Superframe is divided into MAP1 and MAP2 The role of MAP1 and MAP2 is shown as follows.

- MAP1 assigns transmission rights to nodes not subject to interference.
  Even if they try to transmit at the same time, packet collision does not occur.
- MAP2 assigns transmission rights to nodes giving interference.
  This is because nodes giving interference will cause contention on their own BAN and other BANs if they are sent at the same time, so if one BAN is transmitting in MAP2, Other BANs are put on standby.

Figure 3 illustrates this protocol. C1 and C2 mean coordinator.Coordinator1 non-overlapped node (number 2, 3, 4) and coordinator2 non-overlapped node (number 1', 2', 3') are assigned MAP1 and send at the same slot. Since they do not overlap, they can be transmitted in the same slot without interference. On the other hand, coordinator1 overlapped node (number 1) and coordinator2 overlapped node (number 4') are assigned MAP2 and send different slot. Although they overlap, Interference does not occur because only one side transmits in a slot.

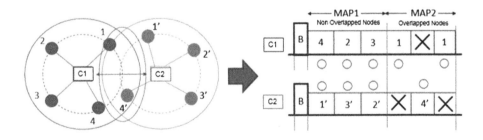

Fig. 3. MAC protocol of MAP

Interference Mitigation MAC Protocol in CAP

Although CAP adopts CSMA/CA, in CSMA/CA, inter-BAN interference occur when overlapped nodes get transmission rights at the same time. Especially, if the user priority of the overlap node is high, the frequency of contention will increase considerably. In order to solve this problem, the protocol of Superframe RAP is as follows.

– If the overlapped node is a non-medical node (UP4 or less), it will not be put in the competition for transmission right
– If the overlapped node is a medical node (UP5 or higher), compete the transmission right as usual

As a point of caution, nodes that are lower than UP of overlapped node did not give transmission right either, in order to guarantee in the order of high UP. Although overlapped nodes may also have transmission rights, and cause inter-BAN interference, if you do not give the right to transmit to the medical node (UP5 or higher), you can not guarantee UP in the order of high UP.

Figure 4 illustrates this protocol. Non-medical interfering nodes do not acquire transmission rights. By doing so, priority control is possible.

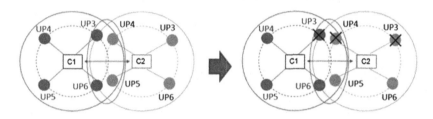

Fig. 4. MAC protocol of RAP

3.3   MAC Protocol to Enable Priority Control

The protocol described so far is a method in which improves average performance of whole UP, but there is no purposeful control such as guaranteeing high UP and sacrificing low UP. Therefore, we propose a MAC protocol that makes a gap between high UP and low UP.

To Make a Gap Between High UP and Low UP in CFP
In order to make a gap between high UP and low UP in MAP, we apply the concept of UP to how to assign packet transmission rights. As a result, high UP will be allocated more and low UP will be allocated less.

To Make a Gap Between High UP and Low UP in CAP
In order to make a gap between high UP and low UP in RAP, the protocol of Superframe RAP is as follows.

– If it is low UP (4 or less) irrespective of interference or non-interference, do not compete transmission right
– If it is high UP (5 or more) irrespective of interference or non-interference, compete transmission right as usual

The difference from the case of average performance is that the distinction between overlapped nodes and non-overlapped nodes is eliminated, which is considered to result in a gap between low UP and high UP as in MAP.

4   Performance Evaluation

4.1   Simulation Model and Parameters

Simulation parameters are based on IEEE802.15.6, as shown Table 2 and simulation model is like Fig. 5. We modeled each BAN by two circles. Solid line circle is communication range. On the other hand, dotted line circle is sensing range. We adopted star topology and there are four nodes each.One node has one priority packet. In order to see the characteristics depending on the traffic volume, we evaluated when the offeredload was varied. Evaluation was performed by simulation under the above settings unsing Matlab as shown Figs. 6, 7 and 8. The contents of the evaluation are as follows.

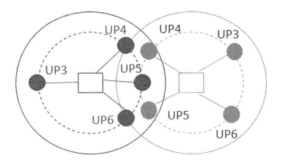

Fig. 5. Simulation model

Table 2. Simulation parameters

Number of nodes	4 (high UP 2, low UP 2)
Data rate	242.9 [kbps]
Payload length	128 [octets]
Number of BANs	2
Superframe length	115 [ms]
Beacon length	1 [ms]
Number of slots	RAP = 5, MAP = 12
Simulation time	30 [s]
Number of trials	100 [times]

- Network overall throughput characteristic
- Throughput characteristic per UP
- Delay characteristic per UP

Each of these was evaluated in two ways, one is average performance for each UP and the other is making a gap between high UP and low UP.

The definition of throughput is as follows.

$$throughput(bit/s) = \frac{Number\ of\ successfully\ transmitted\ packets \times 1024\ [bit]}{Total\ trial\ time\ [s]}$$

(1)

Also, the definition of delay is defined as the time from the occurrence of a packet to the successful transmission of that packet. The conditions for discarding the packet are when the number of attempts for retransmission is 4 or more due to a collision of packets and when the number of packet accumulations is 3 or more.

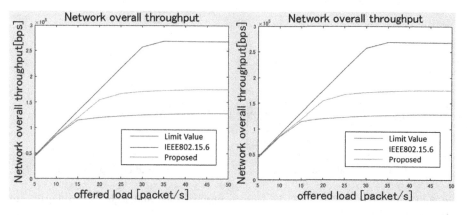

Fig. 6. Network overall throughput (left is average performance and right is making a gap between high UP and low UP)

4.2 Simulation Results

Figure 6 shows overall network throughput comparing IEEE802.15.6 and the proposed method. Left is average performance and right is making a gap between high UP and low UP. The limit value is the throughput of the entire network in the absence of interference. Compared to the standard, the throughput of the whole network is improved in the proposed method. This is because the protocol is changed so that there are less contention using negotiation between coordinators. In addition, we can see that there is no difference between the overall throughput of the network in the case of average performance and in the case of gap between each UP.

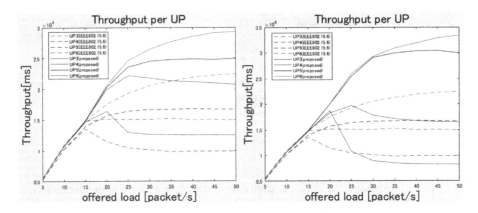

Fig. 7. Throughput per UP (left is average performance and right is making a gap between high UP and low UP)

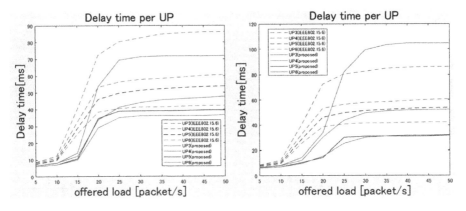

Fig. 8. Delay time per UP (left is average performance and right is making a gap between high UP and low UP)

Figure 7 show throughput characteristic per UP comparing IEEE802.15.6 and the proposed method. Left is average performance and right is making a gap between high UP and low UP. Similarly, the proposed method is superior to the throughput for each UP and the higher UP is, the larger throughput will be because collision can be avoided efficiently. It can be seen that the larger the offeredload is, the better the proposal method will be because the conventional method occur many collisions, if the offeredload is large due to that the number of attempts to send increases. In addition, it can be understood that it is possible to cope with the case of average performance and the case of gap between each UP. This is because the weight of UP was changed between the average case and the gap creation case. Specifically, the difference between the weights of medical packets and non-medical packets is increased.

Figure 8 show delay characteristic per UP comparing IEEE802.15.6 and the proposed method. Left is average performance and right is making a gap between high UP and low UP. Similarly, the proposed method is superior to the delay for each UP and the higher UP is, the smaller delay will be. In addition, it can be understood that it is possible to cope with the case of average performance and the case of gap between each UP. In making a gap between high UP and low UP case, proposed method is inferior at UP3. This is because medical packets sacrifice non-medical packets for high performance. Even in this case, it is necessary to change the protocol so that the performance is higher than the conventional method.

5 Conclusion

We have researched on MAC protocol for interference mitigation in WBAN. The object of comparison is IEEE802.15.6, which is the international standard of WBAN. In this research, as novelty, we proposed a MAC protocol that reduces inter-WBAN interference by negotiating among coordinators and identifying and sharing interfering nodes. As a result, we show that the proposed MAC protocol has improved both the throughput characteristics and the delay characteristics compared with the standard. Also, when the design policy gives in two cases such as average performance for each UP and making is a gap between high UP and low UP, we showed that it is possible to cope with by changing algorithm.

References

1. IEEE Computer Society: IEEE standard for local and metropolitan area networks - part 15.6: wireless body area networks, pp. 1–256, February 2012
2. IEEE Computer Society: IEEE Standard for Local and metropolitan area networks Media Access Control (MAC) Bridges, pp. 1–269, June 2004
3. Movassaghi, S., Abolhasan, M., Lipman, J., Smith, D., Jamalipour, A.: Wireless body area networks: a survey. IEEE Commun. Surv. Tutor. **16**(3), 1658–1686 (2014)
4. Movassaghi, S., Majidi, A., Jamalipour, A., Smith, D., Abolhasan, M.: Enabling interference-aware and energy-efficient coexistence of multiple wireless body area networks with unknown dynamics. Access IEEE **4**, 2935–2951 (2016)
5. Shaik, M.F., Komanapalli, V.L.N., Subashini, M.M.: A comparative study of interference and mitigation techniques in wireless body area networks. Wirel. Pers. Commun. **98**, 2333–2365 (2017)
6. Huang, W., Quek, T.Q.S.: Adaptive CSMA/CA MAC protocol top reduce inter-WBAN interference for wireless body area network. In: IEEE 12th International Conference on Wearable and Implanted Body Sensor Networks (BSN) (2015)
7. Li, N., Cai, X., Yuan, X., Zhang, Y., Zhang, B., Li, C.: EIMAC: a multi-channel MAC protocol towards energy efficiency and low interference for WBANs. J. IET Commun. **12**(16), 1954–1962 (2018)
8. Bhandari, S., Moh, S.: A priority-based adaptive MAC protocol for wireless body area networks. Sensors **16**, 401 (2016)

Pseudo-dynamic UWB WBAN Off-Body Radio Channel Measurements – Preliminary Results

Timo Kumpuniemi$^{(\boxtimes)}$ (iD), Juha-Pekka Mäkelä, Matti Hämäläinen, and Jari Iinatti

Centre for Wireless Communications, University of Oulu, Oulu, Finland
timo.kumpuniemi@oulu.fi

Abstract. This paper presents measurement results on pseudo-dynamic ultra wideband off-body wireless body area network radio channels. The measurements are performed in an anechoic chamber in a 2–8 GHz frequency band by utilizing a vector network analyzer. A dynamic walking sequence was modeled by a test person who took five different body postures which were each measured statically. As a result, when observed together, the five postures can be used to model a dynamic walking sequence as in a cinema film. The antennas were attached on left and right wrist, and left ankle. The off-body antenna node was set on a pole. The work was repeated for two prototype antenna types: dipole and double loop. The mean attenuations of the first arriving paths were noted to lie between $-52\ldots-68$ dB. No large differences were noted between the body postures. The link between left ankle and the pole had the largest attenuation. The averaged channel impulse response durations were noted to lie between eight to nine taps, where one tap corresponds to 0.167 ns in time. The dynamic range on the averaged link types shows values between $17\ldots28$ dB. No clear difference was noted in the performance between the antenna types.

Keywords: Ultra wideband · Wireless body area network · Channel model

1 Introduction

The fast progress in electric circuit technology has enabled increasing computing efficiency in constantly decreasing sizes with better energy efficiency simultaneously. At the same, also the battery technology has improved as well. As a result, small devices with low power consumption have become available in various applications that were not seen a few years ago. One hugely growing area is the internet of things (IoT) concept, which is one of the key areas in the fifth and sixth generation (5G, 6G) wireless systems. 5G is already in implementation phase and is expected to explode the IoT area and the number of sensors rapidly. 6G is currently under research in the academia and industry [1], and it is highly expected that after the deployment the boost on IoT will raise yet to another level.

With the IoT concept, wireless devices or sensors are, or are supposed to be, attached in or on various places in buildings, vehicles, industrial environment, machines and homes. They can monitor various parameters in their surroundings such as temperature, humidity, water leaks or motion. When several sensors are operating

© ICST Institute for Computer Sciences, Social Informatics and Telecommunications Engineering 2019
Published by Springer Nature Switzerland AG 2019. All Rights Reserved
L. Mucchi et al. (Eds.): BODYNETS 2019, LNICST 297, pp. 394–408, 2019.
https://doi.org/10.1007/978-3-030-34833-5_30

together, their data can be collected to a central node to be delivered further in the telecommunication network. Thus, the entity forms up a network, a concept often called as wireless sensor network (WSNs). Especially, when operating in a human, or even animal context, is very often called as wireless body area network (WBAN).

One of the most interesting applications areas for WSNs are particularly using them with animals or humans, as WBANs. The sensors can be attached on the surface of a person's body, a case called on-body communications. Some sensors may be located in the vicinity of a person but off the body surface, called often an off-body case. If a sensor or sensors are situated inside the body, it is called in-body communications. Communication between two or multiple persons each having in- or on-body sensors is often called body-to-body communications [2]. Also hybrid forms of this division may exist. The in-body sensor may communicate with a node at the body surface (in-on-case) or with an off-body node (in-off case). The communication between on-body and off-body is sometimes called as an on-off body situation.

With respect to humans, several fields of usage can be found for WBANs. One quite popular is in the field of well-being and sports. The users can monitor their daily activity and the effectiveness of physical exercise both for professional athletes and fitness enthusiasts. The public sector users, e.g., firefighters, police officers and military troops may find WBANs very useful in increasing the safety in their professions.

The trend of increasing number of eldering people in many countries [3] brings another rapidly developing area for WBANs into the picture. It is the deployment of WBAN in the medical sector. The increasing portion of elderly people sets high demands to organize the healthcare to be available to all citizens at all times, not even to mention the exploding financial costs for the governments to provide these services. With WBANs, the workload and efficiency of medical staff can be eased up. The new technology enables remote monitoring of the patients leading their lives at their homes. The operations of hospitals and medical wards can be decentralized while the patients will be called into hospital facilities only when needed. The quality of life of the patients will be increased. Also the quality of medical treatment will be increased as the central vital parameters of the patients can be followed constantly through the sensors, instead of rarely conducted tests in a laboratory in centralized medical wards and hospitals.

Most solutions on WBANs nowadays are based on narrowband technologies operating most often at the Industrial, Scientific and Medical (ISM) frequency band at 2.45 GHz area. However, with many WBAN scenarios, the radio channels link distances are quite short. This is one reason, why the ultra wideband (UWB) technology is a very suitable solution for WBANs. UWB provides several other interesting features as well. It has a large bandwidth enabling a good performance in a harsh multipath environment. For the same reason, a precise positioning can be obtained, a feature finding several applications within the WBAN area. The tolerance against interference from other co-existing wireless systems is very high. On the other hand, the transmission power of UWB is low, creating minimum interference to other wireless systems, and a low exposure of electromagnetic radiation to humans, measured typically with the specific absorption rate. The transceiver structures are simple providing low unit costs and size, and their power consumption is low enabling long operation time when battery-operated [4, 5].

Real life application areas for WBANs using UWB in the medical field have been proposed, e.g., in [6], where a scenario for monitoring several vital parameters of a patient, e.g. an extensive care is explained. Another practical use case for WBANs is published in [7], which discusses the usage of UWB WBANs in the monitoring of patients suffering from Parkinson's disease.

UWB has been researched for WBANs for over ten years [8]. Quite many papers published are on the on-body communications cases, e.g., [9–11]. However, off-body cases with UWB are to found as well [12–16].

This paper shows preliminary results on pseudo-dynamic measurements in an off-body UWB WBAN scenario. The measured radio channels consist of the combined effect of propagation channels and antennas. The idea is to investigate effects due to the human body, especially on path losses, excluding other influences from the surroundings. For this purpose, the measurements are performed in an anechoic chamber. They are conducted at a 2–8 GHz bandwidth, using a vector network analyzer (VNA). Two prototype antenna types are used: dipole and double loop. The work is a part of a larger measurement campaign consisting of on-, off, and body-to-body cases. Additional results of the measurement campaign in static, pseudo-dynamic and truly dynamic cases are reported in, e.g., [6, 10, 14–18].

The structure of the paper is the following. In Sect. 2, the measurement setup is explained. Section 3 describes the measurement scenario with antenna locations and practical arrangements of the measurements. Section 4 explains the data processing methods together with the presentation of the results. Conclusions and future work plans are covered in Sect. 5.

2   Measurement Setup

2.1   Test Person and the Measurement Environment

A male test person at his late twenties was standing inside the anechoic chamber facing towards the off-body node. He was 183 cm tall with a body mass of 95 kg. He was using a normal cotton T-shirt with jeans during the measurements. Shoes, belt, glasses, rings, jewelry or any other possibly metal containing artifacts were absent during the measurements.

The anechoic chamber had a floor size of 245 cm by 365 cm. It was assembled by using a number of moving absorber blocks. It was located inside an electromagnetic compatibility room with a floor space of approx. 60 m^2, to avoid any excess radiation from other sources entering into the measurement area.

2.2   Test Equipments

A VNA with four ports of the type Rohde & Schwarz ZVA-8 was applied in the measurements. It was located outside the anechoic chamber and connected inside the chamber with eight meter long measurement cables. The VNA was set to sweep the 2-8 GHz band in the frequency domain. 1601 frequency points were recorded, together with 100 sweeps for each measurements. Since a four-port VNA was applied with four antennas in use simultaneously, sixteen scattering parameters were obtained and all recorded. The sweep time was 288.18 ms, with a 100 kHz intermediate frequency bandwidth and +10 dBm transmission power.

The applied antennas were in-house built planar prototype antennas of two types: dipole and double loop. The maximum free space gains have been noted to be approx. +6 dBi, and their operational bandwidth at 2–12 GHz. The reported performances and radiation patterns in free space of the antennas can be found in detail in [18–20].

3   Measurement Scenario

3.1   Rationale for Pseudo-dynamic Measurements

Dynamic UWB WBAN radio channel measurements can be performed by using several methods in time or frequency domain. One very popular technique are frequency domain measurements with VNA as applied in this paper. One problem in dynamic measurements with VNA is the sweep time of the VNA, i.e., the time duration for one single frequency measurement across the frequency band set for the VNA. The sweep time depends on the quality of the VNA and the setting values for the measurements. In order to guarantee the validity of the measurements, the radio channel coherence time must be equal or longer than the sweep time of a measurement. There are several equations available in the literature for the channel coherence time T_0, out of which one of the strictest is defined by [21]

$$T_0 = 9/(16 \cdot \pi \cdot f_d), \tag{1}$$

where f_d is the Doppler frequency, defined as $f_d = v/\lambda$, where v is the relative velocity between the antennas and is the λ wavelength in the propagation media. Assuming propagation in air and the channel coherence time to be equal to sweep time of the VNA, the maximum relative velocity v at exemplary frequencies of 2 GHz and 8 GHz (the measured bandwidth here) can be solved to be $v = 9.3$ cm/s (at 2 GHz) and $v = 2.3$ cm/s (at 8 GHz). The latter sets the limit how fast a person could move in a dynamic measurement. In practice, the velocity should be lower to provide a safety margin between T_0 and the VNA sweep time. It is obvious from the example values, that the dynamic movement can be only very slow in order to guarantee the measurements to be valid, with the sweep time setting used in this work, making it difficult to carry out truly dynamic measurements in practice.

One solution to circumvent the problem is to use the pseudo-dynamic measurements approach, applied in the work in this article and previously in [17]. In it, several static measurements are conducted with different body postures. After combining the results in a sequence, a dynamic movement can be modelled as in a cinema film.

3.2   Antenna Placements

The antennas were placed at the right wrist (RW), left wrist (LW) and left ankle (LA) on the body. The off body node (PO) was installed on a plastic pole at the height of 2 m and at the distance of 2 m from the test person. The locations are shown in

Fig. 1. Combining the antenna position acronyms together, measured radio channels can be defined as the link between the left ankle and the pole (LA-PO), the link between the right wrist and the pole (RW-PO) and the link between the left wrist and the pole (LW-PO). Three on-body antennas and the off-body node were measured each due to the four-port feature of the VNA. The on-body antennas were attached by using elastic bands and painter's masking tape. A 20 mm antenna-body distance was secured by the usage of ROHACELL HF31 [22] material between the antenna and the body. This distance was noted in [20] to provide good characteristics in antenna matchings and channel gain values simultaneously.

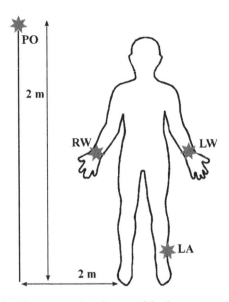

Fig. 1. The antenna locations used in the measurements.

3.3   Pseudo-dynamic Body Postures and Their Measurements

The walking movement of two steps was emulated by the test person by starting from a standing position, facing directly to the pole. Due to practical restrictions in mobility set by the cables, the antennas and the anechoic chamber, the movements of limbs are limited in trajectory. Therefore they are imitating a walk of elderly people or people in a rehabilitation process after, e.g., an accident, a stroke, or a large surgical operation.

The walking sequence was modeled by five different body postures taken by the test person as shown in Fig. 2. At posture 1, the test person is standing at place. At posture 2, a short step with his left foot is taken and his hands start to change position. At next step, posture 3, the initiated move progresses by extending the trajectories of the left foot and the hands further. At postures 4 and 5, similar movement is repeated by starting the step with the left foot of the test person. In all postures, the distance to the pole was kept at two meters. In Fig. 2, also the antenna positions LW, RW, and LA are seen in practice.

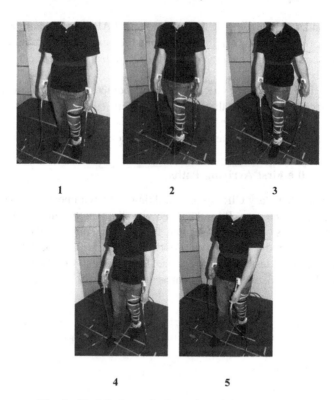

1   2   3

4   5

Fig. 2. Modelled pseudo-dynamic walking sequence.

In order to average out the possible variations in the body positions 1–5 in Fig. 2, they were measured five times. Both forward and reverse radio channels were measured. The same was repeated for antenna types (dipole and double loop). As a result, six off-body channels were recorded, resulting in total 15000 measured channel responses for both antenna types.

4   Results

4.1   Data Processing

The results are examined in the time domain by extracting the corresponding channel impulse responses (CIRs) from the raw measurement data. CIRs are obtained from the frequency domain data by applying the inverse fast Fourier transform algorithm (IFFT) in Matlab software. During the IFFT, no additional windowing was applied, in other words, it could be said, a rectangular windowing was used.

The first arriving paths (FAPs) of the CIRs were observed as a start. Namely, it was noted that the multipath reflections occurring from the human body are decreasing rapidly in power compared to FAPs. In practical solutions, they should however be utilized in RAKE-type receivers. For this reason, also an investigation on CIR duration and the amplitudes of the other CIR taps beyond FAPs was performed. As easily understandable, the reflections originating beyond the human body are minor due to the anechoic chamber, but still visible revealing the unidealistic practical nature of the anechoic chamber.

To find out the FAP in every CIR, all multipath components were observed within a CIR. All components above a threshold value were solved, and the first one was selected to be the FAP. The threshold was set to lie 10 dB lower than the strongest component in a CIR, a value noted as a good choice in practice.

4.2   Results of the First Arriving Paths

Figure 3 presents exemplary CIRs for one walking cycle with postures 1–5 for the link RW-PO using dipole antennas. It can be noted visually, that the attenuation of the CIRs with different postures varies by less than 5 dB giving the result that for the used scenario the human body does not shadow the signal with respect to the off-body antenna in the observed test person positions. The time delays of the FAPs vary due to the changing distance between the antennas depending on the position of the right wrist.

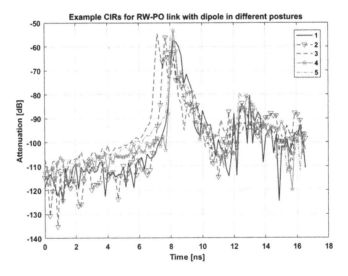

Fig. 3. Example CIRs for body postures 1–5 with RW-PO link using dipole.

To have an insight on the variation on the results between the five repetitions of the walking cycles, the FAP attenuations are next compared between one walking cycle and in the case when the results are averaged over five walking cycles for all off-body links and both antennas. The results are shown in Fig. 4 for one walking cycle and Fig. 5 presents the case averaged over all five walking cycles. Several notifications can be made from Figs. 4 and 5.

Firstly, it can visually concluded, that there is no large difference when comparing the results of one walking cycle to the averaged result over five walking cycles. Therefore, the test person succeeded to repeat the body postures in a similar way in all cases.

Secondly, there is no large difference, generally speaking, between the links LW-PO and RW-PO. This is an understandable result as LW and RW are symmetric locations with respect to the off-body node. In most cases, the difference between LW-PO and RW-PO in attenuation remains within 1...3 decibels.

Thirdly, the LA-PO link shows the weakest performance, with attenuations up to 10 dB higher compared to the wrist links.

Fourthly, a comparison between the antenna types does not show a clear trend in attenuation and no firm conclusion can be made of the superiority between the antennas based on Figs. 4 and 5. This supports the results reported previously in, e.g., [6, 10, 14–18].

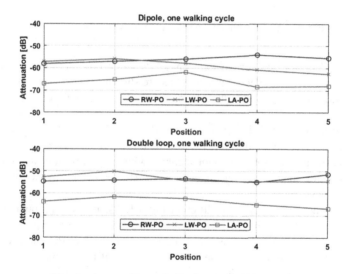

Fig. 4. Attenuation variation in one walking cycle.

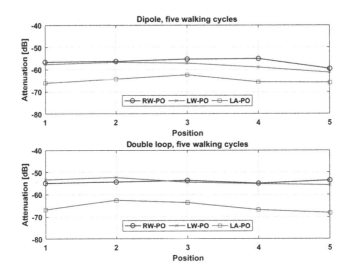

Fig. 5. Average attenuation variation in five walking cycles.

Table 1 collects the numerical data on FAPs when considering all five walking sequences measured. The average attenuations are shown, as well as the minimum and maximum values of them, for both antenna types. The following conclusions can be made.

The mean attenuation values between the different body postures within a single link type show quite small differences, within the range of approx. 1…5 dB. This describes that the applied measurement scenario with the test person facing directly to the pole, does not show a strong effect of body shadowing effect, when examining single radio links.

However, when comparing the different radio links, it is quite apparent, that the LA-PO is the worst link in all positions and for both antenna types. LA-PO has typically approx. 10 dB higher attenuation compared to the LW-PO and RW-PO radio links. A probable reason to this is the relative position of the antennas. The left ankle antenna installation creates a higher body shadowing effect with respect to the off-body antenna. Furthermore, the relative antenna position of LA-PO is different than with the wrist links. As reported in [18], the antenna radiation patterns measured in free space show a high variation with respect to direction and frequency. Even though that the radiations patterns were not possible to be measured as on-body mounted, due to practical reasons, it is highly assumable that the same effect takes place in on-body cases as well.

When comparing the two antenna types with respect to the mean attenuation values, it can be concluded, that generally speaking, in 10 cases out of 15, the double loop antenna shows better attenuation performance than the dipole. However, for the specific link of LA-PO, the dipole performs better in four cases out of five. However, the differences remain within few decibels only, giving a further verification that no clear difference between the antennas can be found out.

The differences between the minimum and maximum attenuations of the separate links, antennas, and body postures lie between 3...12 dB. With the dipole, at RW-PO and position 5, it has the maximum value 13.5 dB. The variations can be explained by the understandable swaying characteristic of the test person while trying to stay in a fixed posture during the one measurement duration of 90 s. Furthermore, all measurements were repeated five times: even one sway of the test person in one measurement and position has a large numerical effect between the minimum and maximum values seen in Table 1.

Table 1. Numerical attenuation results of the first arriving paths for five walking cycles.

	Link	Value	Attenuation per position in dB				
			1	2	3	4	5
Dipole antenna	RW-PO	Mean	−57	−56	−55	−55	−60
		Min.	−53	−55	−54	−53	−54
		Max.	−62	−59	−58	−60	−68
	LW-PO	Mean	−58	−57	−57	−59	−62
		Min.	−55	−54	−56	−57	−60
		Max.	−60	−60	−60	−63	−66
	LA-PO	Mean	−66	−64	−62	−66	−66
		Min.	−65	−63	−61	−64	−65
		Max.	−69	−66	−63	−69	−68
Double loop antenna	RW-PO	Mean	−55	−54	−54	−55	−54
		Min.	−54	−53	−52	−53	−51
		Max.	−58	−57	−58	−59	−59
	LW-PO	Mean	−53	−52	−55	−55	−56
		Min.	−50	−50	−51	−53	−54
		Max.	−59	−58	−59	−61	−60
	LA-PO	Mean	−67	−63	−64	−67	−68
		Min.	−62	−61	−61	−64	−66
		Max.	−72	−64	−66	−70	−70

4.3   Results of the CIRs

This chapter explains the length of the CIRs reasonable to observe as well as the average attenuations for each CIR tap. In this paper, the concept of CIR tap is defined to be one single sample in the CIR, i.e., the time separation between two consecutive taps is the inverse of the measurement bandwidth, $\Delta t = (1/6 \text{ GHz}) \approx 0.167$ ns. The CIR channel taps therefore are not sparse in time.

As noted with the exemplary CIRs presented in Fig. 3, the CIRs have a tendency to decay quite rapidly in anechoic chamber measurements. The threshold to define the limit for CIR taps of interest is defined as follows. Considering the IEEE802.15.6 standard [23], it states that an impulse radio UWB receiver should have a minimum sensitivity of −91 dBm, assuming a receiver noise figure of 10 dB and an implementation loss of 5 dB.

Federal Communications Commission (FCC) from its side sets a maximum transmit power spectrum density limit for UWB in a 3.1–10.6 GHz band to be −41.3 dBm/MHz [4]. For one UWB channel with a bandwidth of 499.2 MHz set in [23], it corresponds to a power of −14.3 dBm. Let us assume an optimistic extra margin of 5 dB for the development in receiver noise figures and implementation. Then, it yields that the CIR attenuation values below −82 dB give only a small contribution to the total signal power, assuming RAKE-receivers, in the scenario under investigation here.

Figure 6 presents an example of the definition of CIR length for links RW-PO, LW-PO and LA-PO for dipole antenna, at body posture 1. They are solved as the average over all five measurement repetitions, all frequency sweeps and both forward and reverse channels. The black vertical line is the −82 dB threshold level. Tap number one is the FAP. The CIR length is defined to be the number of taps when the CIR first time falls below the threshold. Therefore, in Fig. 6, the CIR lengths are 5 (LA-PO), and 6 (RW-PO, LW-PO) taps.

Similar investigation are next repeated for each link, body position and for both antenna types. The results are gathered in Table 2. As noted, the CIR tap lengths vary between five to ten CIR taps. Comparison between link types reveals that on the average LA-PO has one tap shorter CIR duration than the wrist links for both antennas. This is naturally due to the higher attenuation of LA-PO noted in Table 1 as well. Comparison between the antenna types shows, that on the average the CIR tap numbers are 7.0 and 7.2 for the dipole and double antennas. With this respect, no clear performance difference between the antennas can be noted.

As the next step, the average attenuations per each tap are presented for each link and antenna separately. As noted in Fig. 3, the decay slope in the exemplary case is

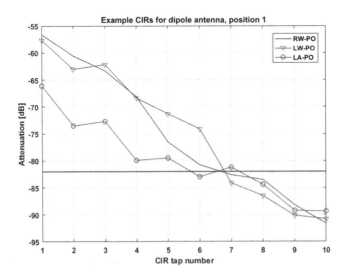

Fig. 6. Example CIR lengths for different links with dipole, body position 1.

Table 2. CIR lengths per link and per body posture.

	Link	CIR length in taps per body posture				
		1	2	3	4	5
Dipole	RW-PO	6	8	9	6	7
	LW-PO	6	6	7	8	10
	LA-PO	5	7	8	6	6
Double loop	RW-PO	6	9	9	7	7
	LW-PO	7	7	7	8	9
	LA-PO	8	5	5	7	8

basically body position independent. Therefore, we average over all body positions to obtain link and antenna specific data to obtain a reasonable number of numerical values to be presented.

Table 3 collects the results with respect to the dipole antennas. As can be noted, the CIR tap lengths in the averaged case extend to seven or eight taps. Due to the higher FAP attenuation in LA-PO links, it has the shortest CIR duration.

Table 4 shows the corresponding results with the double loop antennas. The difference with the dipole antenna is minor, showing only a one tap longer CIR response with links RW-PO and LA-PO.

Finally, one interesting parameter may sometimes the available dynamic range of a radio link. The results are obtained by solving the difference between the first CIR tap attenuations from Tables 3 and 4 and the applied detection threshold level of −82 dB. The dynamic range lies between 24...28 dB for the wrist links and at 17 dB for LA-PO. In two cases out of three the double loop antennas reaches a better performance than the dipole. In practice, the performance with LA-PO is similar, and also the difference in RW-PO and LA-PO is 2...4 dB (Table 5).

Table 3. Average attenuation per CIR taps per link for the dipole antenna.

CIR tap	RW-PO	LW-PO	LA-PO
	Attenuation [dB]	Attenuation [dB]	Attenuation [dB]
1	−56	−58	−65
2	−62	−65	−73
3	−66	−65	−73
4	−67	−67	−77
5	−73	−69	−80
6	−75	−72	−80
7	−79	−78	−81
8	−81	−81	−

Table 4. Average attenuation per CIR taps per link for the double loop antenna.

CIR tap	RW-PO	LW-PO	LA-PO
	Attenuation [dB]	Attenuation [dB]	Attenuation [dB]
1	−54	−54	−65
2	−60	−60	−70
3	−62	−63	−72
4	−65	−65	−73
5	−67	−71	−77
6	−72	−73	−77
7	−75	−79	−80
8	−80	−81	−82
9	−81	–	–

Table 5. Average available dynamic range per link and per antenna in dB.

	RW-PO	LW-PO	LA-PO
Dipole	26	24	17
Double loop	28	28	17

5   Conclusion and Future Work

Pseudo-dynamic UWB WBAN off-body radio are discussed in this paper. The results are preliminary in nature, as only one test person position with respect to the off-body pole is considered. The measurements are performed in an anechoic chamber using a VNA within the frequency range of 2–8 GHz. Pseudo-dynamic approach was used to model a slow dynamic walking sequence. The research is repeated with prototype dipole and double loop antennas.

Considering firstly the first arriving paths of the CIRs, it was noted that their averaged attenuations lied between −52... − 68 dB depending on the body posture, radio channel link, and antenna type. No large differences were noted between the body postures. Considering the channel impulse response durations, they were noted to lie between five to ten taps when examining each link and body posture separately. After averaging the CIR duration data all body postures, the CIR lengths were noted to be eight to nine taps. No clear difference was noted in the performance between the antenna types. The obtained dynamic range within the averaged links vary between 17...28 dB. LA-PO has clearly lower performance compared to RW-PO and LW-PO. Comparison between the antennas shows quite similar performance between the antennas in two links (RW-PO and LA-PO).

As per the future work, a larger variety of scenarios would be interesting to measure. This includes firstly different relative positions of the test person to the off-body pole. Secondly, radio channels in echoic environments should be measured as well.

Acknowledgement. This research has been financially supported in part by Academy of Finland 6Genesis Flagship (grant 318927), and in part by the project WBAN communications in the congested environment (MeCCE).

References

1. 6Genesis Flagship Homepage. https://www.oulu.fi/6gflagship/. Accessed 28 June 2019
2. Hall, P.S., Hao, Y.: Antennas and Propagation for Body-Centric Wireless Communications, 2nd edn. Artech House, Norwood (2012)
3. United Nations: Department of Economic and Social Affairs, World Population Ageing (2017). http://www.un.org/en/development/desa/population/publications/pdf/ageing/WPA20 17_Highlights.pdf. Accessed August 2019
4. Oppermann, I., Hämäläinen, M., Iinatti, J. (eds.): UWB Theory and Applications. Wiley, West Sussex (2004)
5. Ghawami, M., Michael, L.B., Kohno, R.: Ultra Wideband Signals and systEms in Communication Engineering, 2nd edn. Wiley, West Sussex (2007)
6. Kumpuniemi, T., Hämäläinen, M., Yekeh Yazdandoost, K., Iinatti, J.: Categorized UWB on-body radio channel modeling for WBANs. Progr. Electromagn. Res. B **67**, 1–16 (2016)
7. Keränen, N., et al.: IEEE 802.15.6-based multi-accelerometer WBAN system for monitoring Parkinson's disease. In: Proceedings of the 35th Annual International Conference of the IEEE Engineering in Medicine and Biology Society (EMBC), pp. 1656–1659. IEEE, Osaka (2013)
8. Fort, A., Desset, C., De Doncker, P., Wambacq, P., Van Biesen, L.: An ultra-wideband body area propagation channel model—from statistics to implementation. IEEE Trans. Microwave Theory Techn. **54**(4), 1820–1826 (2006)
9. Di Bari, R., Abbasi, Q.H., Alomainy, A., Hao, Y.: An advanced UWB channel model for body-centric wireless networks. Progr. Electromagn. Res. **136**, 79–99 (2013)
10. Kumpuniemi, T., Hämäläinen, M., Yekeh Yazdandoost, K., Iinatti, J.: Human body shadowing effect on dynamic UWB on-body radio channels. IEEE Antennas Wirel. Propag. Lett. **16**, 1871–1874 (2017)
11. Ali, A.J., Scanlon, W.G., Cotton, S.L.: Pedestrian effects in indoor UWB off-body communication channels. In: Proceedings of 2010 Loughborough Antennas and Propagation Conference, pp. 57–60. IEEE, Loughborough (2010)
12. Catherwood, P. A., Scanlon, W. G.: Body-centric antenna positioning effects for off-body UWB communications in a contemporary learning environment. In: Proceedings of the 8th European Conference on Antennas and Propagation (EUCAP), pp. 1571–1574. IEEE, The Hague (2014)
13. Garcia-Serna, R.-G., Garcia-Pardo, C., Molina-Garcia-Pardo, J.: Effect of the receiver attachment position on ultrawideband off-body channels. IEEE Antennas Wirel. Propag. Lett. **14**, 1101–1104 (2015)
14. Kumpuniemi, T., Mäkelä, J.-P., Hämäläinen, M., Yazdandoost, K.Y., Iinatti, J.: Dynamic UWB off-body radio channels - human body shadowing effect. In: Proceedings of the 28th Annual IEEE International Symposium on Personal, Indoor and Mobile Radio Communications (IEEE PIMRC 2017), pp. 1–7. IEEE, Montreal (2017)
15. Kumpuniemi, T., Mäkelä, J.-P., Hämäläinen, M., Yazdandoost, K.Y., Iinatti, J.: Human body effect on static UWB WBAN off-body radio channels. In: Proceedings of the 13th EAI International Conference on Body Area Networks (BODYNETS 2018), pp. 1–10. EAI, Oulu (2018)

16. Kumpuniemi, T., Mäkelä, J.-P., Hämäläinen, M., Yazdandoost, K.Y., Iinatti, J.: Measurement and analysis on dynamic off-body radio channels at UWB frequencies. In: Proceedings of the 13th International Symposium on Medical Information and Technology (ISMICT 2019), pp. 1–5. IEEE, Oslo (2019)

17. Kumpuniemi, T., Hämäläinen, M., Tuovinen, T., Yazdandoost, K.Y., Iinatti, J.: Radio channel modelling for pseudo-dynamic WBAN on-body links. In: Proceedings of the 8th International Symposium on Medical Information and Technology (ISMICT 2014), pp. 1–5. IEEE, Florence (2014)

18. Kumpuniemi, T., Hämäläinen, M., Yazdandoost, K.Y., Iinatti, J.: Measurements for body-to-body UWB WBAN radio channels. In: Proceedings of the 9th European Conference on Antennas and Propagation (EUCAP), pp. 1–5. IEEE, Lisbon (2015)

19. Tuovinen, T., Kumpuniemi, T., Yazdandoost, K.Y., Hämäläinen, M., Iinatti, J.: Effect of the antenna-human body distance on the antenna matching in UWB WBAN applications. In: Proceedings of the 7th International Symposium on Medical Information and Communication Technology (ISMICT), pp. 193–197. IEEE, Tokyo (2013)

20. Tuovinen, T., Kumpuniemi, T., Hämäläinen, M., Yazdandoost, K.Y., Iinatti, J.: Effect of the antenna-body distance on the on-ext and on-on channel link path gain in UWB WBAN applications. In: Proceedings of the 35th Annual International Conference of IEEE Engineering in Medicine and Biology Society (EMBC), pp. 1242–1245. IEEE, Osaka (2013)

21. Saunders, S.R.: Aragón-Zavala, A: Antennas and Propagation for Wireless Communication Systems, 2nd edn. Wiley, Chichester (2007)

22. Rohacell   Homepage.   https://www.rohacell.com/product/rohacell/en/products-services/rohacell-hf/. Accessed 28 June 2019

23. IEEE Standard for Local and Metropolitan Area Networks. IEEE 802.15.6–2012–Part 15.6: Wireless Body Area networks (2012)

Author Index

Printed in the United States
By Bookmasters